Appointment
with
Doctor Death

Appointment with Doctor Death

by Michael Betzold

Momentum Books Ltd.

Cover design and illustration by Jerry Lemenu

Manufactured in the United States of America

1996 1995 1994 1993   5   4   3   2   1

Momentum Books Ltd.
6964 Crooks Road, Suite 1
Troy, Michigan 48098
U.S.A.

ISBN 1-879094-37-1   Hardcover
ISBN 1-879094-42-8   Paperback

Library of Congress Cataloging-in-Publication Data

Betzold, Michael.
    Appointment with Doctor Death / Michael Betzold.
        p.   cm.
    Includes bibliographical references.
    ISBN 1-879094-37-1 (hardcover) : $21.95. -- ISBN 1-879094-42-8
(pbk.) : $14.95
    1. Assisted suicide. 2. Kevorkian, Jack. 3. Pathologists--United
States--Biography.   I. Title.
R726.B46   1993
364.1'523--dc20
    [B]   93-35550
                                                                CIP

To Martie Ruwart

TABLE OF CONTENTS

ABOUT THIS BOOK

I wrote this book because I was placed in the path of a remarkable story. My 1991 assignment to the *Detroit Free Press*'s suburban Oakland Bureau plunged me into the saga of Jack Kevorkian's assisted suicide campaign, a story with national resonance and, eventually, deep personal implications for me.

Happily, this project reunited me with the man who introduced me to the WHOGAS test. Tom Ferguson gave me my start in legitimate journalism when he hired me in 1979 as a reporter for an underfunded Detroit weekly that often beat the big guys to the punch. In ensuing years I found the WHOGAS test indispensable for evaluating stories. WHOGAS is an acronym for "Who Gives A Shit?"

Judge for yourself whether this book passes Tom's test. If it doesn't, Tom is not to blame. For a hectic half-year, he has served steadfastly as my editor, sounding board, assistant reporter, colleague and friend. I am indebted to him for his many talents, his sound judgment, his unfailing wit, his encouragement and his confidence in me. This book has benefitted enormously from his stubborn insistence that journalism is not hyping or massaging news but reporting and writing a good story fairly and honestly and entertainingly.

I also am deeply grateful to Momentum Books for committing its resources to this risky project and for supporting me every step of the way. I thank Brownson Murray and Bill Haney for their invaluable advice.

The forthright contributions of Mary Ruwart, Teresa Ruwart and Karen Swindell have provided depth and humanity to this book; I thank them for sharing their insights with me in a difficult time. In a similar vein, I thank Sharon Welsh and all the others who let me intrude on their personal stories.

For invaluable help in transcribing many tapes and tracking down journal articles I salute Jillian Downey. I also thank Guinevere Voletti, Karen Otterson, Kyle Scott, Judy Davids, Pamela Warrick, Mark Speece, Rebecca Beach, Joel Thurtell, Lori Brasier, Catherine Daligga, Peggy Swift, Shelley Ferguson, Peter Nagourney and Frank Rashid for their sundry efforts. I thank Bob Campbell, my editor at the *Free Press*, for putting me on the Kevorkian beat and supporting my efforts. And special thanks go to Mimi Becigneul and to Ethan Casey for their constant encouragement.

Most especially, I send a huge bouquet to my best friend and life partner, Kathleen Conway, who supported me unwaveringly, body and soul, throughout this demanding project. I salute my wonderful children, Patrick and Bridget, for their patience and understanding.

A word about the section and chapter epigraphs: Notes on the source and the context of the epigraphs can be found in "Notes on Epigraphs," appended. The "Source" section has references to some of the major journal articles, books and periodicals used in preparing this manuscript.

CAST OF CHARACTERS

JACK KEVORKIAN, MD, pathologist, artist, author, inventor, film-maker, entrepreneur, obitiatrist.

GEOFFREY NELS FIEGER, Kevorkian's enormously successful attorney and spokesman, former actor and rock music roadie.

MARTIE RUWART, computer software engineer, environmentalist, assistant book editor and 15th patient of obitiatrist Kevorkian.

DR. MARY K. RUWART, scientist, author, older sister of Martie.

RICHARD THOMPSON, prosecutor for Oakland County, Michigan, tough-on-crime Republican and chief lawman in pursuit of Kevorkian.

LYNN MILLS, anti-abortion activist with experience at garbage-picking who is led to a battle against Kevorkian.

FRED DILLINGHAM, former mortician, leader in the Michigan Senate, staunch Kevorkian opponent, father of a special daughter.

JANET GOOD, longtime feminist and civil rights activist, founder and leader of the Michigan chapter of the Hemlock Society, and frequent contact for people who want Kevorkian's help.

HOWARD BRODY, MD, Michigan State University professor and

chair of the bioethics committee of the Michigan State Medical Society.

NEAL NICOL, medical supplies salesman, Kevorkian's chief assistant and former colleague in cadaver blood research.

MARGO JANUS, Kevorkian's sister, assistant and videographer.

TIMOTHY QUILL, MD, a Rochester, N.Y., doctor who helped his patient "Diane" die and won acclaim from the medical profession.

ED RIVET, legislative director for Right to Life of Michigan and originator of the Slippery Slope flow chart.

CARL MARLINGA, Macomb County prosecutor and man in the middle.

JOHN KELLY, maverick Democratic state senator who found himself typing with monkeys.

MICHAEL SCHWARTZ, the Barracuda on Kevorkian's defense team.

MICHAEL MODELSKI, an assistant to Richard Thompson who wouldn't play ball with Geoffrey Fieger.

MURRAY LEVIN, MD, a respectable doctor who believed former colleague Kevorkian crossed the line.

ARCHBISHOP ADAM MAIDA, Roman Catholic Archbishop of Detroit, who believed in the value of suffering.

JOHN O'HAIR, Wayne County prosecutor, who got Kevorkian to say the magic words.

THE MEDIA, reporting, sensationalizing, lionizing, criticizing, snooping, pontificating, polling and viewing with alarm.

JANET and RONALD ADKINS, Hemlock members from Portland, Oregon, who came to Michigan so Janet could use Kevorkian's suicide machine.

SHERRY MILLER, a woman with multiple sclerosis.

SHARON WELSH, Miller's best friend.

MARJORIE WANTZ, a teacher's aide with chronic pelvic pain.

SUE WILLIAMS, an Avon lady with multiple sclerosis.

LOIS HAWES, a school administrator with cancer.

CATHERINE ANDREYEV, a real estate agent with cancer.

MARGUERITE TATE, a retiree with Lou Gehrig's disease.

MARCELLA LAWRENCE, a nurse with heart disease, emphysema, arthritis and other ailments.

JACK MILLER, a lumberjack with cancer.

STANLEY BALL, a cherry farmer with cancer.

MARY BIERNAT, an Indiana woman with cancer.

ELAINE GOLDBAUM, a woman with multiple sclerosis.

HUGH GALE, a sailor with severe emphysema.

CHERYL GALE, Hugh Gale's wife.

JONATHAN GRENZ, a California real estate broker with cancer.

RON MANSUR, a real estate agent with cancer.

THOMAS HYDE, a construction worker with Lou Gehrig's disease.

WANDA ENDITALL, a figment of Kevorkian's imagination.

THE AUTHOR, a *Detroit Free Press* reporter who became personally connected to his story.

PROLOGUE
THE ABYSS

The artist makes me look down a deep shaft into a dark pit. A man clutches the sheer walls. His mouth gapes in a deep red scream. His arms and fingers stretch pencil-thin from the clinging—in vain, for there is no place to grip. His clawing fingernails leave thin trails of blood on the walls to mark his certain defeat.

Below him is the abyss into which he inevitably must fall. At the bottom are ghastly blue human faces.

I held in my hands a sharp color photograph of this vivid, terrifying painting and wondered:

Whose death—or life—is this? Whose terror? Whose desperate effort to hang on? Whose cry for help, echoing without answer? Whose strange hell below?

The painting is titled Death. *The artist is Jack Kevorkian, MD.*

Like most Americans, I first encountered Jack Kevorkian by reading newspaper accounts of how he helped Janet Adkins die in June 1990. At the time I was a *Detroit Free Press* reporter, but Kevorkian wasn't my beat. In October 1991, just after I was assigned by the *Free Press* to its Oakland County bureau, Kevorkian assisted in the suicides of Marjorie Wantz and Sherry Miller in a state park in Oakland County. In the months to come, covering Jack Kevorkian became one of my major responsibilities. It remained so until I took a leave of absence from the paper on March 1, 1993, to write this book.

Eventually I got to know a lot about the man called Doctor Death. But the deeper I peered into the pit, the more questions I found.

Everyone lugs emotional baggage to the Jack Kevorkian story. The baggage may contain the indelible memory of the agonized face of a dying relative harnessed to hospital tubes and wires. It may include love and affection for a friend who failed at suicide. It may be colored by closeness to a person with special needs. And it almost certainly

1

includes a very personal, deep-seated and unspoken set of intense emotions about death.

My psychological luggage is pretty heavy.

In 1955, a phone call jarred my father awake at dawn on a summer Saturday. Come quickly, the voice said, your wife . . .

My dad arrived at the hospital in time to see my mother screaming and writhing in her death throes.

At age 42, she died from a treatable intestinal blockage, misdiagnosed by a physician subbing for her vacationing doctor.

I didn't go to the funeral. The adults thought it would be too rough on a five-year-old. This was the only explanation I got for my mother's disappearance:

"The angels took her away."

Every night after that, my father would kneel next to me at my bed and together we would pray:

"Now I lay me down to sleep. I pray the Lord my soul to keep. If I should die before I wake, I pray the Lord my soul to take."

Once alone in bed, I would pull the covers over my head to hide from the angels.

Our family never talked about my mother's death. My dad couldn't. I didn't find out exactly how she died until I was 40.

Fifteen years after my mother died, my father remarried. Then he found out he had colon cancer. Operations and chemotherapy followed. The summer I graduated from college, he seemed to be recovering, then suddenly got worse. On the day he left for the hospital, I saw terror in his face.

"I thought I was getting better," he told me.

The doctors had told my stepmother he was about to die. They hadn't told him—or us. And she hadn't, either. He had no time to prepare, and neither did I.

The next time I saw him, his mind was gone. Soon his body was, too. I had no chance to say goodbye.

When Jack Kevorkian was 33, his dad died of a heart attack. A few years later, his mother got cancer. It spread to her bones. For years she lived in constant pain. Her son said it was like "a horrible toothache in every part of your body."

Kevorkian's two sisters asked their mother's doctor to end her suffering.

The doctor refused.

It was years before Jack's sisters told him about their request for euthanasia.

In 1991, Kevorkian told a *Detroit Free Press* reporter that dreams about his parents sometimes still would wake him in the night and start him wondering about death.

"If you don't have any sort of faith, you think of the big nothingness," he said. "And you wonder: What is this brief span of consciousness? What is all this?

"All thinking people go through this—you just don't talk about it. There's no answer, anyway."

In July 1992, when I visited his spare, dingy apartment, I asked the man whose name had been linked worldwide with death what he thought happened after you died.

Without hesitation he replied:

"You rot."

Kevorkian's curt, crude reply fit with the cartoon image the media had concocted for him: the macabre, messianic, misanthropic "Doctor Death." But I was to discover in the months ahead—through interviews and discussions and a sudden, personal shock—that there was more to Jack Kevorkian and the question of assisted suicide than would fit on a television screen or in a tabloid headline.

Shortly after the first use of his suicide machine catapulted him onto the national stage, Jack Kevorkian said in an interview that his life had been a failure. His flamboyant attorney, Geoffrey Fieger, described his client to me as a quitter. But by putting one daring idea into action, the eccentric pathologist with the lackluster career became famous for his audacity, inventiveness and persistence.

His unorthodox one-man crusade had everyone talking about the last remaining taboo: How we die.

The time was right. Modern medicine's powerful technology was working many life-saving wonders but also many previously unimaginable horrors. More hopelessly ill people were being kept alive in some monstrous machine-operated imitation of life.

To the unspeakable terror of death had been added the unfathomable horror of being kept alive while all but dead.

In reaction, scores of hospice programs arose, aimed at keeping the terminally ill well-supported and as comfortable as possible until they died. A series of court verdicts broadened the right to have life-prolonging treatment—even food and water—withheld at the patient's request. The Hemlock Society and other "right-to-die" groups wanted to go much further and push for legalized doctor-assisted suicide.

But until Jack Kevorkian rudely took center stage, most of this was a shadow play, with whispered lines. The Kevorkian-assisted death of Janet Adkins on June 4, 1990, forced the issue. Brazenly, a former nobody named Jack Kevorkian was forcing a reluctant nation to look squarely in the eyes of death.

I

DENIAL

"The so-called health professions have an indirect sickening power, a structurally health-denying effect. They transform pain, illness and death from a personal challenge into a technical problem and thereby expropriate the potential of people to deal with their human condition in an autonomous way."

— Philosopher Ivan Illich (1974)

CHAPTER ONE
THE EYES OF DEATH

The hanged man's bloated bare feet dangle beneath the scaffold's trap door. The artist has us looking up, past the swinging man, at a powder blue sky mottled with white and pink clouds. The painting is by Jack Kevorkian. ❐

Five times the young resident had gotten his ophthalmoscope to a patient's bedside minutes after death. This time, as he wheeled in the bulky mounted camera, he was elated to find the patient still alive. Finally, he could get shots of a cornea before, during and after death. He taped open the sick woman's eyelids and focused his lens.

He had asked to work nights at Detroit Receiving Hospital because more patients died then. His mission was to discover how eyes changed at the moment of death. Jokingly, he called his quest the Death Rounds. For added effect, he sometimes would wear a black arm band. Co-workers called him Doctor Death. He accepted the nickname.

"I was sort of the laughingstock of the hospital," the doctor admitted later in life.

This night, Doctor Death got what he wanted. As the woman went into convulsions and died, the blood vessels in her cornea quickly faded from view. Jack Kevorkian got it all on film.

For the *American Journal of Pathology*, Kevorkian wrote up his research in "The Fundus Oculi and the Determination of Death." It was a fine feather in the cap of a 28-year-old pathologist.

If eyes could pinpoint the moment of death, Kevorkian wrote, doctors would know when resuscitation was useless. They quickly could distinguish death from fainting, shock or coma. It was useful research.

"But really, my number one reason was because it was interesting," he told a reporter years later. "And my second reason was because it was a taboo subject."

❏ ❏ ❏

Everyone who has known Jack Kevorkian first talks about his brain.

"He could tell you any major league baseball player's batting average," his boyhood chum Richard Dakesian told me, his voice tinged with awe. "He probably could have graduated from high school when he was 13 or 14.

"He's the smartest man I ever knew. I think he was born ahead of his time."

In fact, Jack Kevorkian was born May 28, 1928, in Pontiac, then a booming auto industry town north of Detroit. His parents were Armenian immigrants. He had an older sister, Flora, and a younger sister, Margo.

His mother and father had escaped the Turks' "final solution"— the massacre of millions of Armenians in a holocaust the rest of the world mostly ignored.

"I wish my forefathers went through what the Jews did," Kevorkian said later. "The Jews were gassed. Armenians were killed in every conceivable way. Pregnant women were split open with bayonets and babies taken out. They were drowned, burned, heads were smashed in vices. They were chopped in half.

"So the Holocaust doesn't interest me, see? They've had a lot of publicity, but they didn't suffer as much."

Jack grew up in a crowded neighborhood of Armenians, Greeks and Bulgarians. His father, Levon, quit his auto factory job and ran a small excavating company.

"My parents sacrificed a great deal so that we children would be spared undue privation and misery," Kevorkian later wrote. "There was always enough to eat."

Jack played street games such as touch football, jump-rope, tag, hopscotch and kick-the-can until dark. Then he'd go home and read voraciously. He loved to draw, too, especially fighter planes.

School bored him. One day in sixth grade, he was shooting paper wads. The teacher marched him off to the principal's office. The principal told Jack to pack his books—and report the next day to junior high school. He had been promoted for throwing spitballs.

Jack was raised in the Armenian Orthodox faith, but he soon found it to be a fraud. "I realized I didn't believe in their miracles, walking on water, that sort of thing," he said. He quit Sunday school.

Baseball had more wondrous mysteries. His parents' radio could pull in Cleveland games, and Jack preferred Indians announcer Jack Graney's booming voice to the dull tones of Detroit Tigers broadcaster Ty Tyson.

Jack would draw crowds by bouncing a ball off steps and imitating Graney calling all nine innings of a pretend game.

Jack's dream was to go to Cleveland and train under Graney.

"I'd have been a great one—better than Harwell," he once boasted. The Tigers' Ernie Harwell is in the broadcasters' wing of the baseball Hall of Fame. Graney is all but forgotten.

But Jack's parents wanted him to pursue a more serious career.

He had the tools. Dakesian remembered Jack as very studious and uninterested in the social whirl. In the 1945 yearbook at Pontiac High School, he does not appear on the roster of any sports teams or social clubs, but is listed as a National Honor Society special award recipient and a member of the Chemistry-Physics Club. While in high school, Kevorkian learned German and Japanese—the languages of his nation's enemies.

In the fall of 1945, with World War II over, Jack enrolled at the University of Michigan. He quickly finished his undergraduate work and enrolled in U of M Medical School. He graduated in 1952 and decided to specialize in pathology—the study of corpses and tissue to determine cause of death or disease.

As an intern at Henry Ford Hospital in Detroit, Kevorkian one day came upon a middle-aged woman suffering from cancer. In his 1991 book, *Prescription: Medicide*, Kevorkian, in typically purple prose, described the encounter as an awakening for him:

"The patient was a helplessly immobile woman of middle age, her entire body jaundiced to an intense yellow-brown, skin stretched paper-thin over a fluid-filled abdomen swollen to four or five times normal size. The rest of her was an emaciated skeleton: sagging, discolored skin covered her bones like a cheap, wrinkled frock.

"The poor wretch stared up at me with yellow eyeballs sunken in their atrophic sockets. Her yellow teeth were ringed by chapping and parched lips to form an involuntary, almost sardonic 'smile' of death. It seemed as though she was pleading for help and death at the same time. Out of sheer empathy alone I could have helped her die with satisfaction. From that moment on, I was sure that doctor-assisted euthanasia and suicide are and always were ethical, no matter what anyone says or thinks."

In 1953, the Korean War interrupted Kevorkian's career. He

served 15 months as an Army medical officer in Korea, then finished his service on a Colorado mountaintop encampment, where he taught himself to read music and scanned baroque scores by lantern in a tent. He got a little wooden recorder, a primitive wind instrument, and then a flute. Both were good for playing Bach.

Discharged, Kevorkian did residencies at Pontiac General Hospital, in his hometown; at Detroit Receiving, where he pioneered his Death Rounds, and at the University of Michigan Medical Center. It was there, during a seminar in 1958, that an offhand question prompted Kevorkian to research the history of autopsies. Reading journals in German, he found an account describing how the ancient Greeks did medical experiments on condemned criminals in Alexandria, Egypt. The article "shackled me with responsibility to promulgate a profound idea," he wrote later. "Possibilities churned in my youthful and impractically idealistic mind. How simple a solution to so many perplexing problems."

Doing further research, Kevorkian found that 13th-Century Armenians—his ancestors—also had done experiments on condemned men. Doctors gave wine to prisoners to anesthetize them, then cut them up to study blood circulation.

In October, on a day off, Kevorkian drove his 1956 Ford to Columbus, Ohio, the nearest state with the death penalty, on "a righteous crusade" to "challenge profound philosophical viewpoints and clash head-on with enduring and powerful taboos."

Unannounced, he walked in on the warden at the Ohio State Penitentiary and asked to meet with death-row convicts. Kevorkian wanted their reaction to his idea of doing medical experiments at their executions. Amazingly, the warden agreed "without manifesting a trace of the selfish and Machiavellian hypocrisy that fuels much of civilized society."

Kevorkian interviewed two young murderers. One later sent him a letter: "I would gladly give you what you requested of me and in doing so it might help others."

Kevorkian never heard from the other convict, but the one consent was enough: "I knew beyond doubt that the proposal was practical. . . . the crusade was unstoppable."

Elated, Kevorkian wrote an essay outlining his proposal: At the time of execution, put the condemned to sleep with drugs, then do experiments and finally inject lethal drugs to carry out the sentence. The benefits: Millions saved in research costs. New cures discovered.

And, not least of all, a chance to find what makes the criminal mind tick.

He argued that "any human being condemned to unavoidable death for any conventional reason . . . whether justly or not, anywhere in the world should be allowed this choice." He proposed a new specialty of doctors to do the experiments, saying it would be "a unique privilege . . . to be able to experiment on a doomed human being."

Anticipating objections, Kevorkian insisted his proposal was unlike Nazi concentration camp experiments.

"Those medical crimes apparently were such a horrendous discovery for the civilized world that, regrettably, they seem to have blunted reason and common sense with regard to the rational assessment of the use of condemned human subjects for research," Kevorkian wrote. "Medical experimentation on consenting humans was, is and most likely always will be the laudable and correct thing to do."

Professional journals and popular magazines rejected Kevorkian's article outlining his proposal. Kevorkian later admitted his essay "reeked with sophomoric idealism and was highly impractical." But he was able to present it at the December 1958 meeting of the American Association for the Advancement of Science in Washington, D.C.— only because the group's chairman figured the outlandish scheme would turn more people against capital punishment. Kevorkian's speech caused a minor stir in the press, but drew no official support save for a stirring endorsement from an animal rights group, which pointed out that cutting up humans would save the lives of rats and guinea pigs.

The publicity embarrassed the University of Michigan. The chairman of the pathology department asked Kevorkian to drop his campaign or leave. There was a doctor shortage, so Kevorkian confidently quit and found a job back at Pontiac General.

As opposition to the death penalty grew, Kevorkian put his campaign on the shelf. He had experienced for the first time "the enormous force of social, political and historical inertia which makes it almost impossible to implement seemingly radical change, to bridge the wide gap between rational theory and actual practice."

Pontiac General was a busy and loosely run city hospital. Kevorkian had free rein in the pathology department. A colleague told him that Russian doctors were experimentally transfusing blood from corpses. Kevorkian decided to give it a try. He enlisted help from a young medical technologist named Neal Nicol and others.

When a victim of a heart attack or auto accident was brought in, Kevorkian's team would do a quick autopsy, put the body on a tilt table, stick a syringe in the jugular, let the blood drain into a bottle, then give the blood to live patients. It worked.

In 1961, in a paper in *The American Journal of Clinical Pathology*, Kevorkian acknowledged the cadaver blood research "has an ostensible undercurrent of repugnance which makes it difficult to view objectively." But corpses were a free, ready-made source of blood, he wrote. He added that "permission of next of kin is not necessary if corpse blood is to be taken. . . . Routine consent from the recipient is no more necessary than in instances of conventional blood bank transfusions."

Dr. Murray Levin, then an internist at Pontiac General, said Kevorkian's frequent talk about his research unnerved his colleagues.

"Most of us just sort of changed the subject when he got on it," Levin said. "We thought it was inappropriate. We had plenty of blood. We didn't need to deal with cadavers."

After *Time* magazine gave his work a mention, Kevorkian thought of a new twist: To save lives in wartime, why not transfuse blood directly from a corpse to an injured soldier on a battlefield? Not even the Russians had tried to do that.

One day, a stroke victim came in. Kevorkian put the corpse on the tilt table. Neal Nicol, whose blood type was compatible, lay on the floor next to the dead man. Through a transfer device Kevorkian had rigged up, the dead man's blood flowed into Nicol's veins. Nicol felt no ill effects.

Soon after, Kevorkian hooked up a female staffer to an 18-year-old girl who had died in a car crash. Kevorkian went for the corpse's jugular, but her neck was mashed and he couldn't get the needle in. Thinking fast, he plunged the syringe into the dead girl's heart and drew out the blood. The recipient reported a funny taste in her mouth. Kevorkian panicked, wondering if he was poisoning her. After an autopsy, he discovered the dead girl was drunk. He surmised that the recipient had been tasting the liquor.

Kevorkian published his new research in a 1964 article in *Military Medicine*, complete with posed "battlefield" pictures of a corpsman transferring blood from a "dead" soldier to a wounded man. The man playing the corpse looks like Kevorkian.

Kevorkian pitched his idea to the Pentagon, figuring it could be used in Vietnam, but the Defense Department turned a cold shoulder and Kevorkian was denied a federal grant to continue his research. He reacted to the rejection with a more sweeping rejection of his own: "I resolved never again to waste time and effort in futile appeals for support from governmental agencies."

Kevorkian called his years at Pontiac General "the best days of our lives." But the research added to his oddball reputation. "It got me into trouble. Jobs closed down because of that." His resume—full of articles on death-row experiments, cornea photography at death, and cadaver blood transfusions—"scared the hell out of people."

Even his hobbies produced frightening things.

In the early 1960s, Kevorkian took a Pontiac adult education class in oil painting. His classmates were mostly conventional housewives who were painting clowns and kittens and trees.

"Ugh!" he recalled 30 years later. "I just do not like anything banal."

"I says: I'll show them. I'll paint something that will turn their stomachs, and then I'll quit this course."

To his surprise, his staid classmates loved what he drew. To his childhood talent for drawing, Kevorkian had added his extensive knowledge of anatomy and deep interest in deathly matters. The art class painting became the first of 18 striking, gruesome, surrealistic visions full of skulls and body parts and cannibalism and harsh religious parody. Kevorkian executed his canvases with brash directness. The paintings, exhibited sporadically around Michigan for nearly two decades, usually caused a sensation.

"I tire easily of beautiful scenes and portraits, and abstract art has no tangible or intelligible significance for me," he told a newspaper in 1964. "People may wince at some of my paintings, but nobody has yet denied their forceful accuracy."

His art, he said, portrayed "distasteful but widespread aspects of human existence . . . that show how hypocritical we are."

In the painting *Genocide*, a yellowish male torso is seated at a dinner table. Its large arms are holding a huge knife and fork. On a plate on the table is a severed head with an apple stuffed in the mouth. On the table are two gray nuclear warhead-shaped salt-and-pepper shakers, a soldier's upturned helmet filled with bronze bullets and a large dish full of golden crucifixes.

To paint the frame for *Genocide*, Kevorkian mixed outdated blood from blood banks with a little of his own.

"That gets people," he chuckled.

CHAPTER TWO
CHILDREN OF THE '60S

> *"No man has ever been blamed for so much. . . .*
> *He didn't give a hoot for public opinion and only*
> *in his last years did he bother much with church.*
> *. . . He was a crank and a nuisance but withal a*
> *deeply innocent and brave man."*
> —*Arthur Miller,* The Crucible,
> *describing Giles Corey* ❑

Jack Kevorkian was in medical school when the man who would help make him famous was born.

Like me, Geoffrey Fieger was born in 1950 in metropolitan Detroit, the automobile capital of the world and the most impressive manufacturing center in the most prosperous nation on Earth. Fieger was the first-born son of Bernard and June Fieger. His father, a Brooklyn-born Jew, married June, a Norwegian woman, after graduating from Harvard Law School. Like many Jewish families, they settled in the Detroit suburb of Oak Park. After Geoffrey came Doug and Beth.

Bernie Fieger founded Detroit's second interracial law firm and represented several black defendants in celebrated civil rights cases. With other attorneys from around the nation, he went to Mississippi to defend activists jailed in the voting rights struggles of the 1960s. He guided the Michigan Federation of Teachers through several strikes and helped write Michigan's landmark employment relations act. He was secretary-treasurer of the National Lawyers Guild and a member of the American Civil Liberties Union.

Home was a cauldron of ideas, causes and cacophony.

"They were the loudest family in the world. Everything was at maximum decibels," said family friend Roger Craig. "Geoffrey was a precocious kid and a pain in the ass. He always was a bright guy."

Geoffrey's grade school classmates were mostly Jewish, but his only relatives in Michigan were his mother's, so he felt mostly Norwegian. His dad was a non-religious Jew who occasionally took the children to a local Unitarian Church, which went easy on the

God stuff. When Geoffrey transferred in seventh grade to the prestigious private Detroit Country Day School in upscale Birmingham, he was stunned to hear rich kids parroting their parents' anti-Semitic remarks. It was the first time he realized there was such prejudice.

Fieger knew he would be the object of the slurs if his classmates found out his father was Jewish. He never let on. His heritage remained a puzzle—even to him. Fieger mused: "What was I? I don't know."

After ninth grade, Geoffrey had to leave Country Day.

"It was an all-boys school and I hated it. Man, I could *smell* girls. Man, by the time I got out of there it was painful. I was being crushed."

Puberty also fueled Geoff's love for the Beatles. His kid brother Doug had formed a rock and roll band, the Flying Ernies. At school dances, Geoff played guitar wildly and sang an impassioned lead on "Twist and Shout."

At Oak Park High School, Geoff made the varsity football team as a lineman. Between music, girls and sports, he had no time for civil rights rallies or peace marches. He didn't have much interest in his father's causes.

Geoffrey lasted only one semester at the University of Wisconsin. Then he almost got sent to Vietnam—a prospect that never stopped haunting him.

Fieger told me how he had stood in the long line of scared young men at Fort Wayne, Detroit's Army induction center, cursing himself for leaving college and losing his student deferment.

The sergeant at the desk barked out fates.

Fieger stood before him.

"Rejected."

Thank God for high-school football and torn knee ligaments.

Fieger told me: "I would have dreams of being shot at and not being able to see who was shooting you. That's what happened in the fire fights. That's a scary idea."

Sometimes, Fieger said, he still had those dreams of being ambushed by death at a young age.

Escaping the Vietnam trap, Fieger took off for England. Brother Doug had landed him a job as a rock roadie. For a year, he helped stars such as Arthur Brown, whose hit "Fire" was written in the Satanic first person and had the chorus: "Fire! I'll take you to burn."

Fieger later contended that he hated staying up all night and partying.

"I'm a day person," he said. "I've always been into athletics and stuff. There is a strong discordant thing between living a night life and being a healthy person."

Fourteen months after Geoffrey Fieger was born, Martha Ruwart entered the world. A premature "blue baby," she spent a few weeks in a hospital incubator before coming home to her family's modest house in the post-war tracts of Detroit's eastern suburbs. From the start, she was delicate. Everyone called her Martie.

Her father, Bill, occasionally spanked her older sister Mary. But the first few times he spanked Martie, she fainted. After that, he never touched her. If her sisters or brothers accidentally grabbed her, she would recoil.

"We treated her like china," Mary Ruwart recalled.

Once, at a family picnic, Martie fainted and fell out of a tree. Another time, she fainted in church. But she never showed any behavioral problems. She was obedient, good-natured and trusting.

"Mom always said she was a good kid, that something was wrong with her—she was too good," said her youngest sister, Karen.

Martie and Mary loved American pioneer stories, the Revolutionary War, Davy Crockett, *Wagon Train.*

"When we played dolls, our dolls were spies for the American Revolution," Mary Ruwart recalled.

Jean Ruwart encouraged her four daughters and her two sons to go to college. Bright and outgoing, Jean had sacrificed her own career to raise her children.

In high school, Martie was awkward and shy. She couldn't quite get the hang of being cool.

She blossomed socially and intellectually after entering Michigan State University in 1970. The experimental culture of the era suited her curious nature. Her sister Mary, in graduate school at MSU, introduced Martie to the writings of Ayn Rand, a Russian immigrant who championed individual sovereignty.

Martie studied biology and planned to be a nurse. But when she started working in nursing homes as an aide, she found she couldn't handle being around so many terminally ill people.

Instead of finishing her degree, Martie packed her few belongings in the trunk of her '65 Valiant and drove to California with her sister Teresa. They settled in San Diego, near the ocean, and began to frequent a nearby nude beach.

"We weren't hot for the naked part," Teresa Ruwart recalled. "It was more the idea that you could do something you couldn't do otherwise."

When wealthy homeowners tried to close the beach, Martie sold T-shirts and passed out flyers to keep it open. Her side lost.

Like many of her generation, Martie shunned the straight career path. Time and freedom were more important to her than money.

"She didn't want to wear high heels and business clothes," Teresa said. "She didn't want to play the game."

Instead, Martie waitressed and delivered newspapers. Once, she lost a job flipping burgers when she reported her boss to the health department for reselling discarded donuts.

She kept expenses way down. She shopped at thrift stores and food co-ops and had few possessions. She shared modest living quarters with her sister or other roommates. For a while she lived in a garage.

Long before it was fashionable, Martie religiously recycled. She became a strict vegetarian because she believed humans mistreated animals in raising them for food. She even cut out dairy products because she thought milking hurt cows.

"She didn't cheat on vegetarianism," Teresa said. "She believed if you don't like something, you go out and act on it. And if you do something, you do it right."

After his year in England, Geoffrey Fieger decided it was time to get serious. For the next seven years he went to school year-round.

At the University of Michigan, Jack Kevorkian's old school, Fieger majored in theater arts and speech. In *The Crucible*, he played octogenarian Giles Corey—the much-maligned farmer who always was suing people for defaming his character.

With his master's degree in hand, Fieger took stock.

"I was 25 years old and didn't have anything to do," he told me. "I could go to California or New York and be an actor, but that reminded me of what I'd done in England before, that talent isn't a prerequisite to success in the entertainment business.

"I am bright. I liked school. So I said: How can I prolong adolescence? My dad always wanted me to go to law school. I'll try law school."

The law was in his genes. His father had been a Harvard scholar. His uncle was editor of the Harvard Law Review, dean of the University of Utah law school and author of a famous labor law textbook.

Fieger enrolled at Detroit College of Law. DCL, with its gritty downtown concrete-and-brick campus and its large percentage of night and part-time students, lacked Ivy League prestige. But for several generations in the criminal court trenches of Detroit and Michigan, where law is practiced toe to toe, DCL has produced a startling percentage of the best-known attorneys and judges.

Fieger found law was a higher calling than theater.

"Acting is a craft, not an art. The law truly is an art. The real artists in theater or movies are the directors, the writers. The actors are, like Hitchcock said, the cattle you move around. . . .

"Something about the law made total sense to me. . . . I just understood how to play with the clay. . . . It wasn't something that you could teach somebody. . . . Nobody can teach you how to make the statue like Michelangelo or Rodin. You can learn the technique, but you've got to go beyond the technique, and that's where I excel."

In 1979, Fieger graduated from law school and joined his father's firm. His brother Doug, meanwhile, had made it big. His new group, the Knack, had a chart-topping single, "My Sharona," on an album that sold five million copies.

But critics despised the Knack. According to *The Rolling Stone Encyclopedia of Rock & Roll*:

"With their Beatles-like packaging . . . contrived pop innocence and sexist lyrics, the band members were labeled cynical fakes—an accusation heightened by their refusal to do interviews. . . . A 'Knuke the Knack' movement began in the more radical parts of the same LA club scene it started in."

A follow-up album sold only 600,000. Band members fought. A third LP bombed. The band couldn't shake its hype reputation. After a poor tour in 1982, the Knack disbanded. (Doug Fieger in 1992 landed on TV's *Roseanne*, playing Nick, the Conners's neighbor.)

As his brother's rock career flamed out, Geoffrey Fieger became one of Michigan's most successful attorneys, specializing in lucrative medical malpractice suits.

In 1982, Fieger won his first big case. His client suffered from a relatively unknown disorder called tardive dyskinesia. With the help of testimony from a Chicago neurologist, Dr. Harold Klawans, Fieger proved the disorder was caused by a doctor over-prescribing anti-depressant drugs. The case got national attention. For Fieger, it was the first of many million-dollar settlements.

In 1983, Fieger married. He and his wife bought a large house in West Bloomfield Township, one of the richest communities in Oakland County, the nation's third-wealthiest urban county. Fieger joined a recall movement aimed at pro-development township officials and met Michael Schwartz, another attorney-resident who was head of the state's attorney grievance commission.

In 1985, Fieger represented teachers who had been sold expensive life insurance policies promoted as tax-sheltered annuities. He won $2.5 million, then the largest settlement ever awarded under the Michigan Consumer Protection Act.

Fieger's victories made him richer than his father and his rock-star brother. He had enough money for maids at home and work. But he was so compulsive about cleanliness that he would clean up after the maids, order his secretaries to scrub the floor and wash his own dishes at the office.

❐ ❐ ❐

In her late 20s, Martie Ruwart still was searching for her niche. She decided to become a science teacher. But after getting a bachelor's degree in zoology in 1980 from San Diego State University, she lasted only a month as a teacher's aide. Complaining that too much time was wasted disciplining the children, she quit teaching and started taking computer science courses. By 1983 she had another degree and soon got a job as a software engineer. She loved the work.

For environmental reasons, Martie wouldn't buy a car. She biked or took a bus the 10 miles to work. One day, a car ran into her, flipping her over her handlebars. Helmetless, she suffered a broken collarbone and multiple facial fractures. After extensive plastic surgery, her face eventually healed. But her back was never the same.

For years, she battled constant pain. At work, she had to drink as many as eight glasses of wine a day to stave it off.

Eventually, Martie found a therapist who got her on an exercise program. She started swimming, walking and lifting weights. She still had to take anti-inflammatory drugs, but her pain was under control. And her career in computers was blossoming. Employers found she had a rare combination of technical skills and compassionate insight into human problems.

❏ ❏ ❏

After Bernard Fieger died on September 3, 1988, of complications from diabetes, his son and law partner Geoffrey described him as "a brilliant and compassionate attorney who always fought for the underdog."

The younger Fieger kept his dad's name on his firm's shingle. After all, Bernie Fieger had played a big role in Geoffrey becoming a millionaire.

Here is how he explained it to me:

"I got the Jewish guilt but I got this sort of Norwegian arrogance, too. So where my dad was possessed with self-doubt and guilt, probably out of his culture and everything, I've got that, but I've also got a tremendous amount of that WASP-ish quality that exists out in Grosse Pointe. You know how those guys think they're just like God's gift to humanity?"

Also, Fieger told me, his father had instilled in him a constant fear of failure.

"He'd never give me credit for my successes. I'd say 'Look what a great job I did! I won this case!' My dad's reaction would be: 'So what have you done for me today, though, the rest of the day?' . . . I think he did that to himself, too, but he was too hard on himself. He didn't have the self-confidence I had. That's the difference.

"He never allowed me to rest on my laurels . . . so I have a great fear of failing, and that drives me. Also probably in that was a sense of wanting to please my father, to get his approval."

❏ ❏ ❏

Jean and Bill Ruwart talked a lot about death with their children. Cancer was such a frequent visitor there was no avoiding the topic.

Jean Ruwart's mother got cancer when Jean was a young girl. Toward the end, she was so brittle that bones broke when she was turned in bed. For the last six months, her children weren't allowed to see her.

Jean's father later died of cancer. Her younger brother died in his

40s of leukemia. Two uncles and an aunt died of cancer.

Bill's sister had died early, too, at the age of 42.

In 1987, when cancer came to Jean Ruwart, she asked her daughter Mary to research the Hemlock Society's suicide recipes, so she could have a way out if she needed it.

As Jean Ruwart started hoarding drugs to give her some chance to control her dying, no one in the family suspected that Martie, her second-oldest child, soon would be facing the same dilemma.

CHAPTER THREE
THE DOCTOR DEATH DIET

*"A well-balanced sense of humor is a great
defense against hopelessness and reckless panic
which can lead to undue expense, danger, and
psychic turmoil. A well-tickled 'funny bone' is a
prerequisite for keeping things in clear perspective."*
— *Jack Kevorkian,* Slimmeriks
and the Demi-Diet ❐

Like the quills of a porcupine, Jack Kevorkian's principles kept getting in the way of things like a career and a family.

When Pontiac General brought in a new chief pathologist who was enamored with technology, Kevorkian battled the new order, lost and quit. For 18 months, he worked at Wyandotte General Hospital in the downriver suburbs of Detroit. Then he launched another ambitious project. In Southfield, he opened Checkup Diagnostic Center, "a multiphasic diagnostic clinic for preventive medicine examinations." Technicians took histories and did X-rays and lab tests on walk-in clients and provided them with computer print-outs of their medical status. The business lasted only a year and a half because "other doctors felt competition and were frightened," according to Kevorkian.

In 1970, Kevorkian became chief pathologist at Saratoga General Hospital on the east side of Detroit. The job would be the apex of his orthodox medical career.

About that time, Kevorkian was engaged to a young store clerk. But he broke it off. Kevorkian thought his fiancee was not self-disciplined. Marriage wasn't worth it, he decided, if he couldn't find a perfectly compatible partner who shared his values and goals and interests.

He later called his rejection of marriage the biggest mistake of his life.

"That's shirking responsibility as a human being," he said of his refusal to procreate. "From nature's standpoint I'm immoral."

As a bachelor and a loner, Jack Kevorkian had plenty of time for his passions—painting, music and writing. He learned keyboard instruments. He got a concert organ and a harpsichord so he could play his beloved Bach.

For a New York publisher, Philosophical Library, Kevorkian wrote a medical history, *The Story of Dissection*, and a philosophical treatise, *Beyond Any Kind of God*. The jacket of the latter book describes it as an "effort aimed at trying to peer into the Great Unknown" and "to divine a philosophic view as timeless, as totally unchangeable, as the universe with which it deals."

Going from the sublime to the ridiculous, Kevorkian wrote, illustrated and self-published a limerick-laden diet book, *Slimmeriks and the Demi-Diet*.

By way of a biography, Kevorkian offered:

> *The author's official position/ Is not in the field of nutrition/ It wasn't his "dish"/ When at Ann Arbor, Mich.,/ He became a postmortem physician.*

Kevorkian's diet book humor was gentle and silly, not caustic. He opined that "fat people are not jolly" because "deep down they don't like being fat." But he insisted that "I am not on a 'body-beautiful' crusade. It makes little difference to me how you want to look to yourself."

Though a Jack Kevorkian diet eventually would sound like the creation of a David Letterman joke writer, the skin-and-bones pathologist was serious in explaining his personal battle with obesity. That took place in his freshman year at college, when a sedentary life-style and overeating ballooned him to "an unbelievable 162 pounds." In desperation, he started leaving half of all portions on his plate uneaten. That became the basis for his diet philosophy of "controlled nibbling." He also started lifting weights, seeking refuge from the "intimidating cacophony of voices, bouncing balls and thumping feet" in the university gym.

"I just wasn't going to compound my embarrassment and sagging self-esteem by exposing my effete, blubbery body to a gymful of physical fitness buffs," he wrote, explaining his decision to pursue a solitary form of exercise.

The gist of Doctor Death's diet advice, without the limericks: Don't smoke, avoid milk, get moderate exercise and eat whatever you want—just leave half of it on the plate.

Even in a diet book, Kevorkian couldn't resist a dig at death. He sketched a grave digger wiping his brow, resting on his shovel and staring at an enormous bulge in a fresh grave. The accompanying limerick explains:

> A life of profane deglutition/ Can end in a real grave condition:/ How the masses consumed/ Can be fitly entombed/ Will weigh heavy upon the mortician.

❒ ❒ ❒

Many people have wild dreams. Few act on them. But Jack Kevorkian had no family or promising career to hold him back.

As he approached age 40, Jack's big dream was to go to Hollywood and make a movie about Handel's *Messiah*.

Jack wasn't exactly a movie buff. He said he stopped going to movies after seeing *M*A*S*H*, because he found that film full of gory scenes and vile language. His own kind of movie would be more cerebral.

On June 23, 1976, Kevorkian filed incorporation papers with the State of Michigan for a new company called Penumbra, Inc., to produce his movie. He quit his job at Saratoga General, packed all his belongings in his beige 1968 Volkswagen van and drove to Los Angeles. He couldn't find an affordable apartment, so he slept in the van for a while.

Kevorkian talked his way into film studios and worked on his movie late at night. Somehow the lone wolf pathologist managed to complete a full-length, 90-minute film—something that doesn't happen without collaboration and considerable expense. But the film apparently never was exhibited, and it was the only subject in his life that Kevorkian steadfastly refused to talk about when he later became famous.

In 1979, he returned to Michigan and worked briefly at a hospital in Owosso. Soon he was back in California. To make ends meet, he took part-time jobs at the Beverly Hills Medical Center, where he resumed his "Death Rounds" of photographing the eyes of patients, and at Pacific Hospital in Long Beach. In 1981, he took a full-time job at Pacific. His boss, Dr. Fred Hodell, said Kevorkian's work was brilliant.

In 1982, Kevorkian rented a tiny apartment above a garage on Termino Avenue in the Belmont Heights area of Long Beach, an upscale oceanside neighborhood. He lived just above a garage.

"Termino" is Spanish for "the end."

The neighbors didn't care much for the headstrong doctor and his rickety van. One resident on Termino, Jeanne Craven, said Kevorkian always was coming in very late at night and complaining about barking dogs.

"Jack kept weird hours and he creeped up in this dilapidated old van," Craven said. "Naturally dogs are gonna bark."

Down the street lived an architect, Robert Murrin, and his family. Kevorkian tried to get their dog, Doric, impounded for barking at the mail carrier.

After one year at Pacific Hospital, Kevorkian quit in another dispute with a chief pathologist. He "retired" to devote his time to his movie, his research and writing and his reinvigorated death-row campaign.

Kevorkian wrote a comprehensive history of experiments on executed humans. It was published in 1985 in the obscure *Journal of the National Medical Association* after more prestigious journals rejected it. In the article, Kevorkian described in gruesome detail how the 16th-Century Mayans sliced open the chests and pulled out the beating hearts of human sacrifice victims and ate their peeled bodies, how Italians conducted electrical experiments on fresh corpses, and how French experimenters shouted victims' names into the ears of heads severed by the guillotine. Those lurid descriptions later filled many pages in *Prescription: Medicide*.

Kevorkian's research convinced him that modern methods of execution were inferior to the way it was done in the French Revolution or medieval India.

"Lethal injection is probably the most tolerable method on a subjective level," Kevorkian wrote in *Prescription: Medicide*. "But when it comes to technicalities of performance, the guillotine doubtlessly is easier to use, more uniformly consistent, and absolutely certain. And having an elephant squash the victim's head is the quickest of all . . ."

Kevorkian renewed his death penalty crusade. Capital punishment was making a comeback. The Supreme Court reapproved the death penalty in 1976, and the next year mass murderer Gary Gilmore became the first American executed since 1968. At the same time, new strides in transplanting organs provided Kevorkian with a new rationale. Surely no one could object to harvesting organs at execution from consenting convicts, thereby saving several lives in the bargain!

Kevorkian searched newspapers for the names of condemned criminals appealing their sentences. He wrote them letters. Some wrote back. He besieged prison authorities with requests for consent to his proposal. All refused to cooperate.

Kevorkian believed the rationality of death-row organ harvesting and experimentation should be self-evident.

"We wantonly squander priceless opportunities to study ourselves and our living brains, as well as new ways to make us wiser, healthier and happier," he wrote. "We snuff out lives of criminals eager to make amends by donating their organs and helping science unlock some of nature's deepest secrets."

Kevorkian's logic didn't prevail. Legislators in Kansas, Oklahoma, Texas and California toyed briefly with allowing organ donation by death-row prisoners, but the proposals were squashed under the elephantine weight of official disdain.

In 1986, Kevorkian learned that doctors in the Netherlands were helping people die, mostly by lethal injection.

"Then I conceived the idea of expanding my death row proposal to include experimentation on willing patients who opt for euthanasia," he wrote. His new crusade for assisted suicide would be an outgrowth of his lifelong campaign for medical experiments on the dying.

Kevorkian churned out articles about the usefulness of planned death and the benefits of euthanasia. More rejection notes followed. "Are you serious?" editors would scrawl across his manuscripts. The only journal that would print his articles was *Medicine and Law*, published in Germany.

In a 1986 article in *Medicine and Law*, Kevorkian praised Nazi doctors for trying to get some good out of concentration camp deaths by conducting medical experiments. He proposed euthanasia with few restrictions. He questioned whether psychiatrists should have the right to decide whether mentally ill patients were competent to choose suicide. He outlined a system of centers for death-on-demand, calling them "obitoria."

"It's time for a society obsessed with planned birth to consider diverting some of its attention and energy from an overriding concern with longevity of life at all costs to the snowballing need for a rational stance on planned death," he wrote.

At obitoria, research could be carried out on any consenting adult. Patients who did not wish to be anesthetized could remain conscious during some experiments. What kind of research would Kevorkian permit?

"No aim could be too remote, too silly, too simple, too absurd; and no experiment too outlandish. Any magnitude of gain would be better than vacuous death."

CHAPTER FOUR
BY APPOINTMENT ONLY

"Just try it once—that's all we ask."

—*David Letterman's "Top Ten Promotional
Slogans for the Suicide Machine" (#10)* ❐

One day in 1986, Jack Kevorkian's dingy van was gone from Termino Avenue. He had moved back to Michigan and rented a walk-up apartment on Main Street in Royal Oak. Here he seemed even more out of place than he had been in Belmont Heights.

Royal Oak was an older, family-oriented suburb whose down-town was transmuting into a trendy post-punk landscape. Strolling the sidewalks were ladies and gentlemen with multicolored spiked hair, nose rings and tattoos. Beneath Kevorkian's windows were singles bars, sidewalk cafes, nouvelle cuisine restaurants, stylish resale shops and metro Detroit's foremost purveyor of exotic leather lingerie and bondage apparel.

Kevorkian's flat was bare and utilitarian. Living off his savings, he slept on a mattress and worked at a plywood desk surrounded by cardboard file boxes scavenged from alleys. He bought a manual typewriter for $2 at a garage sale. He still had his VW van, but sometimes rode his sister Margo's black one-speed bike to seminars. He was a regular at the local library and the Salvation Army store. He played Bach and sometimes watched cartoons on TV. *Sylvester the Cat* was his favorite.

Kevorkian tried many local hospitals and even the Oakland County Medical Examiner's office, but he couldn't get a job.

"I'm too controversial for most positions," he explained in 1990. "All they have to do is see my publications on cadaver blood and on the condemned prisoner work. That alone settles the issue."

Kevorkian continued his provocative writing. In a 1986 article in the *Journal of the National Medical Association*, Kevorkian argued that only doctors should decide bioethical questions. He called for the medical profession "to reestablish biological order and reassert leadership" by creating a new medical specialty that would combine clinical training with the study of philosophy and religion.

"In the final analysis it is *medical* theory or action that is the crux of any biomedical problem with regard to any patient individually (and collectively through them with regard to society). From this, it follows that the skill and knowledge of a competent physician are more basic and would reign supreme."

Kevorkian acknowledged: "Critics will undoubtedly point out the great danger of concentrating so much power (over life-or-death decisions) in one person and the ever-present threat of abuse of that power." But he said critics exaggerated. Isolated cases of abuse were merely a sign of human imperfection, not any flaw in his proposal, he wrote.

At Michigan State University in East Lansing, Howard Brody, a family practice doctor and an expert in medical ethics, came across Kevorkian's article. Brody was forming a multi-disciplinary committee on ethics, so he wrote Kevorkian a letter offering to put him on the group's mailing list.

Kevorkian shot back a bristling reply. The gist of his letter, Brody said, was: "How dare you put me on your mailing list? I think what you're doing is a terrible, terrible thing. Only doctors should do this. I'm not interested in anything you are doing."

Looking for comrades, Kevorkian in 1987 flew to Amsterdam. Again he found rejection. To his surprise, he discovered euthanasia was not legal but merely tolerated in the Netherlands. And the leaders of the Dutch euthanasia movement considered his proposals for organ harvesting and experimentation so radical they would hurt the cause.

Still, speaking to Dutch doctors who had actually aided in suicides spurred Kevorkian to action.

"I decided to take the risky step of assisting terminal patients in committing suicide," he wrote later. "I could not even consider performing active euthanasia and thereby being charged with murder."

Mulling over methods, Kevorkian recalled a medical school professor who once had remarked that breathing carbon monoxide was the best way to commit suicide. In *Prescription: Medicide*, Kevorkian wrote that the gas is "toxic enough to cause rapid unconsciousness in relatively low concentration. Furthermore, in light-complexioned people it often produces a rosy color that makes the victim look better as a corpse."

In a passage that eerily foreshadowed his most controversial case,

Kevorkian also pointed out a drawback to carbon monoxide: "Some patients, especially those prone to claustrophobia, might suffer discomfort or stress in having to breathe through a plastic mask placed over the nose and mouth." He also speculated: "Popularization of the procedure and the general availability of canisters of the gas could lead to wholesale 'copycat' suicides by others who are in no way terminally or physically ill. That in turn could evoke such a powerful emotional reaction from various clerical and lay factions as to force the voluntary or legal curtailment of supplies of carbon monoxide for that purpose."

Eventually, Kevorkian decided on lethal injection as the best method. He was ready to launch a new career. "To add a touch of dignity and legitimacy to the new specialty, I coined the word 'obitiatry,' " he wrote. He printed up business cards that read: "Bioethics and obitiatry. Special death counseling, by appointment only." He went to hospitals and tried to pass them out to oncologists. Most doctors recoiled.

In June 1987, he placed classified ads in local papers:

DEATH COUNSELING
IS SOMEONE IN YOUR FAMILY TERMINALLY ILL?
Does he or she wish to die—and with dignity?
CALL PHYSICIAN CONSULTANT

According to Kevorkian, the ads brought only two responses: one from a man whose brother had been in a coma for six months, and therefore could not consent, and the second from a rambling young woman whom Kevorkian judged to be mentally ill.

"Maybe the ads were too unobtrusive," Kevorkian mused. "Maybe they were taken to be a charlatan's macabre get-rich-quick scheme or merely the prank of a 'kook.' "

In August 1987, the metro Detroit *Health Care Weekly Review* published an article about Kevorkian's ideas on euthanasia and death-row organ harvesting. George Adams, the story's author and the paper's publisher, had met Kevorkian the previous year. Adams was one of only five students who showed up for a class on medical ethics that Kevorkian was scheduled to teach at Oakland Community College. The class was canceled for lack of enrollment, but Adams and Kevorkian became friends.

Adams's article was the first widespread exposure for Kevorkian, and it generated a lot of angry response from the readers of the weekly, a paper aimed at the Detroit area's medical professionals and administrators.

A follow-up article in the American Medical Association's weekly tabloid, *American Medical News,* got Kevorkian national attention in the medical community—most of it negative.

He was turned down for a lowly paramedic's job at William Beaumont Hospital in Royal Oak. He had crossed the line from being a medical outsider to an absolute pariah.

"I never really fit in," Kevorkian said in 1991. "But I did use to feel at least that I belong to a healing profession. They don't think so any more—and I don't, either."

Casting about for an income, Kevorkian remained inventive.

One day, an eager salesman visited Tim Pendell, public relations assistant for the National Football League's Detroit Lions. The man showed Pendell a prototype of a sun visor cap made from high-grade construction paper.

"It had some pretty elaborate, well-done designs of lions' heads on the front," Pendell recalled. "He had a very high-quality product. It really was a nice item."

The man "had a distinct personality," Pendell said. "He was a pretty good salesman, personably persistent." But the entrepreneur had overlooked one basic fact: the Lions played in the Pontiac Silverdome. Pendell told him that sun visors didn't make much sense in an indoor stadium.

Later on, when the unusual name hit the news, Pendell recalled Jack Kevorkian as the sun visor salesman.

Kevorkian tried to sell his inventive visors to other sports teams. Again he struck out.

In 1990, Kevorkian told *People* magazine that his life had been "a failure":

"If I had married, I'd have had kids—kids and family are everything. Looking back, I would do almost everything differently."

George Adams told me that Kevorkian suddenly dropped out of sight in 1988. For a while Doctor Death was back in California.

One night, Kevorkian called Adams at home after midnight. He reported he was back in Michigan and told Adams he had given up on the idea of working through the system to win support for his ideas.

"I'm just going to have to take the first step to force the issue," Adams recalled Kevorkian saying.

That year, Kevorkian's article, "The Last Fearsome Taboo: Medical Aspects of Planned Death," appeared in *Medicine and Law*. He argued that modern society, facing the longstanding prohibition against planned death, was "subjected to unrelenting paternalistic control based on moral codes that are rapidly becoming obsolete." He called the medical profession "psychically (philosophically) retarded, drifting aimlessly without a coherent or even workable ethical code."

Kevorkian outlined his vision thus: "The acceptance of planned death implies the establishment of well-staffed and well-organized medical clinics ('obitoria') where terminally ill patients can opt for death under controlled circumstances of compassion and decorum. . . . Physician involvement should extend far beyond mere termination of life to permit exploitation of the enormous potential benefit that could accrue from the acquisition of organs for transplantation and the performance of daring and otherwise impossible human experiments under irreversible general anesthesia."

What kind of experiments? Kevorkian provided some hypothetical examples:

● The removal of kidneys, liver and heart from a convict at execution.

● Four days of drug research on another death-row prisoner.

● Implantation of a chimpanzee liver in another prisoner.

● Drug research on a woman with breast cancer who chooses suicide in an obitorium.

● The removal of organs from a "mentally competent 30-year-old man, badly deformed, in great pain, and essentially helpless due to worsening cerebral palsy" who "is granted his wish to die in an obitorium."

● An experimental test of a new technique for removing a pancreas, performed on "a 22-year-old man in robust physical condition" who "certifies in writing and beyond doubt his irrevocable intention of dying" after two years of professional counseling fails to stem his suicidal intentions.

● Four days of drug research on the brain of "a hopelessly incompetent 65-year-old woman crippled by Alzheimer's disease" who enters an obitorium with "proper consent and endorsement from all family members and from designated authorities."

● Drug tests and the removal of the stomach, liver and small intestine from a "full-term infant born with severe spina bifida, paraplegia, and hydrocephalus." The tests formerly were conducted only on rats.

Kevorkian wrote that "obitiatry would make it possible to conduct daring and highly imaginative research beyond the constraints of traditional but outmoded, hopelessly inadequate, and essentially irrelevant ethical codes now sustained for the most part by vacuous sentimental reverence." Such experiments would curtail the use of animals for research, save money and accelerate medical progress, he claimed, but added: "Perhaps the greatest advantage would be the further unshackling of the primal human right of what should be absolute personal autonomy within the bounds of reasonable law."

Critics, Kevorkian conceded, would resort to "unjustified, irrelevant, and occasionally deceitful scare tactics" such as "an emotional resurrection of the Nazi tragedy." But what the Nazis did, Kevorkian wrote, was "merciless killing," not mercy killing.

"Such horrendous infringement of a concept does not necessarily invalidate it," he said.

Kevorkian concluded by saying that "euthanasia"—a "good death"—did not go far enough.

"Such a death still entails complete negativity, no matter how serene. It serves no constructive or positive purpose beyond the bleak aim of extinguishing life. An immense amount of inherent good is thereby senselessly squandered. The aim should extend far beyond a mere 'good' death toward a superlative ideal, which technically might be called 'eutatosthanasia' or *best* death."

On April 4, 1988, Kevorkian called the Oakland County Prosecutor's Office to get a legal opinion on whether obitiatry would be legal in Michigan.

"None was given and there is no statute addressing this issue," wrote Michael Izzo, an assistant prosecutor, in a report. Kevorkian's call prompted an inquiry by the state department of licensing.

State investigator Cathy Svoboda interviewed Kevorkian on August 29, 1988, at a Denny's restaurant in Royal Oak. Kevorkian showed Svoboda a California driver's license and said his residence in Royal Oak was temporary. He gave Svoboda his journal articles and explained his views. Svoboda wrote in a report:

"Dr. Kevorkian indicated he is an ethical researcher and is not permanently employed as an independent physician. . . . Dr. Kevorkian is not pursuing participating in active euthanasia . . . because it is not legal and he does not want to get into trouble. He also said that no oncologists would refer patients to him at this time."

Kevorkian told Svoboda he had planned to assist in a suicide when he was living in California but "there was an attempt to get euthanasia on the ballot and he was asked to refrain from performing the illegal act."

To qualify for his help in dying, Kevorkian said, according to Svoboda, a patient "would have to be terminally ill and would have to be met by the attending physician four or five times" and that "an attempt should be made to dissuade the person." Later in the interview, Svoboda noted "he said it should take only one meeting by a bioethiatrist. The second meeting could last five seconds but at least it would be in the records."

Svoboda noted that Kevorkian "fashions much of his thinking on the way these deaths are prepared for and done in Holland."

"Dr. Kevorkian does not believe laws should rule or guide morality," Svoboda concluded. "Dr. Kevorkian maintains he is law-abiding but cannot agree or condone how law does not represent the consensus of society. He is making every effort to change laws and at the same time fulfill the demands of society. Dr. Kevorkian writes about his opinions—he has not acted on them."

Sometime in 1988, Kevorkian contacted Derek Humphry, the British-born journalist who in 1980 had founded the Hemlock Society with his second wife, Ann Wickett. Hemlock advocated legal physician-assisted suicide for the terminally ill. Kevorkian suggested to Humphry that they join forces and set up an experimental suicide center.

Humphry rejected the proposal. He later told a reporter that the idea of "getting a taxi to a suicide clinic appalled us."

In the summer of 1989, David Rivlin, a 38-year-old quadriplegic who lived in a nursing home in the Detroit suburb of Farmington Hills, publicly asked to be disconnected from life support. Rivlin's spine had been severed in a surfing accident when he was 19, and a failed spinal operation had left him breathing with a respirator. He faced decades of that kind of life. The Oakland County Prosecutor's Office tried to intervene to stop his death.

Kevorkian decided it was time to act. Rivlin—and others to follow—needed help in dying, he believed. But to make the matter as ethically clean as possible and to minimize abuse and coercion, the patient should "pull the trigger."

It took Kevorkian only a few days to work out the design, sketching on the Formica table in his kitchen: Start an intravenous drip of a harmless saline solution. Have the patient press a button to activate a device to stop the saline solution, start a new drip of thiopental and set off a 60-second timer. The thiopental would put the patient into a deep coma. After a minute, the timer's click would send a lethal dose of potassium chloride through the IV, stopping the heart in minutes. The patient would die of a heart attack while asleep.

Quick, painless and easy.

As the summer drew to a close, Kevorkian rummaged around hardware stores, garage sales, flea markets and his own junk piles. Using household tools, toy parts, magnets and electrical switches, he fashioned the death machine. It had an electric-clock motor with a pulley axle, a fine chain and two coils acting as electric bar magnets. He covered it with scrap aluminum siding and fashioned a handle and a stand for the drug bottles. The total cost of materials was $30.

He called the machine the Thanatron—Greek for "death machine."

He then added a device that would allow Rivlin to pull the string with his clenched teeth. But Rivlin rejected Kevorkian's help. A judge refused to intervene. Rivlin went to a friend's home and Dr. Jack Finn, director of the Hospice of Southeastern Michigan, supervised the removal of life support.

Undeterred, Kevorkian decided to test his new machine on a stray dog scheduled to be euthanized. Veterinarians in a local dog pound asked him to get permission from the head of the county health department, who referred Kevorkian to the humane society, who told him the request would have to be put in writing and handled at the next board meeting, four weeks away.

Frustrated, Kevorkian said it looked like he would have to use the machine first on a human being to prove it was safe for killing an animal that was going to die anyway.

He submitted an ad to the Oakland County Medical Society Bulletin:

Doctor seeking patients for new practice of obitiatry.

The submission was passed on to the board of the medical society. One of the board members was Dr. Murray Levin, Kevorkian's old colleague from Pontiac General. The board rejected the ad. But when a TV station found out about the matter, Dr. Jack Kevorkian and his suicide machine flashed into the living rooms of Detroiters for the first time.

Watching were a young woman and her father. She called Kevorkian and arranged a meeting. The man, 47, had inoperable cancer. He said he would rather die while alert than slip into a drug-induced stupor. But he lapsed into unconsciousness before he could try the suicide machine.

Again, Kevorkian tried to place a display ad announcing his services. This time, all the local papers refused it. But he got the kind of publicity you can't buy when first the *Oakland Press*, then the *Detroit News* ran stories about his search for patients.

"I have no fear about what I'm doing," Kevorkian told the *News*. "I'm here to help anybody who's in distress, or thinks he is." He said the machine was "dignified, humane and painless, and the patient can do it in the comfort of their own home at any time they want."

After national wire services picked up the story, Kevorkian, at age 61, finally got the recognition he had sought all his life. Via phone hookups from his apartment, he went on radio call-in shows nationwide. Soon, patients were calling him asking for help. But most were from out of state, and Kevorkian said he would not travel to states where assisting a suicide was a crime.

A local woman with multiple sclerosis called. Kevorkian met with the woman, her daughter and her neurologist. He urged her to try another course of therapy but agreed he would help her die later. After two months, the woman called to say the new therapy had failed and she had more pain than ever and wanted to die. But Kevorkian told her his first patient must be terminally ill. He promised she could be his second patient.

"In order to minimize the passionate (if irrational) storm of criticism certain to be evoked by such a procedure, I realized that ideally it should be in connection with a suffering and indisputably terminal patient—for example, someone dying of incurable and widespread cancer," he later wrote. "I explained how that should blunt condemnation of my assisting her as the second case."

A few weeks later, the woman with MS agreed to hold a press conference at her home to announce her wish to use the Thanatron. But before she could go on the air, a relative whisked her away to a hospital. Kevorkian never heard from her again.

In Portland, Oregon, Ronald Adkins picked up a copy of *Newsweek* and read an article about Jack Kevorkian. On November 13, 1989, he called Royal Oak.

Chapter Five
No Such Thing

> *"People don't like the prospect of sitting in their apartments alone, brewing a (lethal) cup of tea, possibly vomiting everything up and never being found until they are totally deteriorated. If people had a choice of having a nice, kind doctor give them an injection and sit by their bedside until they die, wouldn't that be better?"*
> *— Psychologist Faye Girsch* ❒

When Sharon Welsh was seven, her family moved to the working-class Detroit suburb of Roseville. A girl named Sherry Miller lived two doors away. The two played dolls and dress-up, rode bikes, had childish quarrels and became lifelong friends.

They went to high school together. They double-dated. They went on the same day to the same job interview and worked side by side as clerks at a mall. When Sharon got married in 1967, Sherry stood up at the wedding. The next year, they switched roles. Each had a child in 1971 and another in 1974. Sherry settled in Sterling Heights, Sharon nearby in Clinton Township.

The two women enrolled in the same exercise class. Running on an indoor track, Sherry would jog awkwardly and complain about "my bum leg."

In 1978, Sherry suddenly became unavailable. Sharon would call and Sherry would say she didn't feel like doing anything. When Sharon found out why, she drove to her friend's house and they sat at the kitchen table and cried.

Sherry had multiple sclerosis. It was a hard pill to swallow.

Many people with MS live full and productive lives, but Sherry went steadily downhill. She had to give up family outings, swimming in the backyard pool, painting, ceramics, crochet, needlework. She used a cane, then a walker, than a wheelchair.

Sherry's husband filed for a divorce. He got the house and the kids. Sherry moved back to her parents' house in Roseville.

Sherry didn't talk much about the divorce to her friend Sharon. Sherry never spoke a word of blame. Sharon surmised she still cared about her husband and it hurt her that he wasn't there now that she needed him so badly.

Asking for help was hard for Sherry, but soon it became necessary. There were fewer things she could do for herself.

By the time she turned 40, she was an invalid.

Her parents had to care for her. Physical therapists taught her mother how to massage her legs to keep the circulation going. If she didn't, Sherry's feet would turn purple.

Sherry hated losing her independence. She resented that her parents had to bathe her. She detested being a burden on people.

Occasionally she spoke to her friend about suicide.

"I can't go on like this," she would say. "I can't do anything for myself." Things will get better, Sharon told her friend, but with little conviction.

Sherry thought about driving her car off a cliff. Sharon knew that was just a fantasy. Sherry could no longer drive, there were no cliffs in suburban Detroit, and Sherry wasn't a violent person. But she was becoming a desperate person.

"She cried a lot," Welsh recalled. "She wasn't happy. It was never easy for her to accept what was happening to her."

Sherry asked Sharon to get her a copy of the book *Let Me Die Before I Wake*. When Welsh found it in the library, she was surprised to find it was the Hemlock Society's how-to-die book, with instructions for hoarding drugs for "self-deliverance." Sherry insisted Sharon buy her a copy so she could keep it.

One day, in the spring of 1990, Sherry told her best friend that she had seen a doctor on television who had a suicide machine. She had written the doctor a letter asking for his help. He had written back cordially but non-committally.

Sharon was shocked.

"This can't be true," she told her friend. "He must be some kind of quack. Sherry, make sure you don't give him any money."

Shaken, Sharon went back home. She told her husband. He reassured her that there was no such thing as a suicide doctor.

II

ANGER

"Do not go gentle into that good night,/ Old age should burn and rave at close of day;/ Rage, rage against the dying of the light."

—Dylan Thomas, "Do Not Go Gentle into That Good Night"

CHAPTER SIX
"HAVE A NICE TRIP"

> *"See, it was all theory before. Easy. But when you're doing it, it's rough. I was emotionally drained. It was the hardest decision I've made in my life."*
> — Jack Kevorkian (1991) ❐

Janet Adkins, dressed in a white blouse, a black suit, and a black, red and white scarf, lay still on the bed inside the Volkswagen van.

She stared past the crisp curtains at the towering pines. She watched the nervous little man bustle about her.

"Watch out," she told him when he grabbed a container of liquid. She didn't want another spill.

Finally, he was ready.

He plunged a big syringe into her left arm just below the elbow. But the needle slipped out of the vein. Doctor Death yanked it out.

Janet Adkins had traveled a long way to get here. Now she lay inside a rusted 1968 VW bus at a campsite outside Detroit. She could have stayed in Portland and taken a bottle of sleeping pills. Instead she had placed herself in the hands of this man, who was wearing a gray fishing cap his landlord had given him.

Her final exit, at age 54, was taking a very long time.

Shortly after 9 that morning, the doctor's two sisters had knocked on the door of the Red Roof Inn in Madison Heights, a near-north suburb of Detroit. Janet looked in the mirror, fixed her hair and her makeup and said her last goodbyes to her husband and her best friend. Ron cried a lot. She comforted him. Carroll Rehmke, her friend of 32 years, held her, cried, then pressed a letter into her hand. Then Janet got into the front seat of Margo Janus's car.

The relief Janet Adkins had sought for so many months was at hand. But that last parting from her loved ones had been more than five hours ago.

It took over an hour for Margo to drive to the park. Her sister, Flora, who had timed her visit from Germany to help their brother with Janet's death, rode in the back seat. On the way, Flora told her:

"Janet, you're taking exactly the same path that every human being has to go. You're just going down the path a little sooner, that's all."

After they got to the park and found the van, the doctor made them wait in the car while he tested his machine. Soon he came out of the van and told them he had knocked over a vial of drugs while reaching for a pair of pliers. More than half the thiopental—the drug to put Janet to sleep—had spilled out. Though there likely was still plenty to knock her out, the doctor didn't want to take any chances; and besides, he had left behind some tools he needed. So Margo drove them all back to Royal Oak. Janet remained quiet during the two-hour round trip.

It was after noon before they got back to the park. The day was still chilly and dank, like a June day in Portland. The doctor ducked back into the van and the three women sat in the car.

Flora read Janet her friend Carroll's letter:

"My dear friend —

"My heart weeps for you and for all of us. Keeping this vigil, watching you say goodbye over and over to those you love will change my life forever. My knees shake, my being feels broken and I don't know how to say goodbye . . . except to just say, goodbye, my friend. Shalom, Janet. You leave us with love. Peace to you. I will miss you and there are no words to tell you how very much. You have helped make my life richer. You are leaving us with courage. I am in awe, in pain.

"I love you,

"Carroll."

The doctor anxiously conducted more dry runs. There was a new mechanical problem. Luckily he now had the tools he needed to fix it. Nearly two hours passed with the three women inside the car.

Janet couldn't wait to get out.

Finally, the doctor beckoned her.

"Is it really going to happen?" Janet asked the sisters as she scurried inside.

The van, which looked beat-up from the outside, was tidy inside. On a small bed were clean sheets and a pillow. Crisp yellow drapes covered the windows.

Janet Adkins lay on the bed. She could hardly stand any more delays. The doctor's bony hands cut small holes in her nylon stockings. He hooked EKG electrodes to her ankles. He covered her with a light blanket. Flora stood near the door.

The doctor had a large syringe to make sure he could open a wide hole for the drugs. But her veins were small and fragile. Even a slight movement of her arm would cause the needle to break through the wall of the vein. He tried once, twice, three times on her left arm.

It had been only one summer earlier that another doctor had coldly delivered his crisp judgment, the word cutting through her like a scalpel: Alzheimer's. That doctor told Ron it wouldn't be long before he would have to dress and bathe his wife.

Janet Adkins knew what she wanted. She had played tennis, climbed the Himalayas, traveled around the world, hang glided, played Brahms duets with her husband, raised three sons, taught piano, taught English, learned T'ai Chi, studied reincarnation. Being addled and dependent was not her idea of living.

She and Ron were Hemlock Society members. They started to hoard drugs. Despite the opposition of two of her sons, she set November 30 as the date of her self-deliverance. But every option looked worse as the date neared. She considered jumping out a window or taking pills. "But none of those give you dignity in death," Ron said. "Somebody finds you, or you vomit the drug up." They thought about going to the Netherlands, but then they heard about Kevorkian. His device "in a sense brought the Netherlands to Michigan," as Ron put it.

Ron called Dr. Kevorkian, but the doctor suggested she try another course of therapy. She enrolled in an experimental trial of a new Alzheimer's drug, Tacrine, at the University of Washington. But the drug didn't help.

Finally, Kevorkian asked her to come to Michigan. And now she was in his van, waiting to see if he would make good on his promise.

He decided to try the right arm. Janet Adkins got up from the bed where she had lain down to die, then waited while the doctor moved his device to the other side of the bed.

All the delays were like heavy blocks pressing down on Jack Kevorkian's shoulders. He too had come a long way to get here. By the spring of 1990, nine months after building his machine, Kevorkian had grown frustrated in his search for a candidate. When Ron Adkins called him in April to say the drug therapy hadn't worked, Kevorkian acted quickly. He called Janet's doctor in Seattle. The man adamantly opposed her wish to die and said she had years of quality life left. But that didn't gibe with what Ron Adkins had told Kevorkian on the phone about how fast his wife's mind was slipping away.

In the book he would write later, Kevorkian explained his selection of Janet Adkins:

"Even though from a physical standpoint Janet was not imminently terminal, there seemed little doubt that mentally she was—and, after all, it is one's mental status that determines the essence of one's existence. . . . from Ron's narrative I concluded that her doctor's opinion was wrong and time was of the essence. Because Janet's condition was deteriorating and there was nothing else that might help arrest it, I decided to accept her as the first candidate—a qualified, justifiable candidate if not 'ideal' . . ."

For weeks, Kevorkian searched for a venue. He ruled out his own apartment and his sister Margo's: He didn't want the landlords to be held liable. He inquired at many motels. They refused. Churches, even the ultra-liberal Birmingham Unitarian Church, turned him down. Funeral homes demurred. He got firm rejections from office buildings, clinics, doctors' offices. He investigated getting a life-support ambulance, but found they were not for rent. Even members of the local Hemlock Society refused to let him use their homes. He toyed with the idea of going to Portland, renting a boat and using the machine outside the three-mile coastal territorial boundary.

Finally, in May, a friend agreed to let Kevorkian use his Detroit funeral home. Kevorkian contacted Ron and Janet Adkins. They settled on Monday, June 4, as the date of Janet's exit.

Elated, Janet selected the music and the readings for her memorial service. She arranged for a therapist to mediate final "closure" sessions with her sons. She didn't fear death. A medium had told her she'd lived her last life in Greece with nine children. She already was looking forward to her next life.

A few days before she planned to die, Janet played tennis with her son Neil. She beat him.

In Michigan, the man who owned the funeral home backed out. Now Kevorkian was in a bind. The Adkinses already had plane tickets. His van was the only option left.

Kevorkian called Portland.

"I didn't want to do it in a van," Kevorkian later recounted. "Anything. Anything but the van." But Ron Adkins told him that Janet insisted they proceed.

"She was so distraught," Kevorkian recalled. "I decided I had to do it anyway. For the patient. That's what a doctor is for. To hell with the goddanged ethicists. I'm a *real* physician."

Her husband told him that Janet Adkins didn't care where her death took place. "And she liked Volkswagens," Kevorkian insisted.

He needed an electrical hookup. The owners of a private park refused but suggested nearby Groveland Oaks, a little-used Oakland County park. The spot was remote and beautiful. Kevorkian rented a secluded campsite.

On Memorial Day, Ron and Janet and their sons spent a last day together. Back at their apartment, Janet videotaped final messages to her three grandchildren and wrote a letter to her 82-year-old mother.

On June 1, Janet's son Norman drove her to the airport, so she could have a last ride in his Porsche. She kissed her sons goodbye and got on the plane with Ron and Carroll Rehmke. Arriving in Detroit, they took rooms at the suburban Red Roof Inn not far from Kevorkian's apartment.

Kevorkian and his sisters came there the next afternoon. They had a discussion and Janet Adkins filled out authorization forms Kevorkian had prepared. She couldn't remember how to write the capital "A" to begin her last name until her husband showed her. Then they all went to dinner at Uptown Charlie's and stayed at the restaurant until after midnight, talking and laughing. Janet and Kevorkian found a kinship in their love for Bach. Janet had whiskey before dinner and sat for hours afterwards at the restaurant bar with her friend Carroll.

"It's hard for people to understand," Rehmke said later. "But we had fun all weekend." They went sightseeing, read poetry and had expensive meals. On Sunday, Janet and Ron spent their last day together.

Then came this long day. Janet got back on the makeshift operating table. Doctor Death carefully searched her right arm for a suitable vein. He stuck in the needle and winced as it failed a fourth time.

Exasperated, he tried another vein.

Finally, the syringe held.

As Janet had asked, Flora read her the 23rd Psalm.

"Though I walk through the valley of the shadow of death, I will fear no evil, for Thou art with me."

Now there was a new problem. Kevorkian decided the saline solution wasn't flowing fast enough, so he rigged up a little box and raised the vial onto it to increase the pressure of the flow.

Finally, the anxious doctor was ready to proceed.

"Do you want to go through with this?" he asked Janet. "Are you sure you want this?"

She replied: "Tell me how to hit the switch. Please, show me how."

There was a safety cap on the switch. He showed her how to hit it—three times. She kept saying: "I want it to be right. Is this how?"

Then he took the safety cap off and said: "Are you ready?"

"Yes," said Janet Adkins. She stretched out her arm toward the jumble of plastic tubes and toy parts. With the outer edge of her right palm, she hit the switch on the flea-market science project—once, twice, and a third time for good measure. The thiopental rushed through the tube and into her body.

"Thank you," she whispered, and the doctor bent over her. She rose up—as if to kiss him, the doctor later said. Then her head fell back.

"Have a nice trip," replied Jack Kevorkian.

Janet Adkins turned an ashen gray. Within a few minutes oval waves appeared on the EKG graph paper, indicating the bizarre electrical activity that accompanies death. She made a couple of small gurgles and motions: death rattles. Then the waves tapered off and the machine traced a straight line on the paper. The line went on and on.

The straight line meant Janet Adkins's heart had stopped.

For the first time that day, the sun poked out between the clouds and bathed Groveland Oaks Park.

Later, Kevorkian would write of Adkins's quiet death:

"Flora and I had witnessed an epochal event that will refocus the moral dimensions of purposeful termination of human life, raising it from pointless disputation over merely nihilistic 'mercy killing' or judicial execution to a higher plane of respectability."

Chapter Seven
"Out of Business"

"This is not the time for philosophizing. We've got to try something. The suicide rate is skyrocketing. Elderly are killing themselves by all kinds of violent means. . . . That means the problem is getting worse. It means new action, not old action, not old theories, not old principles. Action, new. It calls for mind over emotions. What distinguishes humanity? The mind. So far emotions are ruling. We need the mind to rule."
—*Jack Kevorkian (1990)* ❐

Sharon Welsh watched the TV in horror. The newscast said a doctor named Jack Kevorkian had used his suicide machine to help a woman die.

It was the doctor her friend Sherry Miller had contacted.

"It was like the bomb dropped," Welsh said. "It became real."

❐ ❐ ❐

One of Murray Levin's secretaries rushed into his office.

"Dr. Kevorkian killed somebody," she told Levin.

"My first thought was: Poor Jack's going to jail. He's really acting out on his thoughts," said Levin, Kevorkian's former colleague."I thought he was more talk than do, at that point. I didn't think he'd do anything that radical.

"I really thought he had gone over the line, and I wondered what had happened to him mentally. This was not cadaver business and harvesting organs from someone killed by the state, this was now something he had done directly.

"He had gone beyond what I would have ever expected of him."

❐ ❐ ❐

After hearing the news about Janet, Ronald Adkins and Carroll

Rehmke went to the airport. Police officers paged Adkins; he did not answer. They went to his gate; he did not step forward. A ticket taker pointed him out; he denied everything. Finally, they pulled him off the plane and questioned him. He said he could not recall the name of the doctor who had helped his wife die. The police let him go.

Back in Portland, Ron Adkins told KATU-TV:

"It's not a matter of how long you live, but the quality of life you live, and it was her life and her decision and she chose."

❐ ❐ ❐

When Janet Adkins died, the leaders of the right-to-die movement all were in the Netherlands for an international conference on euthanasia. By default, Janet Good, the Farmington Hills woman who led the Michigan chapter of the Hemlock Society, became the nation's number one expert on assisted suicide. She logged 144 calls on her answering machine. The *Today* show came to her home.

Good had formed the local Hemlock chapter after reading about Kevorkian's suicide machine. Kevorkian had promised to speak at the chapter's first meeting. But then he asked her if he could use her house for Adkins's death. She had to refuse because her husband, a retired Detroit police officer, was afraid of repercussions. Kevorkian got so angry with her that he canceled his Hemlock appearance.

After Kevorkian took so much flak for using his van for Adkins's death, Good said she felt deep regret about refusing his request.

The day after Adkins died, Good signed up eight new Hemlock members.

❐ ❐ ❐

Jack Kevorkian later recalled how he felt after Adkins died.

"I was so jangled emotionally. You panic because you—is it going well? When I did cadaver-blood work it was the same panic feeling. You know, when you're doing something for the first time and nobody else in the country is doing it, you get scared."

He also told a reporter:

"She was very calm. She dreaded what would have come. I would too. I don't want to die of Alzheimer's—smeared with your own urine and feces, don't know who you are. Come on!"

□ □ □

The adjective "rusty" appeared in the lead sentence of nearly every press account of Janet Adkins's death.

Dr. Howard Brody of Michigan State University said the attention paid to the van's exterior amused ethicists.

"Some of us devised the Ziebart principle of medical ethics, that if the van hadn't been rusty that somehow would have made it morally better."

To critics of the venue, Kevorkian shot back:

"Where was Christ born? The world's worst conditions—in a haystack with manure and animals all around."

Kevorkian admitted: "I took a helluva risk. Don't you think I knew what I was doing? The world's worst conditions—I knew I was going to get heat for it. But for this anguished human being, I did it. Now, that's what a doctor is supposed to do, right?"

Wrong, said Michigan's medical leaders, interviewed for a June 7 *Detroit Free Press* story headlined "Profession Condemns Doctor."

"Any mechanism whereby you overtly end life is unethical," said Robert Paxton, ex-president of the state Medical Society.

Jack Finn, the hospice director who had assisted David Rivlin's death, said that act was ethically superior to what Kevorkian did.

"It was removing a medical device he no longer wanted. He was able to say his goodbyes and tears were shed, photos were passed, his favorite music was played . . . and it was in the home of his dearest friend." Adkins, he said, "died with indignity. She was alone in the back of a van in a park with this machine and this doctor. That's no way to die."

Finn said Adkins "could've lived 10, 20 years. And what bothers me the most is the lethal injection was provided by a physician. That violates our ethical code, the Hippocratic Oath. I would have to say that Dr. Kevorkian's approach is veterinary medicine and that we as human beings are not animals."

Murray Levin told the *Free Press*:

"This is more than can be tolerated. It's contrary to everything we stand for in medicine. We don't go around killing people."

The following day, the *Free Press* apologized for the headline, saying it "should have made clear that members of the medical community, rather than a professional association, are critical of Dr. Jack Kevorkian's actions in helping a woman commit suicide."

❐ ❐ ❐

The nation's paper of record, the *New York Times*, editorialized on June 7:

"Pressing society to weigh the ethics of euthanasia is not outrageous. Dr. Kevorkian's behavior is. This is a time when people are searching for a humane consensus about when to withdraw treatment from the dying. ..."

"But now, here comes a Dr. Jack Kevorkian to publicize himself, his 'Rube Goldberg apparatus' and his willingness to make a martyr of himself. 'They'll be after me for this,' he says.

"They should be."

They were.

Barbara Listing, president of Right to Life of Michigan, warned that if Kevorkian were allowed to continue his practice, the state would be "the place to go for death-on-demand."

Fred Dillingham, a former undertaker who was Right to Life's main man in the Michigan Senate, quickly drafted a bill that would make assisting in a suicide a four-year felony.

Dillingham told me that when he had heard about Janet Adkins's death, "it was like somebody kicked you in the chest and you lost your breath."

Despite a ruling by an acting county medical examiner that Adkins's death was a suicide, Oakland County Prosecutor Richard Thompson launched an investigation.

"It's not the wishes or the desires of the deceased that's important," Thompson said. "It's the acts of the people other than the deceased that are important."

Kevorkian told reporters he wasn't worried about the law:

"There's no law in the first place. Even if there were a law on this, it would still be justified. I have no fear of the law in this society.

"Assisting in a suicide is not illegal in Michigan, so I doubt I'll go to jail. But if I do, then that's all right. Let them make me a martyr.

"I'm not saying you should kill patients or shouldn't kill patients. But it should be a medical service, like it is in Holland. ... If the patient wants to die, it is his right. Personal autonomy is the highest right."

❐ ❐ ❐

A few days after Janet Adkins's death, Sharon Welsh heard on her car radio that a Roseville woman with MS was going to do a TV interview about her desire to have Dr. Kevorkian help her die. When she got home, Sharon, shaking, turned on the TV. There was her friend Sherry Miller. But Sherry had her back to the camera, and her last name was not revealed.

"My main concern was her kids because I didn't think at that point she had discussed any of this with her children," Welsh told me. "What a way that would be to find out."

❏ ❏ ❏

On June 8, Jack Kevorkian stood in Judge Alice Gilbert's courtroom at the Oakland County Courthouse in Pontiac, not far from where he had drawn crowds a half-century earlier by calling baseball games like Jack Graney. Richard Thompson had asked Gilbert, a Circuit Court judge, to issue a temporary restraining order to stop Kevorkian from using his suicide machine again.

The doctor who repeatedly had written that doctors should smash social taboos against planned death now had a chance to convince the government he was right.

He failed, but not for lack of trying. Representing himself, Kevorkian was on the stand for more than two hours trying to explain his ideas and methods. His caustic, often sarcastic questioner was Oakland County Assistant Prosecutor Michael Modelski, a last-minute replacement for another prosecutor who was stuck in a murder trial.

In an opening statement, Kevorkian told the court there was no Michigan law against assisted suicide. He said Adkins's death was "the first concrete step in a long-range plan that I have envisioned long ago. . . . toward true enlightenment, in which we can develop a rational policy of planned death for the entire civilized world. . . . If a rational policy of planned death can be attained, the benefit for society is incalculable."

Kevorkian admitted: "Now, I know that sounds rather self-serving and rather silly, but it isn't."

If Adkins could have donated her cornea and all her major organs, as she wished to do, eight or nine lives could have been saved with her transplanted organs, Kevorkian testified. But "because of that Dark Age mentality born of a taboo, eight to nine people died. . . . That's why I'm so ardent on this project. It's not a personal campaign."

Kevorkian told Gilbert he wouldn't mind an injunction being

issued against his further use of a suicide machine, as long as she would let him "put together a small team of what I call 'Untouchables,' build a little clinic under the supervision of any type of people you want . . . operate it under the same strict supervision with criticism and dialogue until we have what seems to be the most incorruptible system on this tiny scale. . . . . Once that is established, set the guidelines and then use that as a model for the rest of the civilized world."

Modelski put Kevorkian on the stand and asked him if he felt resentful toward the medical establishment.

"I have contempt for their attitude," Kevorkian replied. "They are indoctrinated with Dark Age mentality. And I'm sure if they could do it today they would burn me at the stake."

Kevorkian complained that his articles on planned death had been "stonewalled by the medical press" in the United States "because they want this quiet."

Modelski asked: "So, Doctor, is it true that in fact you sort of want to establish a Domino's [Pizza] of death, where people would just sort of call in, you would deliver with your machine and in your van, is that what you sort of perceive for the future?"

"I'm surprised at the lack of imagination of your question," Kevorkian replied. "Let me put it in two succinct sentences why it was done in the van and what its significance is: No room at the inn. I'm sure you know what that means. And the savior of a major fraction of mankind was born in the most abject conditions possible. . . . It's all I could do. I'm alone . . . a formidable mind in the Dark Ages."

Pressed by Modelski about his ability to evaluate Janet Adkins's condition, Kevorkian admitted he had no expert information on Alzheimer's disease and had never spoken to her before she came to Michigan.

"I probably won't have expert information in the area of many patients who consult me," he said. "I always consult with their doctor first. I don't do it on my own decision, you know. That would be rather presumptuous."

He testified that in May he had called her doctor:

"He said . . . that she could go on probably in a clear mental state and live fairly well for another year." Then, Kevorkian told the court, he asked her doctor: "What happens after she slips into a vegetative state and is no longer available for the service she wants?" Kevorkian testified that her doctor replied: "Well, I'd have her husband shoot her." Kevorkian said he was flabbergasted at the remark.

"I said, 'What?' And he said, 'Sure, right in my own office.' Now, I knew he was lying, first of all; and, second, to make a statement like that as a physician, you're pretty close to insane."

Modelski asked the name of the doctor, and Kevorkian said: "I don't know if I should give it because it's his word against mine."

"Oh, you're saying that he'll probably deny this now?"

"He may. Doctors are very corruptible when their career's on the line."

Despite what Janet Adkins's doctor had told him, Kevorkian said he decided to go ahead anyway because "I've got to take what's best . . . for this patient, considering everything I know about the case, because there's nobody else to help me decide. Nobody. Every doctor would stay as far away from this as they could. So I decided on my own, which is presumptuous, but the only alternative left, if this patient is to get what I think she deserves."

Modelski asked Kevorkian if he would help a 25-year-old in perfect health commit suicide. Kevorkian said no.

"I've had many healthy people call me who are mentally distraught, crying on the phone, begging me to end their lives, miserable, in and out of mental institutions," he testified. "I tell them: Nothing I can do. I only can work with physical diseases at this stage. The rest of it comes when society matures a bit and they can come to grips with this problem."

Kevorkian said there were five criteria for assisted suicide: The patient's needs, the patient's wishes, and the doctor's medical expertise, common sense and logic.

"Now, these last two are lacking in many doctors, common sense and logic," Kevorkian said.

Modelski asked Kevorkian if he was well-versed in the psychological factors involved in requests for suicide. Kevorkian said he wasn't. Isn't that crucial, Modelski asked.

"Not if they have a crippling physical disease," Kevorkian replied. "I don't rely on mental problems. I rely on their physical disease, which then affects the mind. Anybody who's got a terrible crippling disease and is not depressed is abnormal."

Kevorkian admitted it was sometimes hard to distinguish mental from physical problems: "These are gray zones and they're the toughest decision in medicine. That's probably why the profession shied away from it."

Kevorkian said that "in the case of David Rivlin, everybody who saw him said he should die, except a couple of religious fanatics. . . . His doctor came forward and pulled the plug, which is euthanasia. What happened? Nothing. This isn't euthanasia that I'm doing, it's assisted suicide. Euthanasia is illegal in this state. Nothing happened to his doctor, did it? What's this double standard?"

Kevorkian said he repeatedly told Adkins during their dinner at Uptown Charlie's that she could change her mind and back out. Each time, he testified, "her eyes welled up with tears. . . . She was terrified that I was going to back away."

Kevorkian said he chose a public park for the suicide because "it would be a little more immoral to go into a private park than a public park." He said Adkins was in a hurry to die: "Never once did she show hesitation; never once did she show signs of depression. She was anxious to get it done."

Kevorkian said he felt "flattered" when people called him a Doctor Frankenstein: "People who know Frankenstein would know why."

Judge Gilbert asked Kevorkian if he ever had talked to any member of the Legislature about his plans. Kevorkian said that would have been useless.

"I figured the time for talk is over on this. . . . We have ethicists today splitting hairs over cliches and all kinds of silly arguments, so we don't know which end is up, what is ethical and what isn't."

Kevorkian said he didn't help Janet Adkins to get his jollies: "I don't enjoy seeing people die. It was a wrenching emotional experience to me. In fact, the only calm person through this whole thing was Mrs. Adkins. Her husband, her best friend, my sisters and I were sort of emotional wrecks."

Kevorkian made it clear that his real goal was experimentation, "the extraction of medical benefit from imminent death of people who want to get it." Use of his device, he said, was "just the first step trying to break this wide open so the profession is forced to face this problem finally. You can't deny it always. You can't stonewall this. It's in enormous demand out there."

He told the court that if his license were revoked, "I will build another device and use another system because assisting a suicide is not a crime in Michigan. So you can revoke my license and I will still help patients, but not as a doctor."

Modelski also questioned Flora Holzheimer, Kevorkian's sister.

She testified that she and her sister Margo drove Janet Adkins to the park because "there was no other possibility. No human being was brave enough, convinced enough, motivated enough, daring enough, religious enough, genuine enough to take our place."

In his summary, Modelski told Gilbert that Adkins died a "tawdry" death because of Kevorkian's "Keystone Cops" approach.

"He is an irresponsible doctor," Modelski said. "It was an undignified death.

"He sort of revels in the fact that he's sort of an outcast; that he's sort of a maverick, and maybe that he's going to be a martyr."

Kevorkian then admitted to Gilbert: "Almost everything the prosecuting attorney said is correct. I probably am not the best qualified to do it. . . .

"I know it's presumptuous and even looks arrogant for me to get up here and say this. All the arguments that were presented by the prosecuting attorney against me were the same arguments presented against Margaret Sanger when she was trying to establish . . . a rational policy of planned birth. . . . She was persecuted; she was imprisoned for a month; she had to flee the country. . . . She also was considered to be a maverick, doing something in a back-alley way. . . .

"The same thing is happening here. All I'm trying to do is . . . condense the time period between the birth of it and its acceptance, so it's available to everybody in this world.

"Abstractions and medical ethics, philosophy, religion, these are inventions of the human mind. But medicine deals with down-to-earth reality of disease and death . . . When there's a conflict, medicine should prevail. And you are not justified in inventing abstractions . . . to limit the realities of existence. . . . Ethics are always relative or they're ineffective. . . .

"Suicide of the elderly is accelerating at double the rate predicted a few years ago. . . . I have been contacted by elderly patients. . . . Two women, 83, 84 years old, weeping on the phone because for the first time . . . in the last 10 years, they can live comfortably knowing that this option is available if they need it. . . .

"If this service were available everywhere as a legitimate medical service to all the public . . . I know the suicide rate in this country from all causes would plummet . . ."

Citing the suicide of Doctor William Harvey, the discoverer of blood circulation, and the physician-assisted suicide of Sigmund

Freud, Kevorkian argued: "If it's good enough for the elite and aristocracy of society, it's good enough for Janet Adkins, it's good enough for the common people. If only the elite can have this because they have an inside track to the doctors and the drugs and keep it quiet, it's a sick society. Why not a general practice, well-controlled ... for everybody who needs it, no matter what his station in life? That's why I'm doing this.

"If I talk of martyrdom, it's not for me. It's not that I look saintly or want to look saintly. I don't care about that. Have another doctor run it. I'll step back, but do it. Take the step. That's what I'm pleading for. ...

"This Court has the opportunity to show the civilized world how to gain enlightenment. Or do you want to wallow in the Dark Ages for a few more decades while more people kill themselves by jumping off bridges and blowing their brains out and pulling sacks over their heads? ...

"I'm angry. Sure, I'm angry. I'm angry at society. I'm angry at the profession. I'm angry at everyone. Time to end the Dark Ages. Time to move forward. That's what I want ...

"The time has come to take a historic step at least in the controlled circumstances I laid out. There's no danger; it's minimal. It's a little experiment. You have absolute control. Try it. If it doesn't work, we quit. Where's the damage? If it works, you have reached a little further, giant step toward enlightenment, and a victory for the human mind. Thank you."

Gilbert rejected Kevorkian's invitation: "This court is not the forum for the establishment of medical ethics ... or public policy ... or medical practices. Neither is the taking of a life in an old van the proper place to establish medical ethics, public policy or medical practices."

Gilbert ruled that Michigan's citizens could suffer irreparable harm if Kevorkian were allowed to continue, and she issued an injunction:

"The defendant, Dr. Kevorkian, his agents, and employees, and those in active concert or participation with him shall be and hereby are enjoined pending final disposition of this cause from: using, employing, administering, offering, or providing any of his 'suicide machines,' or other similar devices, contrivances, or other modalities or drugs, including nonprescription drugs, on or to any persons seeking to end a human life, or conducting any acts to help a patient commit suicide, regardless of the modality employed."

The judge concluded: "He is causing death through unnatural means, and nothing is more permanent than death."

Kevorkian, who had told reporters he would go to other counties if banned from practicing in Oakland County, was surprised to learn that Gilbert's injunction covered the entire state.

He said he would comply with Gilbert's order.

"I'm out of business," he told the media. "It's the end of Dr. K helping patients die."

CHAPTER EIGHT
"I WANT THE CUFFS"

*"If I go to jail, remember that I am
not immoral. Society is."*
—*Jack Kevorkian (1990)* ❏

On Friday, August 17, 1990, Jack Kevorkian found himself back in Alice Gilbert's courtroom, trying to hack through an unfamiliar thicket of legal procedure by invoking great dead men.

Prosecutor Richard Thompson's office had filed a complaint seeking a permanent injunction against the suicide machine. Kevorkian had not responded to the complaint in the required time. Gilbert ruled he was in default, but gave him 21 extra days to respond.

Still acting as his own attorney, Kevorkian told the court the injunction "was an improper move to begin with, and the default then becomes irrelevant."

Kevorkian tried in vain to submit in his defense a 20-page statement that included "testimony" from Aristotle, Pliny the Elder, Sir Thomas More, Thomas Jefferson and Albert Einstein. In it, he said he wanted to expand his practice of a "rational policy of planned death" for patients with obvious physical diseases who are in obvious physical stress.

"In such cases, medical expertise or specialization becomes irrelevant," he wrote. "Even laymen could readily make the evaluation, and on first contact with the patient."

Gilbert, citing courtroom procedure, did not allow the great minds to speak in Kevorkian's behalf. She urged Kevorkian to get a lawyer: "I recognize that you are an intelligent and articulate person, but now you're in a different forum. You understand?"

"Yes, I understand." Kevorkian responded. "I'm in the machinations of nicety of abstractions, and I know you can get trapped in that."

"You're in the forum of due process."

"Which is a synonym of what I said."

Leaving the fog of the courtroom, Kevorkian told reporters he no longer felt bound to obey Gilbert's temporary injunction and insisted:

"I'm not going to get an attorney because I haven't broken any laws."

That afternoon, attorneys flooded Gilbert's chambers with phone calls. All hoped to get the chance to represent Doctor Death. They failed. Instead, the flamboyant lawyer who once had portrayed the Salem scapegoat Giles Corey stepped forward to defend the modern heretic who had testified the medical profession wanted to burn him at the stake. Within 48 hours of saying he wasn't getting a lawyer, Jack Kevorkian was a client of Geoffrey Fieger.

A former associate of Fieger, who did not want to be named, told me that Fieger solicited Kevorkian. George Adams, Kevorkian's publisher friend, said Kevorkian told him the same thing. Such recruiting of a client would have been regarded as unethical because, while attorneys can advertise on TV, they are barred from pitching their services to individuals.

Fieger told me that Kevorkian just called him up out of the blue. Fieger said he had stopped by the office on a Saturday or Sunday with his wife to cool off after watching a nearby celebrity polo match.

"I think we were having some water or iced tea or something, and I swear to God the phone rang and it was Jack. And he said 'Do you know who I am?' And I said, 'Yeah, I know who you are.' And he said 'I'd like to come over and talk to you with my sister.' "

Fieger said he agreed to represent Kevorkian for free because the case was "interesting."

"I'll tell you this from the bottom of my soul and you better believe me," Fieger told me. "I have never, never done any of this for money."

By every account, Kevorkian was impressed with Fieger's famous performance in the William Beaumont Hospital case. A few months earlier, Fieger had marched into Beaumont, one of metropolitan Detroit's biggest hospitals, with a court order. Outside were a moving van and a forest of TV cameras. If Beaumont didn't pay what it owed his client, he told reporters, he was going to shut the place down.

Fieger had won a $1.25-million settlement against the hospital. Part of that was still unpaid. When Fieger started moving furniture out of an office, a Beaumont official was forced to hand over a check. It was a brilliant PR stunt by Fieger.

"That took gumption," Kevorkian said after hiring Fieger.

❏ ❏ ❏

The same weekend that Kevorkian and Fieger were getting acquainted, Bertram and Virginia Harper and their daughter flew to Michigan from their home in Loomis, California, so that Virginia, who had terminal cancer, could die the Hemlock way. News reports about Janet Adkins's death had led the Harpers, who were Hemlock Society members, to believe assisted suicide was legal in Michigan. In a hotel room in Romulus, near Detroit's Metro Airport, Virginia Harper, 69, swallowed sleeping pills. Then Bertram, 79, put a plastic bag over her head. His wife died of suffocation. Her husband was charged with murder.

Fieger said he bailed Harper out of jail, but much to the attorney's dismay, Harper hired Hugh "Buck" Davis to defend him.

At his murder trial in Detroit, Harper admitted placing the bag over his wife's head.

The jury acquitted him.

❏ ❏ ❏

Assistant prosecutor Michael Modelski said he and Geoffrey Fieger got off on the wrong foot. Fieger called Modelski to ask if he would agree to set aside the default judgment Judge Gilbert had entered against Kevorkian.

"I said, 'First file an appearance as his attorney, and then we'll discuss it,' " Modelski recalled. "He started screaming at me, so I hung up on him. Ten minutes later he called back."

Gilbert set aside the default. Both sides prepared for a trial on Richard Thompson's request for a permanent injunction against the suicide machine, which Fieger had convinced Kevorkian to rename the Mercitron, or "mercy machine."

Kevorkian told *US News & World Report* that he was working on a new version of the machine: "smaller, more sophisticated, smoother looking, very few moving parts. Can't go wrong."

❏ ❏ ❏

From the way they went at it, you'd have thought Richard Thompson and Geoffrey Fieger were two old roosters who'd been scratching each other's eyes out in cockfights for years.

Yet both told me they had never tangled in the pre-Kevorkian era.

Fieger rarely handled criminal cases, so there was no reason for their paths to cross.

Thompson, like Kevorkian the son of Armenian immigrants, for 16 years had been chief assistant to the previous Oakland County prosecutor, L. Brooks Patterson. Patterson, a right-wing Republican, became one of Michigan's most prominent politicians during the Ronald Reagan era. Thompson was elected in 1988 after Patterson anointed him as his successor.

"Some see Richard Thompson as a publicity hound, a less flamboyant version of L. Brooks Patterson, who was Thompson's roommate as a young lawyer," said a *Free Press* profile, which added that Thompson was also "a warm family man."

Thompson refused to allow plea bargains, even in the most minor cases. Thompson's assistant, Gerald Poisson, noted: "The public really does like this hard approach to crime." But many judges—and defense lawyers—said Thompson's policy clogged the court system and was needlessly adversarial. At a 1992 meeting of Young Republicans, Thompson said he trusted "no one who wears a robe."

Donald Tucker, chairman of the county's Democratic party, characterized Thompson as Patterson's "hatchet man": "Their entire modus operandi is geared toward choosing the cases that pander to racist fears, that pander to supermarket tabloid headlines, as in the Kevorkian non-event."

In the late 1960s and early 1970s, Patterson was a lawyer for right-wingers fighting court-ordered busing to rectify segregation in the Pontiac school system.

"Thompson is the successor of a litany of bigots," Fieger told me. "To me that is totally repulsive.

"I think Thompson is really a malevolent fellow. He's not a lawyer. Even though he got a law degree he knows nothing about criminal law other than the same type of thing that Franco or Mussolini or Hitler thought about criminal law. That's his attitude about the criminal justice system and constitutional rights."

After filing an appearance as Kevorkian's attorney, Fieger immediately lit into Thompson. He charged that Thompson was using the civil complaint on the injunction to try to compel testimony from Kevorkian, while at the same time investigating him for murder. To Fieger's way of thinking, it was a way to circumvent the Fifth Amendment protection against self-incrimination.

"He was obviously planning to charge him with a crime and was therefore, without advising him of his constitutional rights under Miranda, taking testimony from a guy he was planning to charge with murder, which is absolutely despicable," Fieger said. "And he was being supported in it by Gilbert, who is a lackey of the prosecutor's office."

Fieger, moving quickly to counter-attack, pulled off the rare feat of compelling a sworn deposition from a sitting prosecutor. Under questioning by Fieger and his partners, Thompson admitted he didn't know much about the law in Michigan on assisted suicide.

Fieger told me that Thompson "picked the two wrong people to play around with. This guy on his best day doesn't come equipped with nearly what he needs to tangle with Kevorkian and myself."

After all, Fieger told me, "I'm the Ty Cobb of plaintiff's attorneys."

Fieger claimed he won eight or nine out of every 10 cases. But his acting training wasn't the reason for his success, he said.

"My ability to speak and think on my feet is a very strong attribute, but it would mean nothing if I didn't have this other quality, which is a crystalline understanding of the law and how it works, and how it needs to be—and don't use this word wrong—manipulated. I'm not talking about manipulating other people. I'm talking about taking all the various aspects and theories of the law and molding them, manipulating them, into something that makes sense to a jury. . . . I'm real good at it. . . ."

Fieger also denied a former associate's characterization that he was a "master of the red herring" in the courtroom:

"That's just bullshit. You can't trick juries. . . . I wish that was true. I wish that I had the ability to trick people. I don't. My ability comes out of the talent I possess and then doing things that I truly believe in, because I've now come to the point at which I never have to take a case I don't believe in."

◻ ◻ ◻

Kevorkian's civil trial before Gilbert was scheduled to start December 4. On the morning of December 3, Thompson called a news conference to announce that he was charging Doctor Death with first-degree murder.

"Doctor Kevorkian was the primary and legal cause of Janet Adkins's death," Thompson contended. "He cannot avoid his criminal culpability by the clever use of a switch. . . . For me not to charge

Doctor Kevorkian under these circumstances would be a corruption of the law and turn Oakland County into the suicide mecca of the nation.

"Doctor Kevorkian is not above the law, and if he wants to change the law he should address the legislative branch of the government. If physicians are to have a license to kill in addition to their license to heal, that license must come from the Legislature, not the prosecutor."

Thompson released a psychological evaluation of Adkins done in June 1989. Clinical psychologist Larry Friedman of Portland Community College concluded that Adkins had memory loss, poor concentration, "severe deficit in abstract concept formation and flexibility in problem-solving" and "mild to moderate deficit in analysis and reasoning, judgment, and visuospatial organization and construction." Friedman reported that Adkins "has expressed concern about her potential quality of life."

Friedman said Adkins "has always made significant contributions to her family and community, and with help she should be able to identify activities through which she can continue to derive a sense of contribution and satisfaction."

Thompson also reported that toxicologist Frederic Reiders had concluded that the suicide machine had not worked as planned. Kevorkian had intended the thiopental to induce a coma, but Reiders said so much of that drug entered Adkins's system that it collapsed her blood circulation and caused death. The potassium chloride intended to stop her heart was not distributed throughout her body but concentrated in a small area around the injection site, Reiders said.

Thompson charged: "Doctor Kevorkian has indirectly attempted to corrupt the decision-making process of this office by characterizing his acts as compassion for a terminally ill, pain-ridden woman. As a result, many people who have seen terminally ill loved ones suffering excruciating pain support his action.

"Janet Adkins was not terminally ill. She was not in any pain. Doctor Kevorkian's sole interest in her was to put her to death and use that death to advance his cause and his machine.

"I have a constitutional duty to faithfully enforce the laws of this state . . . regardless of the tragic and emotional aspects of this case."

Soon after Thompson's press conference, the circus came to town. Thompson and Michael Modelski both told me that Fieger had promised to bring Kevorkian that day to Clarkston District Court, where the arrest warrant had been issued. Instead, Fieger tipped off the media that he was going to the county courthouse. Cameras trailed as he brought Kevorkian to Judge Gilbert's chambers.

Fieger told me that the prosecutor's office called him after Thompson's press conference and ordered him to bring Kevorkian to the state police within a half-hour. "I said: Fuck you, I'm takin' him to court and showing what a fuckin' bogus piece of shit you are, because I've been saying through this whole civil action that this was a ruse to try and criminalize and now you've violated his rights, and besides that we're supposed to start this trial tomorrow. So I took him to Gilbert's courtroom for what I thought would be some meting out of justice."

In vain, Fieger tried to get Gilbert to stop the arrest on the grounds it would interfere with his client's civil trial.

State police went to the courthouse. Kevorkian confronted the officers and demanded they handcuff him:

"It's a charade. Let's make the charade right to the letter," he shouted. "I want the cuffs. I want the cuffs."

He didn't get cuffs, but was arraigned before District Court Judge Gerald McNally in Clarkston. Kevorkian was taken to the county jail late in the afternoon and released that evening after a $50,000 bond was posted.

The *Free Press* story the following day had five paragraphs quoting Thompson's press release before Kevorkian was quoted for the first time, in the 18th paragraph:

"I don't take this seriously. This is all immoral anyway. . . . What happens to me is immaterial. The time has come for this thing."

Fieger is first quoted in the 27th paragraph, calling the murder charge "a moral and legal outrage. The suggestion that Doctor Kevorkian as a deliberative act killed a person with premeditation is totally and utterly ridiculous."

Under Michigan law, the penalty for first degree murder is life in prison without parole.

CHAPTER NINE
THE WORD FOR THE END

*"I'm supposed to tell an intelligent person
she should go to a day-care center and learn
to play with blocks? Learn to wear a diaper?
She didn't want that."*
—*Ronald Adkins* ❏

More than two-thirds of the states in the United States have laws against assisted suicide.

Michigan had a legal conundrum.

In 1919, a Michigan farmer named Frank Roberts mixed a deadly poison in a cup and placed it on a nightstand next to the bed of his wife, Katie. Multiple sclerosis had so ravaged Katie that her weight had dropped from 143 pounds to 67. She previously had tried to commit suicide by taking carbolic acid. Katie drank the cup of poison and died. Her husband was charged with murder.

The case went to the Michigan Supreme Court, which in 1920 found Roberts guilty even though his wife wanted his help in ending her life. Roberts was the only man ever convicted of first-degree murder for assisting a suicide in Michigan. The governor commuted his sentence to four years, and Roberts went free in 1923.

In 1967 and again in 1979, the state Legislature rejected efforts to make assisted suicide a lesser crime than murder.

In September 1980, 22-year-old Steve Campbell of Goodells, Michigan, caught his wife Jill in bed with his best friend, 20-year-old Kevin Basnaw. Campbell slapped his wife, then spent the evening drinking beer and taking mescaline with Basnaw. Late that night, he told his wife he was going to get even with her and Basnaw.

A few nights later, Campbell and Basnaw were drinking heavily. Basnaw complained about his bad luck and said he wanted to kill himself. Campbell encouraged him to do so and offered to sell him his gun. They left and returned with a sawed-off .22 rifle. Basnaw told his girlfriend and Campbell to leave so he could kill himself.

They left. Basnaw was found the next morning in a pool of blood with a suicide note to his mother beside him.

Campbell was convicted of murder. But the state appeals court reversed the ruling. The Michigan Supreme Court declined to hear the case, saying incitement to suicide is not a crime. It noted that even in states where assisted suicide is a crime, the penalties imposed are much milder than for murder. It urged the Legislature to act to clarify the matter.

In bringing charges against Jack Kevorkian, Richard Thompson argued that *Roberts* was still the law in Michigan because no court had overturned the 1920 Supreme Court ruling. Thompson said the Supreme Court's refusal to hear the Campbell case meant that it had chosen to let *Roberts* stand.

Geoffrey Fieger would argue that the *Campbell* court had ruled that *Roberts* no longer was the law, and the Supreme Court's refusal to hear the appeal meant that it concurred in the opinion that assisted suicide was not a crime.

With the murder charge against Kevorkian pending, Judge Alice Gilbert held a hearing on December 4, 1990, on Thompson's request for a permanent injunction against the Mercitron.

At Fieger's advice, Kevorkian refused to answer any questions. Fieger said the murder charge made it necessary for his client to invoke the Fifth Amendment.

Outside the courtroom, Kevorkian had something to say:

"This is something that has got to be addressed by the medical profession. I'm not going to commit wholesale suicides."

Fieger tried to get the civil trial stopped because of the murder charge. He also said Thompson and Gilbert were conspiring and should be charged with prosecutorial and judicial misconduct.

No dice.

Then Fieger brought out the Barracuda.

Michael Schwartz, a former assistant prosecutor in Brooklyn, New York, had gotten the nickname while heading Michigan's Attorney Grievance Commission from 1979 to 1988.

"He earned that name because of the vicious way he carried out the duties of the office," Fieger told a reporter. "He made a lot of lawyers cringe in fear."

During Schwartz's tenure, more than 750 lawyers were disciplined—more than the number sanctioned in the entire previous history of the state bar.

Fieger said he wanted Schwartz's experience in criminal law.

"We complement each other," Fieger said. "He's very deliberate, very judicial. I'm more likely to react. We're perfect foils for each other."

Fieger and Schwartz called a press conference and held up a torn piece of paper. They said it was the top of an internal memo from the prosecutor's office. The memo, they said, reported that assisted suicide was not against state law.

Schwartz charged that Thompson "knows and has known full well that the acts . . . that Doctor Kevorkian is alleged to have committed are not and have never been violations of statutory law in the state of Michigan."

Thompson said he knew of no such memo.

"It's just another blatant lie," he told reporters. "It's a grandstand play to shift the focus away from the real issue here, which is the legal application of the law to Kevorkian.

"There has never been a memo that I have seen in this office that's held that physician-assisted suicide is legal.

"If Mr. Schwartz was Pinocchio, he'd have to have plastic surgery on his nose right now."

The next day, Thompson gave the press a one-page memo that stated assisted suicide was illegal. He said that opinion was written after Kevorkian called an assistant prosecutor in 1987 asking for a ruling on the issue.

When I interviewed him for this book, Thompson opened his drawer, looked in it and read from what he said was the memo, written by the assistant prosecutor Kevorkian had called:

"The man wanted to come in and talk about a matter of a delicate nature . . . he wanted to know if it was against the law to help someone commit their own suicide. I told him yes. He got upset and said he had already checked with the Detroit College of Law and they told him there was no law against it."

When I asked Fieger about what Thompson had read to me, Fieger said: "I promise you that she was told to write that after she had told Thompson that it is not a crime in Michigan."

Why did Fieger have only the top part of a memo?

"I don't remember, but I didn't have all of it."

◻ ◻ ◻

On December 12, Judge Gerald McNally began a preliminary exam on the murder charge. Amber Wells, an investigator for the state licensing bureau, testified that she had interviewed Kevorkian on August 6 and asked him what he would have done if the drugs had not killed Adkins.

"He stated he would have to break the law and finish it himself," she said. Fieger vehemently objected to the question, and the judge ordered it stricken. But Wells's statement led all the news reports of the hearing.

"He was not concerned about what the law was," assistant prosecutor Modelski told the court. "He was going to finish it himself. His intent all along was that she die."

Margo Janus, Kevorkian's sister, stood up in the back of the court and shouted at Modelski: "Liar! Liar!"

Dr. Jacob Chason, a neuropathologist, testified that Adkins's brain tissue showed she had a severe case of Alzheimer's—more diseased than all but one of the thousands of brains he had examined.

The next morning, prosecutors showed a videotape of Kevorkian's discussion with Ron and Janet Adkins, taken at the Red Roof Inn on Saturday, June 2. The tape had been seized under a search warrant in Kevorkian's apartment.

Each side claimed the videotape supported its case.

On a TV interview a few days earlier, Fieger had said the tape showed that Adkins wanted to die.

"Janet Adkins says explicitly, 'I see my life ending. I know that I will end up in a nursing home confined to a bed, tied down, not knowing who I am, what I am, or where I am. . . . I wish to end it now while I'm cognizant.' "

In fact, Adkins makes no such explicit statements in the taped interview.

Thompson said most of the tape consisted of "self-serving statements" by Kevorkian and Ron Adkins, and that they made the tape to absolve themselves of blame.

I didn't see the tape in court that day. It would not be until a year later that I would be assigned to the Kevorkian story. But when I did see the tape while working on this book in the spring of 1993, I fully understood how ambiguous it was and how both sides could claim it supported their contentions about Janet Adkins.

In the tape, Kevorkian, Janet and Ron Adkins sit facing the camera left to right. Janet Adkins wears round glasses. Her brown hair is pulled back into a thick ponytail. She is wearing a peach-colored blouse with a big bow in front. Her husband, in a bow tie, white shirt and sports coat, sports a salt-and-pepper mustache and goatee and smaller round glasses. He looks more like a college professor than the investment broker he is.

Kevorkian asks when they first noticed a problem. Ron does most of the talking. He says two years earlier Janet started having trouble sight-reading music and playing the piano. She started having difficulty spelling and writing numbers. Ron had to help her grade papers for her English classes.

When her doctor "dropped the bomb" on June 12, 1989, he suggested some experimental therapies, but "she didn't want to be a guinea pig," Ron says.

Kevorkian asks Janet what bothers her about living.

"My life before was wonderful," Janet says animatedly, "because I could play the piano, I could read. I can't do any of those things now. . . . It's too taxing."

Janet says she still can play tennis, though she can't keep track of the score. Kevorkian asks how good she is, and Janet laughs and replies: "Fantastic."

"Oh, sort of the Steffi Graf of Portland?" Kevorkian jokes, and Janet laughs again. "Almost," she replies.

Kevorkian asks whether she is in pain and Janet looks a little confused, then says she is not.

"Do you find this is so incapacitating that it destroys the balance of life toward the negative side?" Kevorkian asks.

"Oh, absolutely," Janet replies. "It's not the way I want it at all."

Ron explains that Janet "has been the light of our lives"—a woman full of mental curiosity who has kept her family intellectually stimulated. He says it is hard for everyone to be "seeing things she loves taken away from her."

"Tennis is about the only thing she has left," Ron says.

Kevorkian asks: "Now, Janet, you don't want to go on?"

"No, not at all," she says.

"And it's your decision?"

"Yes, it's my decision."

Her voice is insistent but sounds like a petulant child's.

Kevorkian asks Ron how he feels about it.

"I am for what she wants to do," Ron replies. "I love her and I want her to have what she wants. If I were in her position, that's what I would want."

"In other words, we're talking autonomy and self-determination?"

"That's right," Ron replies, "to not have to suffer and to have a rational way to do it."

"Of course you realize that she is not terminal."

"Not in a physical sense, but mentally she is."

"Close to it, anyway. How would you characterize her mental state?"

"I think she's rational and she's able to make decisions on her own and exercise her own free will."

Kevorkian then asks Janet Adkins:

"Janet, are you aware of your decision and the implications of your decision?"

"Yes."

"What does it mean?"

"That I can get out with dignity." She pauses. "Maybe." She giggles.

"What are you asking for? Can you put it in plain words?"

"I don't know."

"Just—what is it you want? What is it you want?"

"I would like to . . ."

"Put it in simple English."

She wipes an eye with a finger.

"Self-delivered and . . ."

"No, simpler, simpler than that."

"I don't know." She looks confused and turns to her husband. "Can you help me?"

"Do you want to go on?" Kevorkian asks.

"No, I don't want to go on," she says, again sounding like a plaintive child.

"You don't want to go on living."

"*I don't.*"

"Do you know what that means?"

"Yes, I do."

"What does that mean?"

"That's the end of my life, but whatever is next I don't know . . ."

"What's the word for that?"

She hesitates. "Euthanasia?" she ventures, looking at Ron.

"No. What is the word for the end of life? What happens when you stop living?"

"You're dead." She laughs.

"Is that what you wish?"

"Yes."

"That's the word I want. You understand the implications of that? Do you understand what that means? What the word 'death' means? It means the end of life."

"Uh-huh."

Kevorkian asks her how her sons feel about her decision.

"They said, 'Go with peace, mom.' That's what they said." For the first time, she begins to cry softly.

"Why do you want your life to end?"

She is at a loss for words, then starts to reply, but Kevorkian cuts her off.

"Because what's coming—now I don't want to put words in your mouth now—because what's facing you is worse than death?"

"I've had enough."

"Enough?"

"I've had enough."

"What does that mean? For example? That you lived well?"

"Yes, I did."

"That you lived a whole life?"

"Yes, very, very . . ." She wipes her eyes.

"Are you in agreement with everything she says, Ron?"

"Yes, yes I am."

Kevorkian asks if her disease is getting worse. Ron says it is. He says he has to call her to remind her when it's time to leave the house to play tennis. He says she keeps leaving her purse behind.

"These are things that are slipping away," Ron says.

Kevorkian continues: "You know what you're asking me to do?"

"Yes," Janet Adkins replies.

"You want help from me?"

"Yes."

"You realize you push the button?"

"Right."

"You can stop any time. You don't have to go on."

"Right."

Kevorkian confirms that the suicide is planned for Monday.

"You realize that Janet's decision is going to be harshly criticized," he comments. "Have I encouraged you in any way to do this?"

"No," says Janet.

"Absolutely no," says Ron.

"You understand of course that I prefer that she do change her mind and go on, because it's a tragic event at best, and the end of human life is never desirable. You know that."

Ron says Janet had drugs available, but that she prefers "this option" because it is "a much more humane way."

"I did not suggest to you that this is the best way to go?"

No, says Ron: "Your name came up in an article in *Newsweek*, and I called you."

"I'm helping mainly for one reason," Kevorkian says. "The highest, the top ethical principle for me is having individual self-determination. . . . So even if I find it repellant or distasteful to help you do this, it becomes of secondary importance to the main principle of the physician doing what's best for the patient in front of him. It's a tough decision, and I think more doctors should make it, because they're in a position to do so, nobody else.

"And therefore I'm doing this, even though it's a disagreeable action on my part, because it's rational and correct. . . . And that's why I'm doing this, you see, not because I like to see people die, you understand that?"

He points to the camera.

"People are looking at this out there. Some say you're correct. Some say you're not. Some say you're doing the wrong thing. What do you tell them?"

Janet replies: "That I just"—she sighs—"I want to get out." She looks at Ron and then at Kevorkian. "That's the way I feel."

"What would you say if they say that you're doing the wrong thing?" Kevorkian insists.

"I'm sorry, I just still want to get out?" Her voice rises at the end as if asking a question, and she looks at both men.

"Ron, what would you say to someone who would say that Janet is taking the wrong course?"

"I would say that it's her decision and she's made it. And she has the right to make her own decision on it, and it's her life and it's her dignity."

"Right," says Janet.

Kevorkian continues: "I would say that these tough decisions have got to be made. And who's in a better position than physicians, because life and death are in their domain? And they're abrogating their responsibility by dodging the issue.

"If this is going to be kept incorruptible—which everyone is going to bring up, the corruptibility, the Slippery Slope, sliding into license . . . it calls for the deepest and the most serious and hardest thinking on the part of doctors. . . . They've got to do this, no matter how distasteful to them. . . .

"Well, Janet, I'll go along with you to help you out because I see that you're a very intelligent woman from a very intelligent background and a good and loving and intelligent family. . . . And I can empathize with you with what's facing you with this diagnosis. The day may come when what you have can be cured. Unfortunately for you, I don't think it will come quick enough for you and your family."

"That's right," Janet says.

"I then agree to help you in the spirit of Hippocrates—this is probably what they would say in his day, many doctors did it despite what people say today—in the spirit of Hippocrates and disregarding my personal feelings and all the emotionalism that's going to swirl around what you want. In the name of human rationality which you're beginning to lose, I've decided to help you on two days hence, on June 4, on the morning of June 4. Ron, how does that sound?"

"If that's OK with Janet, that's fine with me."

"Thank you," Janet says, and laughs.

"Don't thank me. I think the world one day will thank you and Ron because what you're doing is a historical move. I don't think it's ever been done officially since the days of classical Greece. So I think the world will thank you one day."

The tape ends with the three staring into the camera.

After seeing the videotape, Judge McNally went to lunch. When he returned, he dismissed the murder charge.

The judge said *Roberts* did not apply to this case and the state needed a new law to cover assisted suicide.

"The Legislature has a responsibility, and I would hope they would step out and meet it," said McNally, and invited an appeal. "I certainly hope it doesn't end with my decision."

Grinning at the verdict, Kevorkian said he would not use his suicide machine until the injunction was overturned. He called on the
medical profession to work with him to devise guidelines for assisted
suicide.

"I'm going to work with the authorities and within the system,"
he told reporters. "I'm not going to break laws."

Despite Judge McNally's invitation, Richard Thompson did not
appeal his decision. Instead, he urged the Legislature to act.

"As a prosecutor I have a natural abhorrence of judges making
rules, inventing law," Thompson explained to me later. He also said
he feared that after years of appeals, "we could have come to the
same place that they did in the *Campbell* case: The court says we
don't want to hear the case."

Besides, he said, Kevorkian had promised he wouldn't violate the
injunction.

Health Care Weekly Review named Jack Kevorkian its Man of the
Year for 1990. Readers revolted at the selection. About 100 of the
paper's 1,000 or so paid subscribers canceled their subscriptions.

CHAPTER TEN
VILE HARANGUE

> *"Frankenstein was benevolent, a dedicated*
> *researcher and doctor. He created this monster*
> *because he was interested in life and death. The*
> *monster was very loving. But he was shunned*
> *everywhere he went, so he lashed back.*
> *Society treats my creation the same way they*
> *treated Frankenstein. Evil! Terrible! Immoral!"*
> —*Jack Kevorkian (1990)* ❐

Geoffrey Fieger had blocked one legal behemoth. To get his client into the open field, he now had to neutralize Judge Alice Gilbert. Fieger believed the best defense was a good offense. On the eve of the civil trial before Gilbert on Richard Thompson's request for a permanent injunction, Fieger told reporters:

"I intend to try Mister Thompson."

The real battle would be between Fieger and Mike Modelski, the assistant prosecutor who had made a thorough study of Kevorkian's writings and career. Modelski, in a more understated way, was as rabid pushing his viewpoint as Fieger was in defending Kevorkian. There was no love lost between the two.

Fieger once told reporters: "Modelski's not in my league."

Citing that comment, Modelski told me: "I don't want to be in his league."

Modelski waged psychological warfare. When Kevorkian entered Gilbert's courtroom on January 4, 1991, he saw his suicide machine on the prosecution's table. Next to it was a big pile of books. On top of the pile, in clear view, sat a thick, black volume. It was *The Nazi Doctors: Killing and the Psychology of Genocide*, by psychologist Robert Jay Lifton.

For two days, Modelski kept leading doctors and ethicists right past the big black book to the witness stand.

One of the first to testify was Janet Adkins's doctor, Murray Raskind.

"I don't think that a person with her degree of Alzheimer's would be able to give informed consent," Raskind told the court. "Judgment is one of the first abilities to be impaired in Alzheimer's disease. Her judgment was certainly impaired in the time I saw her." Raskind said that he told Kevorkian in their May phone call that Adkins "was the wrong person for a test case" because she had seven to 10 years of life left.

Fieger lit right into Raskind. Hadn't he told Kevorkian that he would urge Ronald Adkins to shoot his wife if she became a vegetable?

Raskind insisted he'd never said such a thing. And Raskind steadfastly maintained that Janet Adkins was not mentally equipped to decide her fate.

"She'd been incompetent for a year," he told Fieger.

"Then why do you commit malpractice?" Fieger asked.

"How dare you!"

"But you did."

"Never."

"And treated her illegally, with wantonly illegal behavior. You tell us she has been incompetent for one year, yet nine months ago, you allowed her to sign the consent form for medical experimentation. Here in Michigan, that's illegal. Isn't it in Washington? To say nothing of unethical and immoral."

After Raskind left the stand, Amber Wells again testified. She submitted a letter Kevorkian had sent the state licensing bureau on January 24, 1990, outlining his new "practice":

"Candidates for the service must be alert and mentally competent, and their underlying condition must be physical (not psychiatric). The service entails more than one consultation with the patient, their close family members, and their personal physicians. The suicide is accomplished in a painless, fast, and dignified way by means of a device I invented last year. . . . In every instance the local medical examiner will have been given prior notice."

Wells testified that Kevorkian had told her on August 8 that he would need to take refresher courses in medicine to continue his practice. He admitted he had never before used the drugs he used on Adkins, and he was unsure how effective they would be. She said Kevorkian told her he had no back-up plans, and if there were any problems he might have to break the law and finish things himself. Wells also said Kevorkian told her that in the future he wanted to help assist the suicides of healthy young adults who had long felt a desire to die.

Next came to the stand a parade of anti-Kevorkian medical ethicists. Dr. Leon Kass of the University of Chicago testified that patients wouldn't trust doctors if doctors helped patients die. "This is the deepest violation of the meaning of being a healer," he said. And Kass said it would be impossible to determine whether patient requests for assisted suicide were voluntary and informed.

Dr. Arthur Caplan of the University of Minnesota, author of a syndicated column on medical ethics, said Kevorkian's role in Adkins's death was unethical because Kevorkian had a conflict of interest in testing and promoting his suicide machine, because Kevorkian bought the drugs and hooked up the machine, because he did not know Adkins well enough to determine if her consent was informed, and because Adkins was not terminally ill.

During his cross-examination, Fieger surprised Caplan by blurting out: "Are you a Nazi?"

Fieger wanted to counter Modelski's experts with one or more of the 12 doctors who had written a 1989 article in the prestigious *New England Journal of Medicine* advocating assisted suicide in some cases. But none of the authors he invited was willing to risk testifying.

So Fieger brought no "expert" witnesses—just lay "experts" on suffering. His star witness was Sherry Miller. Her testimony would complete her amazing transformation from an intensely private person into a public figure. In many radio and TV appearances, Sherry had spoken openly of her desire for Jack Kevorkian's help.

"Maybe she felt going public would help her chances to have him help her," said her friend Sharon Welsh. "Her goal could have been to make it clear that dying was her choice, that she was pulling the strings."

In court, Miller testified she had waited too long already.

"I'm no longer able to care and do for myself," she said on the stand. "Everything has to be done for me. Look at me. I can't walk. I can't write. I can hardly talk. . . . I should have done something sooner. I should have ended my life when I was capable of doing something on my own. I can't take a bottle of pills. I can't get to them. I need help with everything."

Fieger asked Miller if Kevorkian was egging her on.

"I'm the one who is making the decision," Miller said. "Nobody else.

"I want the right to die and I want the right to have help."

In his cross-examination, Modelski asked Miller if she would want to die if she didn't feel she were a burden to others. She paused and said she couldn't answer hypothetical questions.

Modelski later told me: "People say they want to die. But dig deep down and find out why. It could be because people tell them they're a pain in the ass, you're wasting all our assets, you're being really selfish. How do you check for that?"

During a break on the third and last day of the trial, Fieger tried to move the *Nazi Doctors* book so a photographer could get a clear shot of the suicide machine. Modelski told him he couldn't touch anything on the prosecution table. Kevorkian walked up and confronted Modelski. Why, Kevorkian asked, was that book there in the first place?

"Guys like you are in that book," said Modelski, who is of Polish heritage. "My family suffered at their hands."

"Oh really?" Kevorkian replied. "I didn't know the Nazis did *animal* euthanasia."

The anecdote was reported in *Vanity Fair* by Ron Rosenbaum, who flew in to cover the trial. Rosenbaum, author of *Travels with Doctor Death* (a book not about Jack Kevorkian), took Fieger and Kevorkian to lunch or dinner at expensive restaurants every day of the trial, then wrote an article critical of Kevorkian.

After the close of testimony, Kevorkian was morose, Rosenbaum reported. Over dinner, he quarreled with his attorneys when they ridiculed his latest idea: That anyone sentenced to more than three years in prison get the option of assisted suicide instead.

At the bar of the Radisson Plaza Hotel in Southfield, Rosenbaum reported, Kevorkian started talking about going to another state. He also brought up the advantages of using carbon monoxide.

"The gas itself offers a simple, painless, odorless death," he told Rosenbaum. "Better than that, it leaves the body looking good. Your complexion looks beautiful and pink. Gives your corpse a lovely, rosy glow."

When I had first read that description in *Prescription: Medicide*, I left open the possibility that Kevorkian was joking. When I read *Vanity Fair* and discovered he had told Rosenbaum the same thing, I realized Kevorkian was serious.

Within little more than two years after Kevorkian's meals with Rosenbaum, more than a dozen people would get that rosy glow after an appointment with Doctor Death.

❏ ❏ ❏

On February 5, Judge Gilbert unleashed her decision. As the *Free Press* indelicately put it: "An Oakland County circuit judge pulled the plug on 'Dr. Death.' "

Gilbert said Kevorkian was not qualified to diagnose or treat Janet Adkins and never did a thorough evaluation and diagnosis of her. The video didn't make it clear that she wanted to die, the judge wrote: "The interview conveys the impression that Doctor Kevorkian was rather anxious to try his invention that he had advertised, and Janet Adkins appeared as a likely candidate."

Gilbert concluded: "The rights of privacy and self-determination do not encompass the right to direct another person to kill, or the right of a third person to participate in the killing. Patients cannot confer a right upon a doctor to assist a suicide."

Gilbert allowed: "There is reason to condone dying with dignity, but it mandates a controlled environment that can be properly and professionally monitored by competent persons and in a manner that is acceptable to society." Kevorkian was not the man for the job, she said:

"The multiple eccentric, unorthodox, and controversial remarks made by Doctor Kevorkian provide convincing evidence that he has a flare for flamboyancy, a propensity for media exposure, and seeks recognition through bizarre behavior. His arrogance coupled with unabashed disregard and disrespect for his profession and its current professional and ethical standards reveal that his real goal is self-service rather than patient service. The reasons why Doctor Kevorkian has been unable to find employment in any accredited hospital are made patently clear to the Court. . . .

"Doctor Kevorkian envisions himself as a charitable maverick, destined to revolutionize the practice of medicine. His peers look upon him as a menace that threatens the existence of the medical profession and those creeds that have endured since the time of Hippocrates. This Court finds it hard to believe that the physicians of the past 2,000 years have been blind to need, and only Doctor Kevorkian has the vision to lead them out of the darkness. At the present time, patient self-determination does not encompass self-extermination effectuated by a physician."

Outside the courtroom, Kevorkian told reporters he was astonished by Gilbert's "vile harangue."

"Everything she said was said in the past with every new advance in society," he said. "Persecution is always prelude to an advance."

Janet Good, the local Hemlock leader who attended the entire trial, said the ruling was tragic.

"I have personally talked to 19 dying people who will be in despair today," she said.

Kevorkian again told reporters he would not violate Gilbert's injunction.

But the very next day, Fieger called a news conference to announce that Kevorkian had disobeyed Gilbert. Kevorkian had told a dentist suffering from terminal bowel cancer how to use a suicide machine the dentist had built with Kevorkian's guidance. Fieger and Kevorkian would not say who or where the dentist was.

"Furtiveness is foreign to me," Kevorkian told reporters. "I decided that I've got to tell the world what I'm doing or else I'm betraying my own principles."

When a reporter asked why Kevorkian had broken his previous day's promise not to violate the injunction, Fieger responded: "I can't let him answer that question. What's in the news release is in the news release."

Fieger said he planned to sue in federal court claiming that Kevorkian's free speech rights had been violated.

But—as the *Free Press* put it the next day—"the Oakland County Prosecutor's Office said he was dead wrong."

"He can advocate his ideas. He can explain what he said. He can write a book about it," said assistant prosecutor Gerald Poisson, prophetically. Those things, Poisson said, did not violate Gilbert's injunction.

Poisson added: "The press conference was a desperate attempt to create sham issues and grab more headlines. . . . This stunt clearly indicates that Doctor Kevorkian and his lawyer care more about media coverage than they do about respecting the court or the law."

Fieger said Gilbert had tried to impose her personal morality on society.

"It's scary. This is a civil rights matter on the scale of the Scopes trial," Fieger told a magazine reporter, referring to the famous early

20th Century trial in which a teacher in Tennessee was convicted of the crime of teaching evolution. Fieger would use that analogy relentlessly in the months ahead.

"Here is an elected judge who all of a sudden tried to enforce morality," Fieger said. "If a judge can do that, another judge can issue an injunction against teaching birth control or wearing long hair. It's ridiculous."

In an editorial titled "Dr. Arrogance," the *Free Press* applauded Judge Gilbert and excoriated Kevorkian:

> Jack Kevorkian, MD, by his self-assured pronouncements that he would lead the way to a brave new world through physician-assisted suicide for the terminally ill, reminds us of someone who believes that only his view of reality is worthy of consideration.
>
> In point of fact, Doctor Kevorkian arrogantly and unacceptably went beyond what the law and medical ethics permit by assisting the suicide of Janet Adkins. Oakland County Circuit Judge Alice Gilbert wisely is trying to brake his hubris with a permanent injunction. . . .
>
> Doctor Kevorkian Wednesday vowed to persevere in his nefarious activities, boasting for the cameras about "professional duty." However intelligent he may think he is, he has missed the point.
>
> Sure, many Americans agree that medical technology at times keeps people alive when many of us might prefer to die. But, perhaps blinded by his unseemly glee at being in the spotlight, Doctor Kevorkian has failed to see that he and he alone gave himself the authority to redefine so recklessly the role of physicians. . . . it remains incumbent upon the Legislature to make clearer what physicians can and cannot do. Few things could make that more imperative than the prideful advent of Doctor Death.

A few months later, the *Free Press* ran a long letter to the editor from Dr. Herbert Bloom, identified as an official of the Michigan

Cancer Foundation. Bloom scorned "the grotesquely ludicrous behavior of Jack Kevorkian, a physician suffering from an obvious obsession with death." Bloom lauded Judge Gilbert's restraining order. He called Kevorkian "a dangerous menace" and said: "Kevorkian's bizarre behavior closely parallels that of his attorney, Geoffrey Fieger, whose primary method of defending his client is heaping verbal abuse on those who challenge his points of view. They really deserve each other."

The next day, the paper ran a clarification: "Doctor Bloom is the husband of Gilbert and should have been so identified."

◻ ◻ ◻

Fieger never carried out his threat to sue in federal court over Gilbert's injunction, but he did appeal her decision. By mid-1993, the state appeals court still had not heard the case.

Authorities returned Kevorkian's van, which took up seemingly permanent residence in a public parking lot behind his apartment at 223 Main Street in Royal Oak. The suicide machine he had pieced together from scrap materials and used on Janet Adkins stayed in an evidence locker at the county courthouse while the appeal remained pending.

◻ ◻ ◻

Right to Life of Michigan, one of the state's most powerful lobbying groups, put all its muscle behind Fred Dillingham's bill to outlaw Jack Kevorkian. On February 26, 1991, Doctor Death went to Lansing to testify before a Senate committee. He told senators the bill was immoral.

"To make it a blanket felony so it's out of discussion—you are in the Dark Ages, and you have not solved anything," Kevorkian said.

Dillingham's bill easily passed the Republican-controlled Senate. It then journeyed to a committee in the Democratic-controlled House, where it was studied to death for nearly two years.

CHAPTER ELEVEN
PAINFUL CHOICES

*"Suffering can be lessened to some extent,
but in no way eliminated or made benign, by the
careful intervention of a competent, caring
physician . . . to think that people do not suffer in
the process of dying is an illusion."*
—Dr. Timothy Quill ❐

Even though Jean Ruwart's large breast mass and other tumors were receding, she was in trouble. She had been given at least one extra treatment of adriamycin, a chemotherapy which can be toxic at high doses. While on anti-depressants she had doubled her weight, and the chemotherapy had made her diabetic. She was having difficulty breathing. She was hospitalized.

Her daughter Martie flew to Michigan from California. All her children came to her bedside. Jean had told her family she didn't want to be kept alive by artificial means. The family asked that life support be disconnected. As the breathing pump gradually slowed, Jean woke up. Her husband and six children talked to her until she died on March 15, 1991.

"It made her death easier that we were all there and we were well connected to her," Mary Ruwart recalled.

❐ ❐ ❐

A week earlier, on March 7, the *New England Journal of Medicine* published a remarkable first-person account of a doctor-assisted suicide.

Timothy Quill, a Rochester, New York, physician, wrote about how he had given a patient pills to end her life. "Diane," a longtime patient of Quill, was a recovering alcoholic who had struggled with depression but had put her life in order when she learned she had acute leukemia. Diane decided not to undergo extensive chemotherapy and painful bone marrow transplants, which would have given her a 25 percent chance of recovery.

Quill, a former hospice director, wrote that he was "a longtime advocate of active, informed patient choice of treatment or non-treatment, and of a patient's right to die with as much control and dignity as possible." When Diane told him she wanted to go quickly rather than waste away, Quill suggested the hospice program of pain management and "comfort care."

"Although Diane understood and appreciated this, she had known of people lingering in what was called relative comfort, and she wanted no part of it. When the time came, she wanted to take her life in the least painful way possible. . . ."

Quill said he believed Diane's fear of a lingering death would get in the way of the rest of her life. "I feared the effects of a violent death on her family, the consequences of an ineffective suicide that would leave her lingering in precisely the state she dreaded so much, and the possibility that a family member would be forced to assist her, with all the legal and personal repercussions that would follow."

Diane's husband and adult son supported her wish to die. Diane asked Quill to prescribe barbiturates to help her sleep.

"I made sure that she knew how to use the barbiturates for sleep, and also that she knew the amount needed to commit suicide."

Two months passed. Diane told Quill she was going to end it. Two days later, she told her husband and son goodbye and went into her living room with the pills. She told them to wait an hour to enter. When they did, they found her dead, and called Quill.

Quill certified that Diane had died of acute leukemia.

"I said 'acute leukemia' to protect all of us, to protect Diane from an invasion into her past and her body, and to continue to shield society from the knowledge of the degree of suffering that people often undergo in the process of dying."

Quill concluded: "I wonder how many families and physicians secretly help patients over the edge into death in the face of such severe suffering. I wonder how many severely ill or dying patients secretly take their lives, dying alone in despair."

The *New York Times* editorialized:

"Doctor Quill's courageous action allowed his patient to die with dignity."

A Rochester district attorney launched an investigation. He presented his case against Quill to a grand jury. It refused to indict him.

CHAPTER TWELVE
TOO MUCH FUSS

"I feel like a 42-year-old baby, and I hate it."
—Sherry Miller ❏

Sherry Miller kept calling Kevorkian. Kevorkian kept insisting she wasn't ready to die.

"Maybe he felt she would change her mind," Sharon Welsh said. But never once did Miller waver.

At Kevorkian's request, Miller went to see a psychiatrist. She had sessions with her parents, and another with her children. The psychiatrist prescribed an anti-depressant. Sherry tried the drug but stopped.

She told her friend: "The only thing that works anymore is my head, and these drugs cloud up my head, make me dopey, then nothing works. . . . He can't help me. He can't change the fact that I have MS."

Months dragged on. Sherry kept getting worse. She was confined to her bed and wheelchair. She could not use her legs or her right arm and had only limited use of her left arm. She did not want to go into a nursing home.

It got harder to take Sherry out. She was limp, all dead weight. She had no motorized wheelchair, no van, no lift. Her parents and Sharon used slide boards to get her in and out of cars. Though Sherry weighed well under 100 pounds, Sharon Welsh feared she would drop her friend.

Pain was not the issue. When Sharon bent Sherry's legs to get her into a car, she asked "Did I hurt you?" and Sherry replied: "I wish I could feel something."

"She was not in physical pain, but she was in a lot of emotional pain," Sharon said. "I saw her say on a TV show once: 'I could be having a good day with a friend visiting'—and I'd imagine it was me—'and if Doctor Kevorkian would come to my door and say "Are you ready?" I would be.' "

Sherry would stay up late at night with her dad, watching TV. Frequently she told her friend: "I hate to go to bed at night because I know I have to get up another day."

On September 4, Sharon Welsh drove Sherry Miller to Royal Oak to have lunch with Kevorkian. They parked on Main Street, and a wiry man came bounding up. Smiling, he swept Sherry out of the van. The three went to a sidewalk cafe.

Sharon Welsh was surprised how warm, personable and unaffected Doctor Death was.

"I felt comfortable with him," Welsh recalled. "He fussed over Sherry. It was a genuine concern and caring for her. I could see that caring. That was important to me."

They talked for a couple of hours—mostly about the two women and their kids. Jack Kevorkian said he regretted never marrying.

Kevorkian asked Sherry to reach across the table and squeeze his hand as hard as she could. Sharon realized that he was trying to see if she had enough strength to activate the suicide machine. Then, for the first time, Kevorkian clearly said he would help Sherry Miller die.

He asked Sherry if she would mind dying with another woman, Marjorie Wantz, who lived in western Michigan and suffered from severe pelvic pain. Sherry said that would be fine.

Kevorkian asked Sharon if she would be with Sherry at her death. Sherry had never asked her friend that. Sharon said: "If it's something that she wants me to do."

Kevorkian told the women to go home and think about it and he would get back in touch. Their drive home passed mostly in silence.

"That was the first time I realized that it was really going to happen," said Sharon Welsh.

Two weeks later, Sherry eagerly called Kevorkian, hoping he would set a date for her death. But he wasn't that far along.

On the last Sunday in September, Kevorkian and his sister Margo Janus came to Sharon Welsh's house. Kevorkian said he was trying to get the drugs and construct a machine that could handle both women. He was looking for a place for the double suicide. He had been checking into offices for rent, but no luck. Sherry had ruled out her parents' home. Kevorkian asked if Sherry had relatives out in farm country. She didn't.

Margo Janus impressed Welsh.

"You could see the caring. She's just a nice lady. She could see the pain that Sherry and I were going through. She said we were lucky we had each other."

Kevorkian and Sharon both told Sherry that she had to tell her parents the specifics of her plan to die.

"I remember saying I can't just pick you up at your house some morning and get in your car and drive away and not bring you back," Welsh recalled. "She wanted it to be quiet. She didn't want a big fuss."

Sharon now realized Sherry wanted her to be there when she died.

"It was something I knew I had to do. If I had said 'I can't be a part of this,' it would have been something I would have regretted all my life. Sherry didn't ask a lot of me."

In her final weeks, at age 43, it was hard for Sherry to speak. She had trouble breathing and talking at the same time.

In between all the confusing preparations for Sherry's death, the two childhood friends spent a lot of time reminiscing. Sharon, who as a child had always been envious of Sherry's store-bought clothes, discovered Sherry had envied her homemade clothes. Each woman confessed she had secretly coveted the other girl's bike.

"We got to say the things we wanted to say and got to share feelings that a lot of people don't get to share before they die," Welsh said.

On October 12, Sharon Welsh came over to Sherry's house and sat down at the kitchen table with a pencil and paper. Sherry Miller dictated letters to her two children.

Though her children knew she wanted to die, Sherry couldn't bring herself to tell them face-to-face that she had made the final decision and set the date.

"It was just too hard," Sharon Welsh explained. "Everybody said to her: 'Shouldn't you say something to them?' And she would say: 'I can't. I can't.'

"I think that was the hardest thing she had to do, writing those letters."

Sharon typed the letters and promised her friend she would give them to Sherry's children after Sherry died.

Kevorkian called to say he had found a place: a rental cabin in a state park north of Detroit. They set a date: Wednesday, October 23.

Three days before she planned to die, Sherry Miller called her two brothers and one sister, who lived in Texas, to tell them. To her dismay, they all insisted on flying in. Now there would be a big commotion.

The night before Sherry Miller and Marjorie Wantz were to die, they met with friends and family and Dr. Kevorkian at Sherry's parents' house. Margo Janus rolled the video camera.

I later saw the remarkable footage in Geoffrey Fieger's office. Once again, Kevorkian's "counseling" session raised a host of questions.

"We're here to discuss what's called physician-assisted suicide," Kevorkian announced. "We're here to discuss the wishes of Sherry Miller and Marjorie Wantz.

"Sherry, have you thought this over a lot?"

Sherry, her dark hair in a short bob, sat in her wheelchair and spoke slowly and softly. It took obvious effort for her to form the words.

"Yeah, I have. I thought about it for a long time, a long time. I have no qualms about my decision. I could do it tonight."

"You realize of course the implications of your decision?"

"There's no turning back. I want to die, and there's no turning back. This is not an overnight decision . . . I waited too long. . . . I cannot do it by myself."

"Are you afraid at all? Do you have any fear?"

She looked down and shook her head.

"No, no. None," she said, and smiled.

Marjorie Wantz, 58, sat on a couch next to her husband Bill. Heavyset, with graying hair, she looked haggard, beaten. Her eyes were sunken and had dark circles under them. Her voice was flat. She wore a cross on a chain around her neck.

"I wish we could have done it a year ago, two years ago," she said. "I'm a little nervous because I've been waiting so long. Waiting a week seems like you're waiting a month. Three days seems like three months when you're hurting and going crazy."

Wantz said her pain was unremitting. Heavy doses of painkillers were not helping. She said she sometimes took four or five of the pills at a time, hoping they would slow her heart down. "That would be a blessing," she said.

Wantz said nothing could lift her spirits.

"People say, 'Hang in there. Go out to restaurants and eat.' When you're in such misery . . . all you want to do is go to bed and take pain pills. When you're in a situation like this, when you're in my shoes, then you tell me what to do. Until you are, don't tell me what to do . . .

"I would give anything in the world just to be able to go to a store, just a grocery store. People should realize how lucky they are to go into a Kmart."

Wantz's monotone voice sounded rational. Yet it told incredible stories. She said she had tried several times to end her life. Once, she went in the garage, closed the door, put a hose in the tailpipe, stuck the hose through the window of her car, and got in the car and turned on the engine.

"Nothing happened," she said. "I didn't get sleepy. I stayed in the car for three hours and I didn't get sick, there was no nausea. Nothing happened."

Twice, she said, she took 120 Halcion tablets. Nothing happened.

"I tried everything short of a gun. I tried loading a gun, but I don't know how to load one, and Bill says I probably wouldn't have succeeded, and I would be in worse shape than I am now.

"It's got to be done right . . . no mistakes. You do it yourself, you don't know what you are doing."

Wantz said every surgery had made her worse. The last time, she claimed, the doctor left a needle deep inside her vagina. She said the doctor told her: "Go home and live with it."

Bill Wantz grabbed his wife's hand.

"I don't want to lose this one, but I see her in pain every day," he said. "I told her on the way down: 'If you don't want to do it, we can go back home.' I don't want to lose her, because when I lose her, I'm alone."

They said that once, when she tried loading a gun, the gun went off and shot a hole in the couch in their mobile home.

Kevorkian started talking about how people who chose assisted suicide eventually would have the option of donating their organs or consenting to experiments. In the middle of his explanation a cuckoo clock struck the hour.

Kevorkian asked his two patients if they would choose either experimentation or organ harvesting if given the chance. Each said no.

Marjorie Wantz insisted she wanted a detailed autopsy to reveal the medical horrors that had been inflicted on her: "I want an extremely, extremely thorough autopsy. I want to be cut like 10 ways." Kevorkian assured her it would be very thorough.

That led to a discussion of who would take the bodies. Kevorkian said the authorities would handle everything.

Kevorkian talked about the site: "It's a beautiful setting on a little lake in a little woods." He said he picked a spot in Oakland County to annoy Richard Thompson.

Kevorkian assured them no friends or relatives would get in trouble if they stayed in the cabin during the suicides, as long as they didn't help.

(Sharon Welsh later told me the session had alleviated some of her fears about police reaction. "We were reassured that there wouldn't be any problem," she said. "I'm glad I didn't know what was going to happen.")

Bill Wantz said he had a plane ticket to Utah to see his new grandchild. He wasn't skipping town, he said, he just didn't want to go home to his mobile home in Sodus and have the media hound him.

Kevorkian beamed as he explained how his new device would work for both women and how it ran without electricity, making assisted suicide possible in a rustic cabin with no power.

"There's no whirring noise," he said. "They can't say 'machine' anymore."

He said the drug he planned using "is twice as fast as pentothal" and predicted each woman would be unconscious within 15 to 25 seconds and dead in less than six minutes.

"How are your veins, by the way?" Kevorkian asked Wantz. "I know Sherry's veins are excellent."

Kevorkian said there were plenty of bunks in the cabins and he planned to pile four or five mattresses atop one another for each woman. He would clamp his device on a stool between them.

"I have all the linen ready and it's all immaculate," said Margo Janus from behind the camera.

All the while the others discussed what to do with her body and what the authorities would do after her death, Sherry Miller looked down into her lap and said nothing. After the taping ended, she remained very quiet. Sharon Welsh knelt down by her and said: "It will be OK." Her friend started crying.

"I just don't want all this fuss," she said.

CHAPTER THIRTEEN
NIGHT ON BALD MOUNTAIN

"Kurt Vonnegut had earlier envisioned 'ethical suicide parlors' being set up around the country to encourage people to end it all. The parlors were tended by beautiful young women who talked with you, brought you your last meal, played your favorite music, and, upon your request, induced death by lethal injection."
—Medical ethicist George Annas ❐

It was early in the morning when the teacher told Sherry Miller's son to go to the school office. His dad was on the phone. The boy gathered up his books and left school in a hurry.

His sister got a call at work from her grandparents.

Sherry's two children spent the day at their grandparents' house in Roseville, watching TV and waiting for the news that their mother had died. They expected to hear something by noon.

The news was a very long time coming.

❐ ❐ ❐

At 7:07 p.m. on October 23, 1991, the Oakland County Sheriff's Department got a phone call.

"This is Jack Kevorkian," a voice said. "I want to report a double doctor-assisted suicide."

A few minutes later, Sheriff's Deputy Donald Smith drove up the dirt road to the cabins at Bald Mountain Recreation Area. A man greeted him at the gate.

"I'm Jack Kevorkian," the man told the officer.

Kevorkian directed Smith and other officers to the cabin. Inside, illuminated by candles, the bodies of two women lay on cots. The woman closest to the door had a mask over her face. Tubes led from the mask to a tank labeled "CARBON MONOXIDE." A yellow-handled screwdriver was taped to the nozzle of the tank. The other woman had an IV tube running from her right arm to three connected bottles.

91

Other bottles, syringes and lanterns were on a table next to the bed.

Kevorkian refused to tell police the names of the women.

Outside the cabin on a picnic table sat Sharon Welsh and Bill Wantz. Police put them in a squad car, and Kevorkian in another. They sat there for hours.

The remote park turned into a Fellini movie set. Kleig lights glared. Police cordoned off the area. A crowd of the curious stood behind the yellow tape and peered into the dark, hoping to catch a glimpse of Doctor Death.

Geoffrey Fieger took command.

Fieger told the media that Marjorie Wantz died at 5:05 p.m. with her husband at her side and that Sherry Miller died at 6:15 with her best friend Sharon Welsh beside her. Wantz used the suicide machine and Miller inhaled carbon monoxide, Fieger said.

"She just breathed it and went to sleep."

Reporters asked Fieger if he expected Kevorkian to be charged with a crime.

"No, that's silly, because it's everything he stands for and it's everything he's involved in. It's a humane, ethical, medical act and certainly this is no different."

◻ ◻ ◻

"My feeling is we need to punch Kevorkian's lights out right now. He has proved himself to be an imminent danger to the public." Fred Dillingham was indignant.

"We're looking at somebody who wants to be Doctor God. It's a very scary concept. He violated a court order, violated medical ethics, then turns around and broadens it to the chronically ill. It makes me wonder what's next if we don't get him checked in this state."

Dillingham's Senate bill to make assisted suicide a felony was still languishing in the House Judiciary Committee. Dillingham accused the committee chair, Democratic Representative Perry Bullard, of refusing to hold hearings.

"We've got two brazen people here—Doctor Kevorkian and Representative Bullard," Dillingham said.

Bullard lashed back, calling Dillingham's bill "a hastily drafted, meat-cleaver criminal law that does not deal with the nuances of the problem." Better to bring in experts to explore what guidelines were needed, he said. He promised to appoint a subcommittee to study things further.

The head of Right to Life of Michigan issued a call to action to her legions of members: Contact your legislator.

"How many more deaths do we need?" Barbara Listing pleaded. "Doctor Kevorkian's aim is to establish suicide clinics. Maybe we have to wait until he's selling franchises before that bill gets out of committee."

Arthur Caplan wondered in print whether a "banner carrier for euthanasia" could be a dispassionate judge of candidates for assisted suicide.

"He is a man with a cause, and the cause is immoral, unethical and very dangerous," Caplan wrote.

Even allies in the "right to die" movement spoke out against Kevorkian.

Cheryl Smith, attorney for the national Hemlock Society, said Miller and Wantz fell outside Hemlock's guidelines for physician aid-in-dying because they weren't terminally ill and certified competent by psychiatrists.

"This type of *ad hoc* assistance in suicide for the dying is wide open to abuse, because there are no ground rules and no criteria," Smith said.

Kevorkian could not respond to these charges, because Fieger was doing all the talking.

"I certainly don't want him making statements to anybody," Fieger said. That irked prosecutors.

"The only witnesses are people who won't talk and two ladies who are dead," Michael Modelski said. "It would make things easier if Kevorkian and the others told us what they observed, but they're not."

Fieger said that Kevorkian had been counseling each woman for about two years but had refused to help them previously because Miller's parents and children opposed her suicide and because Kevorkian wasn't satisfied Wantz's pain couldn't be relieved. Fieger said Kevorkian aided both women on the same day because he didn't want to leave either one stranded if he were arrested.

Fieger produced a suicide note from Wantz. In it, she said she was afraid of trying to kill herself and failing, and wanted Dr. Kevorkian's help so it would be done "properly."

"After 3 1/2 years I can no longer go on with this pain and agony," Wantz wrote. "I'm so glad there is Doctor Kevorkian to help me. . . . If God won't come to me I'm going to go to God."

❏ ❏ ❏

When Sharon Welsh came home from work on October 24, she was greeted by a horde of reporters. She told them she had no comment. Then she drove back to the Oakland County Sheriff's Department to pick up her car, which had been confiscated the night before at the cabin. To her dismay, police had taken maps, mileage receipts, a get-well card she was going to send to a friend who had surgery scheduled a few days later—and the letters Sherry had dictated to her children.

Nothing was ever returned. A few days later, Welsh's friend who was having surgery got calls from reporters.

Back home, Welsh frantically sifted through bags of garbage hoping to find the original drafts of Sherry's letters to her children. Finally, she found them in a desk drawer.

❏ ❏ ❏

On October 28, reporters and camera crews swarmed Fieger's office for a press conference, hoping to see Jack Kevorkian. Instead, they saw the video of the October 22 discussion at Miller's parents' house.

Fieger released a letter from Kevorkian calling for a blue-ribbon commission to establish guidelines for assisted suicide. About Miller and Wantz, he wrote: "I am sure that wherever they may now be, the radiant light of their souls' freedom from the disease and pain which ravaged their earthly bodies shines brightly to illuminate a world yet emerging from the dark."

Fieger demanded that the prosecutor return the letters Miller had written to her children. He also accused Thompson of harassing the Millers' neighbors by telling them a grand jury might question them if they didn't cooperate. He called Thompson a "certified raging loon" and a right-wing religious fanatic "on a mission from God" to enforce his own morality.

Thompson rejoined to reporters:

"I've noticed that almost every day we have a three-ring circus going, being conducted by the other side, and almost every day they have a new act that they are highlighting."

Thompson said Fieger's antics were hurting Kevorkian's cause and alienating his supporters. And he got in an "I told you so."

"I told people when Doctor Kevorkian used his suicide machine to kill Janet Adkins last June that the Legislature should take some action. Nothing happened. Now we have a macabre scene of two people being killed in a cabin, or killing themselves. Is that the beginning of the assembly line? We know that Doctor Kevorkian has said he has 50 or 60 more people lined up. We need some direction."

Carl Marlinga, the prosecutor of neighboring Macomb County, said that if it were shown that Kevorkian hooked up the machine, turned on the gas or helped in any physical way, Thompson should charge him with murder.

❏ ❏ ❏

When Wantz and Miller died, Washington was two weeks from becoming the first state to allow physicians to help terminally ill people commit suicide. A Tacoma newspaper poll showed the initiative leading 61 percent to 27 percent.

On November 5, voters in Washington turned back the proposal by about 55 percent to 45 percent. Why the sudden shift in sentiment? Many supporters blamed a multi-million-dollar TV and radio ad blitz bankrolled by Right to Life and Catholic groups. But some blamed Kevorkian for sabotaging their dignified campaign with the deaths on Bald Mountain.

CHAPTER FOURTEEN
ALL IN HER HEAD?

"Once this gets going as a practice for physically debilitated people, the psychiatrists are going to have a whopping job, because it is going to be up to them to decide how this fits into their field."
—*Jack Kevorkian (1993)* ❐

Marjorie Wantz was Kevorkian's most controversial suicide patient. Was she sick? Was she crazy? Was she both?

Clearly, she was not terminally ill. Kevorkian's willingness to help her die fanned the flames of criticism. Defenders of Wantz's choice said much of that criticism might be sexist. Her case history underlined all the difficulties inherent in separating physical from mental distress—problems Kevorkian had blithely dismissed in his statements before Judge Alice Gilbert.

Records show this much:

Marjorie and William Wantz married in December 1986. She was 53, he 59. Each had two grown children from a previous marriage. Marjorie was a teacher's aide, Bill a security guard. They lived in a mobile home in Sodus, near Benton Harbor in the southwestern corner of Michigan.

In May 1988, Marjorie Wantz had laser surgery at the University of Chicago Hospital to remove painful, non-cancerous growths inside her vagina. The doctor told her afterwards that about one-third of the growths remained, and that they could be removed in the future if they caused her any pain.

In 1990, the Wantzes filed a malpractice suit, claiming she had suffered third-degree burns and scarring in her vaginal tract because of the surgery. They documented $30,000 in medical bills from doctors in her area, at the University of Chicago, the University of Michigan, the Cleveland Clinic and the Mayo Clinic. The Wantzes said Marjorie had undergone nine or 10 surgeries to try to control the vaginal pain.

Because of her pain, both Wantzes quit their jobs. Court documents also alleged that "Mrs. Wantz's personal relationship with her husband has also suffered" and "her ability to perform various conjugal duties has been hindered" and Bill Wantz's "social life has ceased to exist."

Bill Wantz said a doctor who examined Marjorie at the University of Indiana told her: "I've never seen anybody this bad."

Marjorie Wantz would scream through the night, her husband said, and needed sleeping pills to escape the pain. In fact, she became dependent on Halcion, the controversial drug suspected of contributing to suicidal depression in some people.

Marjorie Wantz got in contact with Jack Kevorkian shortly after he started advertising his services in 1989. In 1990, when she was in Sinai Hospital in Detroit, Kevorkian visited her and recommended she go to the Cleveland Clinic. She asked a doctor there to cut her spinal cord, but the doctor told her even that might not stop the pain. Kevorkian also suggested acupuncture and hypnotism. And he referred her to Hospice of Southeastern Michigan, headed by Dr. Jack Finn, the man who had helped David Rivlin die but had called Kevorkian's treatment of Janet Adkins "veterinary medicine."

In court, Bill Wantz testified that Finn's prognosis was: "pain, pure and simple . . . all the medicine he gave her wasn't taking care of it. His statement to me was it would be better off to be cancerous; at least in six months you might be dead."

Her pain was so bad even wearing panties hurt her, Bill Wantz said. She could rarely leave home, and when she rode in a car she had to lie down in the back seat.

In June 1991, Wantz's physician reported that he had talked with Dr. Kevorkian. He reported that he had told Kevorkian that she was "not a candidate for suicide machine . . . Patient has not exhausted therapy modalities."

On August 5, Wantz was admitted to Sinai Hospital for more tests. She left the hospital August 15 to appear with Kevorkian on a local TV show. She refused to return to the hospital.

Psychiatrist Linda Hotchkiss of Sinai tried to get Wantz committed. She reported that Wantz "has not completed a course of available non-narcotic medication therapy at appropriate levels. She refuses hospitalization or other treatment for treatment of her depression which exacerbates her pain."

Dr. Gerald Shiener of Sinai told Wayne County Probate Court that Wantz was suffering "major depression." The basis for his determination: "Patient insists on killing herself."

Dr. Ronald Trunsky, another psychiatrist who examined her at Sinai, said Wantz had "severe depression" and "somatization syndrome." He said: "Patient feels no one understands the severity of her pain—it is unremitting. She refuses proven treatment plans for medical pain relief programs."

Wantz left the Detroit area and went home. The Berrien County prosecutor, Gregory Cleveland, took up the case. He ordered Wantz examined by two psychiatrists at Mercy-Memorial Medical Center in St. Joseph, Michigan. They disagreed on whether she should be committed, so she was sent to Kalamazoo Regional Psychiatric Hospital for a third opinion. Dr. M.B. Mehta examined her there. He said Wantz was well-oriented and coherent and did not exhibit signs of delusion or paranoia.

"According to her, half of her vulva had third degree burns. She states that she was told that she had human papilloma virus, which was causing severe pain and burning. She states that she has been to Mayo Clinic and was told that there is no evidence to suggest that she has that viral infection. . . .

"She denies having an urge to commit suicide. . . . 'I am still here and I have not done it. I will not do it to hurt my husband or my children.' . . . She states that she is willing to try any reasonable treatment which is expected to help her."

The authorities let her go back to Sodus. Two months later, she lay dead in the cabin at Bald Mountain.

"Would it have made a difference if they were MEN?" asked the headline in the *Free Press* The Way We Live section on November 4, 1991. Subtitled "Feminists deplore second-guessing," the article sought reactions to what it called the "second-guessing" that "began almost immediately after the two women committed suicide in a wood-side cabin." Feature writer Antoinette Martin described the second-guessing thus:

"They . . . had sought the assistance of Doctor Jack Kevorkian because the women saw him as a father figure.

"They had looked for a passive way to die.

"They didn't really know what they were doing."

To these contentions—raised mainly by male psychiatrists and observers interviewed by the media—psychotherapist Micki Levin reacted: "It really made me mad. How patronizing!"

To the suggestion that Marjorie Wantz was fantasizing her pain,

Carol King, executive director of the Michigan Abortion Rights Action League, countered:

"Just like Anita Hill was supposed to be fantasizing her emotional pain at being harassed by Clarence Thomas!"

King likened the judgments about Wantz's condition to the Freudian "hysteria" diagnosis of women with emotional pain. King told Martin that it reminded her of being a teenager, writhing on the floor from menstrual cramps, and being told, "It's all in your head."

Martin, almost editorializing, said King now finally "got it: Deciding how and when to die when terminally ill or riddled with unending pain is an issue of choice. Just like abortion!"

Janet Good, who had been enshrined in the Michigan Women's Hall of Fame a few days after Wantz and Miller died, "was way ahead of King on that road to realization," Martin wrote.

"Would any of this have come up if it was a man suffering from prostate cancer?" Good asked. "No. And most women know that, and that's part of why they're getting involved.

"Self-determination! That's what it's about—taking charge of the rest of your life."

King concluded:

"Kevorkian was not a father figure. A pioneer perhaps. Not a father figure. That is insulting to these women who thought this out, made plans, took great pains to see that their points of view would be seen and heard by people by leaving notes and videotapes. I respect them for their courage."

In a court brief filed months later, assistant prosecutor Michael Modelski wrote: "the autopsy . . . revealed there was nothing physically wrong with Marjorie Wantz and . . . her pain was all in her head."

The October 1991 issue of *Today's Woman*, out when Miller and Wantz died, included an article on chronic pelvic pain. Dr. Robert Reiter of the University of Iowa, an obstetrician-gynecologist, reported that "pelvalgia"—chronic pelvic pain without a plausible physical cause—was a widespread complaint. Some experts had identified organic causes such as pinched nerves, hernias, irritable bowels, postoperative adhesions, endometriosis or ovarian cysts. Others saw it as psychological—a "somatization disorder, a condition in which the patient has become preoccupied with a broad range of symptoms and complaints."

At a University of Iowa pelvic pain clinic, experts discovered support for both theories, finding 75 percent of patients had something wrong physically and 65 percent had something wrong mentally. One startling finding: Half of all women with chronic pelvic pain reported major childhood sexual abuse, compared with seven percent of the pain-free population.

In a 1985 article in the *Journal of the American Medical Association*, titled "Somatization Disorder: One of Medicine's Blind Spots," a physician wrote that patients with that disorder were frequently unrecognized, misdiagnosed and subjected to scores of useless medical procedures. A better solution, the physician-writer suggested, was a long-term relationship with a primary doctor who would treat the patient and her symptoms seriously and respectfully.

"These patients use symptoms as a way to communicate, express emotion, and be taken care of," the doctor contended.

The doctor who wrote the article was Timothy Quill.

CHAPTER FIFTEEN
CLOWNING AROUND

"You've got to give Fieger credit for really mobilizing the media. He's attuned to what the media wants—a nice punchy sentence or two, a quotable quote, and the more outlandish the better.
"Our office sort of let him have the field. Fieger had this beautiful vacuum, so he could say almost anything he wanted. And unless it was a direct shot at this office, we didn't respond.
"And the media—they were always good at finding some lady who wanted to die next week—and that played well, the emotions of it."
—Michael Modelski ❏

"I am the best there was or ever will be."

Geoffrey Fieger said that to a TV reporter who asked how good a lawyer he was, the *Free Press* reported in a 1991 profile.

"Geoffrey Fieger doesn't believe in modesty, not when television cameras are nearby," wrote reporters Robin Fornoff and Joel Thurtell.

Roger Craig, a former law partner of Bernard Fieger, told the *Free Press* that the younger Fieger "has this marvelous quality of really believing his own hype."

In the unedited version of the story, Craig didn't say "hype," but "shit."

Craig also said Fieger could see only his own side in a trial:

"I think he's like that because he was spoiled a little as a child. You get used to having your own way and you come to think of the world and the things in it as your toy to be manipulated as you please."

That quote didn't make the paper at all.

Checking records, *Free Press* reporters found Fieger had been convicted of drunk driving for a 1986 incident in Saline, near Ann Arbor. When questioned about it, Fieger flew into a rage.

"I thought that was a character assassination," Fieger later told me. "Come on, 1986, I get a fucking drunk driving ticket and that has to do with me? Come on. I mean, that's just bullshit, OK? Yeah, if I was some kind of like heinous criminal out there, but you know, five years before I get a drunk driving ticket and you're going to use that as somehow indicative of me?"

Before the story ran, Fieger called at least one editor at the *Free Press* and raised hell.

"I said, if you're going to do a story on me, do a fair story," Fieger told me. "What the fuck does a drunk driving ticket have to do with me representing Jack Kevorkian?"

Much of the long Fieger profile was trimmed before it reached the paper. Stories often are cut because of space limitations.

The version that ran included a truncated report on the drunk driving conviction. A jury convicted Fieger in 1987 despite a defense that included seven attorneys, among them a retired state Supreme Court justice. Fieger appealed the case twice to the state's top court and lost both times.

Washtenaw County Prosecutor Lynwood Noah said Fieger "wanted me to dismiss the drunk driving case because he's an attorney." Noah said Fieger testified that he had gone to meet a friend "and got lost and was out there eating cheese and drinking wine by himself."

Fieger told me: "I was arrested walking to my car by a policeman who said I must have been drunk driving because I was drunk coming back to my car. I never denied that I was drunk, but I wasn't drunk driving."

Noah said: "I've never seen anyone fight drunk driving so hard."

❑ ❑ ❑

On November 20, 1991, the Michigan State Board of Medicine summarily suspended Jack Kevorkian's medical license, declaring him a "threat to the public health, safety and welfare requiring emergency action." The vote was 8-0.

Board chairman Dr. Norman Bolton, who was absent, had urged his colleagues in writing not to revoke the license because such an action would be "precipitous, unnecessary" and "would only add to the circus atmosphere at this point."

Bolton said "it is far-fetched to consider him an immediate danger to the health of the people of the state of Michigan."

The board acted just after Attorney General Frank Kelley, a Democrat and the longest-tenured elected state official in the nation, issued a press release reporting he had requested the suspension.

"Regardless of his motives, Doctor Kevorkian's actions appear to be beyond the law," Kelley stated. "Under our system, people are not allowed to take the law into their own hands."

Kevorkian's opponents cheered.

"It removes some of the veneer of respectability he had in which he could hide behind his medical license," Michael Modelski told a reporter. In Lansing, Fred Dillingham was quick to drop the "Doctor" from Kevorkian's name.

"Mister Kevorkian can continue to do what he's been doing unless the prosecutor's office finds a way of stopping him," Dillingham said.

It took only a week for Fieger and Schwartz to sue the attorney general in Oakland County Circuit Court. The license suspension, the suit alleged, took place "without even the semblance of due process of law and without the slightest concern for the constitutional rights" of Kevorkian and was "the apparent product of political manipulation."

Kevorkian, the suit said, learned he had lost his license by listening to the radio. His attorneys found out when a reporter called.

Fieger and Schwartz charged the board buckled under pressure from an unnamed senator who had threatened to punch Kevorkian's lights out and to stall a bill beneficial to doctors.

The suit was assigned to Circuit Judge John N. O'Brien. On December 9, Fieger made a motion to disqualify O'Brien. Fieger said O'Brien's wife had told him months earlier that she and her husband opposed Kevorkian's work on religious, moral and personal grounds.

O'Brien refused to step down from the case, and the court's chief judge refused to disqualify him.

On December 6, Michael Modelski testified before Representative Lynn Jondahl's subcommittee as the assisted suicide law continued its glacial creep through the Michigan House. Modelski said the perception that the government could not prosecute Kevorkian could lead to more deaths soon.

"I don't know what Doctor Kevorkian is going to do as his next step. He'll probably have more candidates after the Christmas season" because of post-holiday depression, Modelski said.

Modelski also suggested that the Wantz and Miller deaths were timed to promote sales of *Prescription: Medicide*, which was released in September.

"It's an odd coincidence" that after the book came out "we had the big show with two people in October," Modelski said.

Fieger told reporters: "Michael Modelski is a lunatic, a certifiable lunatic."

❐ ❐ ❐

On December 19, Oakland County medical examiner Dr. Ljubisa Dragovic ruled the deaths of Miller and Wantz were homicides.

"All the evidence indicates these deaths were brought about by another person," Dragovic said.

Fieger responded: "These women took their own lives. Everybody knows that. . . . Anybody who thinks that Sherry Miller or Marjorie Wantz were murdered by Doctor Kevorkian is a certifiable lunatic and ought to speak to their families."

Fieger later said of Dragovic: "He wrote a phony report and should be convicted of a crime. . . . He would have been an excellent medical examiner for the KGB."

The day after Dragovic's ruling, Richard Thompson announced he would put Sharon Welsh, Bill Wantz and other witnesses before a grand jury to investigate the deaths at Bald Mountain.

In response, Fieger called a press conference. Kevorkian was there, but Fieger kept him muzzled. Fieger charged Thompson had acted illegally in bringing the case before a previously impaneled grand jury which had been charged with investigating unsolved crimes.

In front of the TV cameras, Fieger held up a picture of Thompson and placed a red balloon on his nose. He then referred to the prosecutor as "a first-class buffoon" and an "arch-Machiavellian manipulator."

"Nobody in Oakland County is asking for Jack Kevorkian to be charged with murder," Fieger said.

Thompson said he would "handle this like any other unsolved homicide, despite the absurd, ridiculous and slanderous remarks of Mister Fieger."

Fieger later told me how he came up with the clown nose: "I said I have to come up with some way to crystallize. People remember visuals better than they remember words. . . . And to me that picture crystallizes, putting the nose on his face. I never called him a clown. . . .

I just put the nose on this picture and referred to him as 'the man with the red nose.'

"I thought it was fun. I remember we were laughing hysterically, Jack and Michael and I.

"Everybody remembers that, including everybody who ever looks at Thompson."

Thompson wasn't laughing. He later told me that Fieger's constant attacks on him hurt Kevorkian's cause.

"He became so obvious about it that it really had no effect at all. The legal profession got a black eye from it. People were surprised that a professional person would go through the antics Mister Fieger was going through. The statements were so far-fetched, they were so personal in nature that I didn't think people would really accept that."

◻ ◻ ◻

Martha Ruwart had rented a room in a beautiful oceanside house in Cardiff-by-the-Sea, an upscale California community. She had a good job but still lived frugally. Her compassion grew wider. If someone acted angrily, she often would say: "That person must be in a lot of pain." Her co-workers appreciated her kindness and intelligence.

Martie had never married because she hadn't found the right man. She believed a strong, independent woman didn't require a man to complete her. Approaching her 40th birthday, she was peaceful, confident and making great progress in healing her back. Weight-lifting had strengthened her frail body.

Though thousands of miles away, Martie was closer than ever to her sister Mary. In 1987, Mary, a senior scientist at the Michigan-based Upjohn Co., had launched an ambitious personal project: Combining insights from her longtime activism in the Libertarian Party with Christian and New Age philosophies in a book that would tackle the world's economic and social problems.

Since their childhood days of pretending their dolls were Revolutionary spies, and through their days at Michigan State studying Ayn Rand's philosophy of objectivism, Mary and Martie always had shared political ideas.

"She was the only person who understood what I was trying to accomplish with the book," Mary recalled. Mary started sending her drafts, and Martie would provide helpful comments. For five years Martie encouraged her sister to keep going on the book.

"Martie gave me the courage to go on," Mary said. "She told me this was my mission is life. Without her I might have dropped the book."

As Martie came home to Michigan for Christmas 1991, Mary's book *Healing Our World: The Other Piece of the Puzzle*, was ready for publication by Sun Star Press. It was the family's first holiday without their mother Jean.

At Christmas dinner, Martie complained that spicy food was giving her indigestion. She didn't eat much.

Martie feared she had an ulcer.

❏ ❏ ❏

Jack Kevorkian was walking to the post office on the morning of February 5, 1992, when two cars screeched to a stop near him. Three men came at him.

"I thought I was going to be attacked until one of them, while he was running, flashed a badge," Kevorkian said.

Pictures of Kevorkian in handcuffs dominated the TV news.

Thompson was going to try again. The grand jury had handed down an indictment: two counts of open murder and one count of delivering a controlled substance—the lethal drugs Kevorkian "delivered" into Marjorie Wantz.

"We have testimony that it took Sherry Miller over 10 to 15 minutes, and they heard noises from inside the cabin," Thompson said. "What concerns us is that if Sherry Miller had changed her mind, there was no way that she could take the mask off."

Fieger assailed the charges as part of "a moral and political persecution . . . of Doctor Death and his mercy machine." He said officials pursuing Kevorkian were "truly malevolent, sick people, acting like some kind of *Terminator* cops." He said there was "not one iota, one scintilla, one speck of evidence that Doctor Jack Kevorkian murdered Sherry Miller and Marjorie Wantz."

Fieger said grand juries—"17 poor slobs who know nothing about the law"—always carry out the will of prosecutors.

Fieger was ready to battle the man with the clown nose.

"I'll be kicking Dick Thompson's ass until my legs are tired," he boasted.

Kevorkian appeared before Circuit Court Judge Richard Kuhn, who released him on $1,000 bond. A condition of the bond was that he not assist in more suicides.

Asked by reporters if he felt guilty, Kevorkian replied: "I would feel no more guilt than any physician who performs a medical service." In a TV interview, Kevorkian said: "I keep constantly reminding myself that it's the suffering patient that counts. Nothing else."

National Hemlock Society leaders blasted Kevorkian. Hemlock attorney Cheryl Smith told me Kevorkian was bad for the "right-to-die" movement "if people think he's the kind of doctor who would be involved in these assisted suicides." Smith said Hemlock wouldn't offer him any support:

"He's out on his own. I think he's got his own movement."

Even Bertram Harper, who had put a bag over his wife's head in Romulus, weighed in against Doctor Death: "I don't agree with what he did at all. Everybody should have the right to make that choice to die themselves and have a doctor assist them, but . . . we should try to limit that to someone who is terminally ill."

Thompson, saying it would be tough to get a jury to convict Kevorkian, admitted to the *Oakland Press*: "Normally, murders are committed against someone who doesn't consent to their death and we have clear evidence on the face of it that these people consented to their death."

At Prometheus Books, spokesman Michael Powers was excited by the bad news about the company's prize author/pathologist. Powers told a Detroit reporter: "Any time an author gets in the news, it's going to help sales, no matter if the news is good or bad."

CHAPTER SIXTEEN
THE FINAL TRIP OF DOCTOR GAS

"If you're not dead in 30 minutes—it's free!"
—David Letterman's "Top Ten Promotional
Slogans for the Suicide Machine" (#2) ❑

When 10 minutes passed, then 15, Don Rubin got scared. His best friend, Gary Sloan, still had a pulse. The newspaper clippings Dr. Kevorkian had sent said the potassium chloride should kill him in six minutes. Did they have the dosages right? Rubin thought of calling Kevorkian, but he'd never talked to the man, it was 3 a.m. in Michigan, and Rubin didn't have his phone number.

So Rubin called his ex-wife.

"If I run out of this stuff and he wakes up, he's going to be really pissed," he told her. "What am I going to do?"

Finally, 20 agonizing minutes after the drugs were started, Sloan was clearly dead. Rubin heaved a sigh of relief, then gathered up all the drugs and tubes and threw them into the garbage.

Gary Allen Sloan had met Don Rubin in Cambridge, Massachusetts, in the 1960s. The pair lived in communes and experimented with drugs. Sloan was a dentist. Sometimes when Rubin visited him at work, Sloan would strap him in the chair and give him laughing gas. Sloan became known by the acronym "Doctor GAS."

Sloan pioneered and franchised a preventive dental health program called "Smiles." Rubin became a free-lance writer and devised a weekly syndicated word game, "The Puzzle," which spawned several game books.

Colon cancer had killed Sloan's father at age 39. Just before he turned 39, Sloan found out he had the same disease. Over the next five years, he had five surgeries. He also tried magnets, crystals, wheat grass, coffee enemas, and urine extracts that cost hundreds of dollars. He moved to Florida, ran out of money and cashed in his life insurance policy. He drifted around, sleeping in his Jeep and working for other dentists. He always slept with two pistols and a "suicide bottle" full of prescription drugs.

In June 1990, Sloan called Rubin and said: "Guess who I just

spoke to? Doctor Kevorkian. Yeah, you know, Doctor Death. He said
he'd do me."

Sloan wrote Kevorkian a letter dated June 28:

> I now have a large metasis to the liver. An attempt was
> made by one of Boston's top liver surgeons to resect. It
> was inoperable. . . .
> I don't seem to be coming back from this operation as I
> did in the four previous ones I've endured. I lack vitality,
> strength and mobility. I have no energy for the things that
> have made life important for me: work, bicycling, running
> with my dog, playing my guitar, having dreams for the
> future, being appealing and of interest to a pretty woman,
> you know, the small but important components of life. . . .
> I don't know how long it will take before I begin to deteri-
> orate beyond what is acceptable to me. Months? Years? I
> would expect it (the pain) to get worse, not better.
> I write for your help. So I can plan for the future.
> Having "control" is important to me! . . .

In July 1990, Kevorkian sent Sloan newspaper clippings, including diagrams of his suicide machine drawn by *Free Press* staff artists.
Kevorkian wrote:

> The enclosed diagrams will give you a general idea of
> how my device is constructed. There are several ways that
> details of the internal structure can be worked out satisfac-
> torily. All it takes are a couple of solenoids and switches, a
> timer, and a couple of small valves. . . . I'm sure you could
> put it all together yourself, especially if helped by a friend
> who is good with his hands or is an engineer. As you told
> me, you yourself could obtain the drugs. . . .

Late that summer, Sloan moved to Los Angeles to live out his
final days with his friend Don Rubin. Sloan contacted the Alcor Life
Extension Foundation about having his head frozen in hopes of a
future cure. But the $41,000 price tag cooled him to cryogenics.

Sloan joined a local hospice program but kept calling Kevorkian.
Kevorkian prescribed amounts of drugs and discussed how to
administer them. With Rubin's help, Sloan built a crude delivery

device adapted from Kevorkian's model but designed so it didn't look so much like an electric chair to Sloan.

Sloan used his dentist's license to get the drugs—sodium pentathol to induce a coma and potassium chloride to stop the heart. He saved valves and tubing from the mountains of paraphernalia delivered by the hospice.

After McNally dismissed murder charges against Kevorkian, Sloan wrote again:

> Congratulations on being "cleared." I hope your battle hasn't been too depleting for you. Pioneers pay a price. I'm sure you've had your share of stress, lawyers and grief.
>
> I am "failing." Have about 25% of my liver left. Chemo hasn't helped. My Calif. "D." says I've got weeks to months.
>
> As I may have mentioned, I have been preparing for my own "machine" and I'm ready (I think). Have a few mechanical questions ...

In February 1991, Sloan and Kevorkian talked by phone for the last time, going over in detail the procedure for using the suicide machine. Rubin listened in on the call. The next day, Fieger called the press conference to announce that Kevorkian was violating Alice Gilbert's court order by counseling an unidentified dentist.

On February 15, Sloan signed a document giving Rubin the power to make medical decisions for him. By then, Sloan was so sick that he was sleeping 18 to 20 hours a day. His weight had dropped from 170 to 125. He couldn't hold down food, except 7-Up.

The night of March 4, Sloan collapsed in the bathroom. Rubin saw he was jaundiced—a sign that his kidneys had failed and the end was near. Sloan said "What are we waiting for?" and insisted Rubin help him prepare the suicide machine.

"This was the moment of truth," Rubin said. "At this point if I had let him down or stepped aside, I would have failed him."

Rubin mixed the drugs. He gave Sloan small doses of the pentathol to test its effects. When Sloan was ready, Rubin opened the valve and delivered enough of the drug to knock out Sloan. Then he released the potassium chloride and waited nervously.

When it finally came, Sloan's death was peaceful and apparently painless—"as good a death as you could expect," Rubin said.

Kevorkian never called back to find out what had happened to

Sloan. Rubin stewed a long time. Finally, nearly a year after his friend had died, Rubin called the *Free Press*. I happened to pick up the phone. Rubin told me his story.

Rubin said he had mixed feelings about Kevorkian. He was grateful he had helped his friend but disturbed at Doctor Death's seemingly casual attitude.

"It took 20 years of knowing this guy and knowing him as a brother to know I was doing the right thing," Rubin said. "How could Kevorkian from Royal Oak in a couple of phone calls make that decision? . . . What if Gary had just been going through a depressive episode?"

Rubin said he was haunted by the idea that the death could have been botched.

"We had no other choice," Rubin said. "I wish we had someone else. He's turning this into a circus."

Fieger seemed genuinely surprised when I called him and told him about Rubin's phone call and Sloan's death.

"He took his own life?" Fieger said. "Wow, interesting."

Fieger said Kevorkian didn't make any decision for Sloan.

"Kevorkian had to take him at his word. If he wasn't a doctor, he couldn't get the drugs anyhow. And the machine is a worthless piece of junk if you can't get the drugs," Fieger said.

After Rubin went public, California authorities investigated the incident, but did not charge Rubin or Kevorkian. Under California law, assisting in a suicide was a felony.

Larry Bunting, an assistant Oakland County prosecutor, saw danger in Kevorkian's phone advice: "He doesn't know if this is a sick patient or someone bent on killing someone. He's gone from dealing with terminal patients to someone he doesn't even know."

In Lansing, Fred Dillingham reacted: "Kevorkian is scary and he's out there without any constraints. There's no one he has to report to. He's completely on his own."

But Fieger said it was much ado about nothing: "Certainly Doctor Kevorkian talking to another doctor about the drugs that another doctor is able to get under law is not a danger."

Fieger said Kevorkian was still counseling several people, including a Detroit area surgeon who was terminally ill. Judge Richard Kuhn was not happy when he heard that. Kevorkian's bond forbade such counseling, Kuhn said.

"He's not supposed to carry out any of these activities," Kuhn said.

CHAPTER SEVENTEEN
LIKE A COMMON CRIMINAL

A nude figure stands in a cell. Its face is a theatrical mask, divided into a brown right side and white left side. The body is also split into brown and white sides. The brown side has a complete right arm and leg. The white side has an arm that ends in a stump and a leg cut off above the knee. The brown hand is holding the white forearm and hand. The broken lower leg, severed into two parts, is lying beside the stump. On the bare wall, hanging by a chain, is a large gray internal organ. The painting is another Kevorkian original. ❏

In prosecuting Jack Kevorkian a second time, Richard Thompson faced an uphill battle. In a poll conducted by Market Opinion Research for the *Free Press*, Oakland County residents by a 10-to-1 margin said they would acquit Kevorkian of murder charges if they were on a jury. The margin statewide was 5 to 1.

Sixty percent of Michigan residents polled would back a law to let doctors help a terminally ill patient commit suicide.

Pollsters were astounded at Kevorkian's name recognition—94 percent statewide and 98 percent in Oakland County. They found that almost everyone was eager to talk about the topic.

"Everybody has one thing in common, and that's dying," noted pollster Steve Mitchell.

Kevon Kirk of Walled Lake told pollsters: "I give the guy a lot of credit. He's taking on the entire government basically. . . . If you want to look at it in a different light, Jesus himself had a form of suicide. All he would have had to do to stop it is say the word."

Fieger explained the poll results by saying: "People have decided that Doctor Kevorkian isn't some madman or a crazy scientist." He also said his recent arrest brought Doctor Death sympathy. "He was stopped on a Royal Oak street and slammed into a patrol car, like he was a common criminal."

Thompson said the poll oversimplified a complex case.

"I think the poll does not accurately reflect the facts in this case," Thompson said. "In any case, I can't conduct my whole administration of justice on the whims of public opinion."

In a *Detroit News* profile, Kevorkian said of Thompson:

"It boggles the mind to think that this man could do this alone. I'm convinced that he's being pressured by very powerful forces behind the scenes to do this. Organized medicine's against this. Much of the religious groups are against this." Kevorkian explained that he was pursuing his crusade "because it's right."

"You've got to do something with your life," he added.

There were other discouraging signs for Thompson. The case was assigned to District Court Judge James Sheehy, a bitter foe of Thompson. Sheehy, unhappy with Thompson's no-plea-bargain policy, had dismissed dozens of drunk driving cases. Thompson had filed suit to reverse 48 of Sheehy's dismissals.

Thompson asked Sheehy to disqualify himself from the Kevorkian case. Sheehy refused. Thompson asked Dennis Drury, the district's chief judge, to disqualify Sheehy. Drury said no.

Fieger told reporters he would ask Sheehy to dismiss the case and appoint a special prosecutor to bring charges against Thompson and medical examiner Dragovic. Assistant prosecutor Larry Bunting, heading the prosecution team, shot back:

"Fieger uses words like Saddam Hussein used Scud missiles. They are inaccurate and they have no bearing on the outcome of the case."

The *New York Times*, CNN and other national media sent reporters to Sheehy's small courtroom in Rochester Hills.

On the first day of the trial, Valentine's Day, Kevorkian, dressed in a gray suit and tie, joked with friends and supporters and signed copies of his book. Sheehy quickly dismissed Fieger's motions, and Bunting started calling witnesses.

William Wantz took the stand. He insisted his wife's pain was real: "She said it was like sitting on a bonfire all the time."

The testimony of Wantz, Sharon Welsh and Karen Nelson—another friend of Miller's who was at Bald Mountain when she died—provided a detailed account of the events of October 23.

The day had started smoothly. Marjorie Wantz shared some of

her Halcion pills with Sherry Miller to relax her. Kevorkian set up the equipment.

Then Kevorkian inserted a needle into Miller's right arm to start the IV. The night before, he had remarked about Miller's "good veins." But, as with Janet Adkins, he could not find a vein to hold the syringe. The autopsy revealed three needle punctures to the crook of Miller's right arm and one to the back of her right hand.

Abandoning his plan to use lethal injection on both women, Kevorkian left before noon with his sister Margo to return to Royal Oak and pick up a canister of carbon monoxide and a gas mask—a backup plan they had prepared in advance.

Kevorkian and his sister didn't return until after 3. Margo had retyped the consent forms to change the means of death. Welsh sat next to Sherry and read her the paper. Welsh helped her make a small "X" as her signature.

The two-patient machine had to be modified to work just for Marjorie Wantz. Then Bill Wantz and Kevorkian set up the tank of carbon monoxide and Sherry tried to turn the valve. She didn't have the strength to do so. So the two men attached a screwdriver for a makeshift lever. Miller was able to pull the screwdriver down.

At about 4:45 Kevorkian hooked up Marjorie Wantz. He had no trouble inserting the needle. He attached the tubing to her arm, which was taped to a board. He tied two strings to her other hand. The strings led to clips clamped over the tubing. Welsh and Nelson left the cabin.

Bill Wantz testified: "I heard Doctor Kevorkian say, 'You don't have to do this for me. You can stop.' Then I said, 'Marge, you don't have to do this. We can go home.' But she indicated no, she wanted to go on."

Wantz said goodbye to his wife and left the cabin as she was trying to pull the string. As he left, he heard Kevorkian say: "Marge, you have to hold your hand up." Only Kevorkian and Margo Janus remained in the room.

Welsh and Nelson and Bill Wantz were all outside when Margo came out 10 minutes later to tell them that Marjorie was dead.

Sharon Welsh went back into the cabin. Karen Nelson and Bill Wantz stayed outside. Sherry Miller was lying on a cot a few feet from the door and not far from Marjorie Wantz's body. Kevorkian told her:

"Sherry, this has been a long day. You could change your mind. We'll just do it again another day."

Miller raised her hand and said:

"Next!"

Welsh saw her friend pull the screwdriver toward her. Welsh heard a hissing sound, then quickly left because she was afraid the carbon monoxide might leak.

Outside the cabin, Welsh looked at her watch. It read "5:26." She and Nelson walked around and periodically checked back at the cabin. Most of the time Kevorkian was on the porch. At one point, 15 or 20 minutes after she had left the cabin, Welsh could hear irregular breathing through the door. Kevorkian told her Miller was still alive. Welsh found it too hard to listen, so she walked away. It was somewhere between 6:15 and 6:30 when Margo finally came out and said: "Sherry's gone."

Dragovic, the medical examiner, testified that Miller was malnourished and had multiple sclerosis plaques throughout her brain and spinal cord. But, he said, she had sufficient tissue quality in her internal organs to have had a good chance of relatively long survival.

"Her body had a cherry-pink coloration characteristic of poisoning by carbon monoxide," Dragovic testified, confirming Kevorkian's observations about how the gas colored a corpse.

Dragovic said Miller's death was homicide because she was too frail and weak to rig up the equipment. He said it didn't matter who pulled the screwdriver.

Fieger asked Dragovic if he were aware that the news media had established that Miller turned on the gas. Dragovic replied: "No, and I don't make my determinations on the basis of news reports, because news reports were generated basically by you."

Dragovic testified that Sherry Miller would have died even if she hadn't pulled the screwdriver because the gas mask would have suffocated her. He said the air holes in the mask were too small.

Dragovic said Wantz, like Adkins, apparently died from an overdose of anesthetic, not from the potassium chloride intended to stop her heart.

Sheehy refused to let medical ethics columnist Arthur Caplan take the stand for the prosecution. Fieger called no witnesses. Sheehy adjourned on February 17 and promised a ruling by the end of the month.

Afterward, Bunting told a reporter:

"We don't know where Kevorkian is going next. . . . What's going to stop him from helping a 35-year-old woman who is depressed because she can't feed her kids to kill herself? Or a 22-year-old woman who is pregnant and not married? He's uncontrollable."

On February 28, before a huge bank of television cameras and reporters, Judge James Sheehy read a puzzling opinion. Almost all of it backed Kevorkian. He referred to public support in polls and cited favorable legal opinions on the right to die. He said Kevorkian "treated the deceased in clearly a physician-patient relationship."

But Sheehy said "the question as to who caused the deaths and who is legally responsible has not been answered by the evidence presented." He said only Kevorkian and Margo Janus were present when the devices were activated and the deaths occurred.

Sheehy dismissed the count of drug delivery but ordered that Kevorkian stand trial for murder.

Fieger objected that Sheehy had made a factual error, but the judge gaveled him down.

Sharon Welsh was flabbergasted.

"Bunting asked how far she had pulled the screwdriver, and I testified that I was in the cabin and saw her doing it," Welsh said.

Kevorkian smiled elfishly as Sheehy read his decision. He then sank into a knot of supporters and reporters. I heard him say to Michael Schwartz as they left the courtroom: "Geoff's sad, you're sad, everybody's sad. Why?"

Outside the courtroom, it was a media melee.

"There is no doubt with the evidence we have that we will be able to prove he's guilty of homicide," Bunting said, but added: "It will be an uphill battle. This is not a typical murder."

About Wantz, Bunting said: "We found out from the evidence that the only problem with her is that she had a mental illness and she needed mental health treatment."

Bunting also told reporters: "We're opening the door to Pandora's Box if we claim that doctors can decide if it's proper for someone to die. We can't have Kevorkian running wild dealing death to people."

Fieger and Kevorkian stood side-by-side. Fieger did most of the talking. He said that he was prepared to have Kevorkian and Janus testify at the upcoming trial.

"I welcome another chance to go after the prosecutor," Fieger said. "The jury will never convict Doctor Kevorkian."

Kevorkian said he wasn't surprised at the judge's ruling.
"I expected it," he told the crunch of reporters.
Fieger then passed out a statement by Kevorkian:

> I am a physician, unconditionally dedicated to the honorable and ethical practice of alleviating hopelessly irremediable physical suffering. Any mentally competent adult who, after protracted and thorough reflection and professional consultations, rightly considers his or her continued existence to be devoid of any possibility of qualitative life worthy of the essence of humanity, should have access to relief. No other consideration is of equal importance in fulfilling this fundamental medical obligation for two groups of humans.
>
> The first group consists of victims of devastating physical disease. From down-to-earth practical experience I have proposed a model as a foolproof way to implement this sorely needed medical service. . . . All prior and currently proposed legislative bills and initiatives do not seem to me to be the correct way to proceed. If every doctor is allowed to perform this service, abuse and corruption may soon follow.
>
> From my practical experience, assisted suicide is least often requested by terminal cancer patients, whose mental anguish and panic disappear when I consult with them.
>
> On the other hand, victims of chronic, progressive and terribly incapacitating afflictions may choose not to endure years and decades of intolerable suffering.
>
> The second group who should be permitted this service is comprised of healthy men and women now awaiting execution as a result of criminal convictions. Through interviews and correspondence many of the condemned tell me that they want the choice of dying under general anesthesia (induced at the exact time set for execution) so that their organs can be transplanted to patients who otherwise would die. A single condemned donor could save from four to eight patients! I know of at least thirty-five condemned men in six states who want to donate their organs to save the lives of innocent victims of disease who

are otherwise doomed. ...

Those in government, organized medicine, and organ procurement agencies who would prevent innocent victims of disease from obtaining these vital organs would snuff out the lives of the very people whom they claim to protect.

CHAPTER EIGHTEEN
THE STORY OF WANDA ENDITALL

"The medical profession made a mistake when
they ostracized me. I have no career any more.
This is the substitute."
—Jack Kevorkian (1990) ❏

At last, some professionals were taking Jack Kevorkian seriously. The *American Journal of Forensic Psychiatry* devoted an entire issue to his 36-page article "A Fail-Safe Model for Justifiable Medically-Assisted Suicide ('Medicide')" and commentaries on it by 13 psychiatrists.

Many times, Fieger had told the press that Kevorkian was no seat-of-the-pants experimenter.

"He's laid out a system that includes the most assiduous controls, the most comprehensive safeguards against abuse," Fieger said over and over. "It's all in his journal article."

But few reporters who covered Kevorkian bothered to read it.

In the article, Kevorkian detailed what he called "a mandatory and intricate interplay of cross-checking consultations and unabridged documentation involving patients, kin, friends, physicians, and other paraprofessional experts." He insisted that the "true Hippocratic spirit" required doctors "to ameliorate or end pain and suffering as well as to preserve life." He noted: "Almost fanatically committed to preserving life at all costs (which have just about reached their limit today) physicians sometimes override patient autonomy and not only cause pain and suffering but also magnify it to horrendous proportions."

Kevorkian said physicians shouldn't blindly follow bad laws: "The 'ethical' doctors in Nazi Germany were guilty of obeying obviously immoral laws." And, he argued, religion had no place in medicine: "Medicine is a purely secular profession, like engineering and many others. . . . It is as absurd for a theologian to dictate medical ethics as it is for a doctor to dictate religious ethics."

Kevorkian admitted: "The overriding concern of most citizens is the fear of potential abuse, or society going down the so-called Slippery Slope." Safeguards to prevent that abuse "need not imply an overly cumbersome system. Surely the collective intelligence of the medical profession is equal to the task, provided there is the will to do so."

In an aside, Kevorkian acknowledged that the term "medicide" would translate properly from Latin as "killing a physician," but "it is appropriate as a shorthand label using the first and last syllables of the phrase 'medically-assisted suicide.' "

Kevorkian said only specialists should help people die: "It is easy to imagine . . . the abuse, tragedy, and chaos which would result if every physician—no matter what his or her talents, experience, and attitude—were allowed to practice euthanasia and assisted suicide."

At first, "pioneers" with experience would be certified. They would design and administer post-graduate training programs. The specialty would have its own competency exam and journal. Training would include study of philosophy, religion, psychology and the law, practical experience in hospitals and clinics and partici- pation in religious rites.

To illustrate how his system would work, Kevorkian divided Michigan into 11 obitiatric zones, with five obitiatrists in each zone. All requests for medicide, he said, would have to come in writing from a personal physician to zone headquarters.

This writer of limericks and sometimes sophomoric wordsmith then presented the hypothetical case of "Wanda Enditall, a 45-year- old female afflicted with multiple sclerosis." Wanda lives in Wayne County. Her physician, Frieda Blaime, is opposed to assisted suicide but conveys her patient's request to zone headquarters—in Kevorkian's hometown, Pontiac. Dr. Will B. Reddy, assigned to the case, visits Enditall, her parents and Dr. Blaime. After a discussion, Enditall signs a consent form: Document A, "Request for Medically-Assisted Suicide." The form is witnessed by nurse Vera Feier.

Document B, "Patient Data," lists Enditall's religious advisor, I. Ammon Abbott, and family members: husband Frank Lee Enditall, parents Flo N. and Justin Tiers, sister Sheila Byde, brother Barry Grieph, and 19-year-old daughter Dawn Enditall.

Form C, "Initial Clinical Assessment," includes the patient's med- ical history, physical condition, diagnosis, and the results of special tests and consultations.

Dr. Reddy conducts a consultation with Enditall, her doctor and her nearest relatives. He fills out Document D, listing those present and summarizing the discussion. Reddy notes: "There was much understanding and almost unanimous agreement. The only opposition to Wanda's decision came from her daughter, Dawn, who tearfully begged her mother to change her mind."

Psychiatrist Lotte Goode examines Enditall and finds her mentally competent. Sociologist Sharon Tydings attests that there are no family disputes except that "Dawn is not fully in agreement . . . Dawn is to graduate from college next year, is very close to her mother, and the absence of the latter, she feels, will impair her ability to complete her course of study." Neurologist Sarah Brumm reports that there is no hope of a cure. I. Ammon Abbott, the Episcopalian priest, reports that "Wanda's religious orientation apparently is not strong enough to override her decision to act in a way which many would consider to be sinful." Eight months later, another psychiatrist, Sy Keyes, reviews her case and finds no change. All the consultants fill out Document E.

Enditall reviews all the reports with Dr. Reddy. Kevorkian noted: "This cross-check maximizes honesty and objectivity, instills confidence in the patient, and serves as control against oversight and abuse. If in any of her reviews Wanda manifests *any degree* of ambivalence, hesitancy, or outright doubt with regard to her original decision, the entire process is stopped immediately, and Wanda is no longer—and can never again be—a candidate for medicide in the state of Michigan."

The "Final Joint Consultation," summarized on Document F, includes a meeting between Wanda, Dr. Blaime and an obitiatrist. Dr. Reddy meets with family members and reports: "Dawn now tearfully agrees fully with her mother's wish." Finally, all parties meet in a joint session. Reddy reports: "No reason to deny medicide."

Reddy then takes all the documents to a meeting of all five zone obitiatrists. They all must agree for the suicide to proceed. They fill out Document G indicating their consent.

The case passes to one of the "action obitiatrists"—Dr. Shelby Dunne. He takes Wanda's original consent (Document A) to her for review and she verifies her wish to die by signing a final informed consent on Document Z, at the bottom of the same page.

After Document Z is signed, medicide must be performed within 24 hours. If not, the consultations must be repeated.

In some cases, "when death is imminent or the disease fulminating, there may be time for only one joint consultation," and Document D would be marked "final." All consultations should be videotaped, and all documents and tapes filed at headquarters.

As for procedure, Kevorkian said that "The optimal choice is lethal injection . . . activated by the patient. . . . All that is required is extremely light pressure on a hair-trigger switch."

The site of medicide could be the patient's home, another home, a hospital or nursing home or a small clinic at the obitiatric zone headquarters. Wanda chooses to die at home.

At the suicide, an official observer must be present. Dr. Dunne carries out the lethal injection and fills out Document H, listing all people present, start and end time, and a summary of the details of the procedure.

Kevorkian noted "the crucial distinction" between euthanasia and assisted suicide: "On the one hand (euthanasia), the physician is obligated to be the direct agent of killing, and on the other hand, is merely the indirect agent abetting the killers—the patients themselves—and consequently less vulnerable to moral censure."

Kevorkian asserted: "The aim of obitiatry for the future goes far beyond the mere termination of human life. . . . obitiatry alone is capable of making death positively meaningful to human life—of extracting from inevitable and justifiable medicide incalculable benefit for all of humanity."

Kevorkian argued that not only terminally ill people should be eligible: "Physicians in the Netherlands have wisely expanded their perspective also to include patients facing many years of excruciating and severely incapacitating illnesses, such as crippling arthritis or emphysema, severe pneumonia and bronchitis, progressive degenerative neurologic diseases, and stroke. . . . From personal experience I know that the Dutch scope is the best approach."

Medicide would lower the suicide rate, Kevorkian predicted: "The mere availability of competent medicide will reduce the need, desire, and incidence of suicide among ill patients and elderly healthy individuals by relieving the sense of hopelessness in their panic-stricken minds."

Kevorkian reported he had gotten requests for help from about half a dozen people ranging in age from late teens to early 40s who "complained of a perpetual desire to have their lives ended even though they denied any sort of significant depression or specific illness." One woman wrote him: "I am 20 years old and have always wanted to die my whole life. I am not a bad person. I am not sick or depressed. I have never been in trouble with the law, have never taken drugs or anything like that. I don't have any problems. I just feel this way and always will until someone helps me accomplish what I want."

"Here is where I draw the line," Kevorkian asserted. "And here is where it should be drawn—until this kind of fail-safe model has been finely honed by years of experience. Only then might medicide be expanded for the benefit of patients apparently tortured by other than organic diseases; and that expansion will be the sole prerogative and duty of psychiatrists. . . . such an expansion can be fraught with immense potential uncertainty, and therefore will be contingent upon exhaustive and penetrating research and experimentation into the human mind and psyche while medicide dealing with organic diseases is carefully implemented, expanded and refined."

Kevorkian—who charged no fee for assisting in a death—said the procedure should be free and obitiatrists should work for a small set salary to curb "the potential of abuse by eliminating the incentive for inordinate pecuniary gain which might occur with remuneration on a per-case basis." Obitiatry would be funded by charitable donations and fund-raisers, he speculated.

Kevorkian concluded: "The only state law needed for the proposed practice is one which makes assisting any suicide a felony for everybody except obitiatrists." Infringement of the law should be a felony with maximum punishment. The medical profession would regulate the practice.

Kevorkian envisioned the end of the circus: "The legitimized and routine practice of obitiatry as outlined above eliminates the current situation in which an assisted suicide is accompanied by sensationalized and frantic responses and investigations . . ."

❐ ❐ ❐

A range of reactions followed the article, with some psychiatrists giving their qualified approval of Kevorkian's idea and others blasting it.

U.S. Navy staff psychiatrist Kenneth Karois called Kevorkian a "pioneer" but said: "Doctor Kevorkian's obviously well thought out proposal leaves me cold. . . . the bureaucracy he has proposed seems truly horrifying. If such a monster were created, it would probably kill its clients through frustration and boredom."

New York City forensic psychiatrist Douglas Anderson ridiculed the term "obitiatrist":

"Why not simply call the person an 'Assisted Suicide Specialist,' as Doctor Kevorkian originally describes him, or ASS for short? . . .

"Let's look at the potential of this thing while we're at it. For one thing, we're going to save a heck of a lot of tax dollars that are currently being wasted on medical research. At a stroke, Doctor Kevorkian has discovered the means to end the pain and suffering of all but the most masochistic of patients. So we shall no longer need to fund any more research into cancer, AIDS, multiple sclerosis, or cerebral palsy. Just think of it: No more telethons!"

California psychiatrist John Ravin voiced support for Kevorkian but predicted: "Those who oppose medicide will rise up and violently oppose this last freedom of choice and Doctor Kevorkian. They will attempt to force their religious views and philosophy on us . . . Waving the Ten Commandments and the murder statutes, the opposition will engage in a battle involving every significant politician in America. A vote for medicide will be equated with a vote for Satan! . . .

"So begins the fight—and make no mistake there will be a fight. Despite Doctor Kevorkian's well-reasoned approach, he touches on 'sacred subjects' and there will be no reasoning with many on the other side . . ."

CHAPTER NINETEEN
HOUSE CALL

"With this doctor, if you want it, you get it.
Kevorkian comes across as a very strong kind of
guy with very little doubt about what he's doing.
He'll give you what you ask for."
—*Sociologist Ronald Maris* ❐

Martie Ruwart didn't trust doctors. Her family believed doctors may have contributed to her mother's death by prescribing too much medication. Doctors hadn't helped her own painful back; it got worse after one chiropractor's treatment. When it came to her own health, Martie had learned to be self-reliant and cautious.

When she returned to the San Diego area after her Christmas vacation in Michigan, Martie sought treatment for an ulcer. But weeks later, she was vomiting frequently. She could hold down only potatoes.

Doctors wanted to put an endoscope into her stomach. She balked. Weeks passed, and she got worse. Finally, she gave her consent. Doctors put the scope inside her and found a golfball-sized tumor in her duodenum. She went into the hospital, and her sister Mary came from Michigan to be with her.

Martie searched for an alternative to surgery. She found out about the Gerson Clinic in Mexico and its cancer-fighting juice diet. Martie asked Mary to find out more. The Gerson people told Mary that Martie couldn't take its cure if she couldn't hold down any food. They recommended surgery.

But Martie didn't want to lose her entire pancreas. She asked the doctors to get Mary's consent if, during surgery, they decided to take out the pancreas. They refused, and recommended a specialist in Sacramento who did pancreatic resections. But the surgeon had scheduled a three-week speaking tour and could not cancel his plans. Martie, who normally weighed 110 to 115 pounds, was down to 90 pounds and was being tube-fed. But she decided to wait another three weeks. Mary got set to return to Michigan.

They discussed her options. Martie, though optimistic, wanted to be prepared for any eventuality. She told Mary:

"If it gets too bad, I can always call Doctor Kevorkian."

◻ ◻ ◻

Dr. Kevorkian was busy battling the law.

On March 12, 1992, he was arraigned before Oakland County Circuit Judge David Breck on charges of murdering Marjorie Wantz and Sherry Miller. Fieger moved the case be dismissed. Breck took that under advisement, and continued the bond prohibition against Kevorkian assisting in any more suicides.

On April 14, a federal judge dismissed Fieger's suit seeking to overturn the suspension of Kevorkian's medical license. The next day, Oakland Circuit Judge John N. O'Brien heard arguments from Merry Rosenberg, an assistant attorney general, and Michael Schwartz on yet another challenge to the license revocation.

Rosenberg told O'Brien: "Doctor Kevorkian maintains quite assiduously that there is no threat to the public health, safety and welfare, but the State vehemently opposes that position. . . . He is clearly out there advertising his services. He is clearly out there ready and willing as soon as he is able to have his license back."

Schwartz countered: "Doctor Kevorkian did nothing more than what his patients asked him to do."

O'Brien refused to take over the case, ruling the state medical board had jurisdiction.

◻ ◻ ◻

As May began, Martie Ruwart flew to Sacramento for a major, 10-hour operation. Doctors found cancer in her small intestine and about half her pancreas. They removed about a quarter of her stomach and the cancerous half of her pancreas. There was no cancer in her lymph nodes, a hopeful sign.

After six weeks of recovery, Martie turned down an option of limited radiation and chemotherapy. She was not holding down foods well, and she feared chemotherapy would compromise her digestion even further. And the limited treatment would not be of much use if the cancer had spread, she figured.

Before leaving the hospital, she requested a copy of the results of a post-operative CAT scan. But patient copies take a long time to get through hospital bureaucracies.

Martie went to Texas to spend the summer with her brother Bill and his family.

□ □ □

Clawson is a small, undistinguished Detroit suburb where big news rarely happens. But when I arrived on South Marias Street on the calm, sunny spring morning of May 15, the sleepy neighborhood was crawling with reporters and cops. A crowd was gathering on the sidewalk in front of a small, tidy house with a pot of red begonias on its front porch.

Inside the house, former Avon lady Susan Williams lay dead in her bedroom. At age 52, she had ended her 12-year struggle with multiple sclerosis. When police arrived, they found her four sisters and her son sitting in the kitchen munching doughnuts and drinking coffee. Kevorkian and his sister Margo were there, too. Sue Williams's 81-year-old husband, Leslie, who had a fragile heart, was not.

This was no dark cabin in the woods, no rusty van. This was kids on bikes and neighbors gossiping over fences. This was respectable, middle-class suburbia. This was Anytown, USA.

Every so often, Geoffrey Fieger would emerge from the front door, stalk the porch, promise sound bites later, and duck back inside.

Around noon, cameras rolled as a small man, head bowed, left the back door of the house and got into his attorney's car. Police cleared a path down the driveway for Doctor Death. He seemed incredibly tiny in the huge luxury car.

Fieger took up a spot on the lawn just in time for the noon news. Kevorkian, he said, would not cooperate with any prosecution. If sent to jail, he would become a martyr.

"He will starve himself in prison," Fieger told the camera crews and the scribblers. "I promise you that."

Fieger said Kevorkian hadn't violated the terms of his bond because he had only counseled Williams. She had put on the gas mask and released the flow of carbon monoxide, Fieger said. Kevorkian hadn't even supplied the gas, Fieger said—a statement that turned out to be wrong.

Later that day, Fieger released a letter from Susan Williams dated May 14:

I have never had a remission from multiple sclerosis since I was first diagnosed in 1980. It has been downhill ever since. I don't want to live in this condition any longer and feel I have the right to end my own life. The quality of my life is just "existing"—not living. The only time I was able to leave my home in the last year or so was to go to the Doctor and I can't even do that anymore. I am completely incapacitated and am unable to do anything for myself.

After counseling with Doctor Kevorkian for several months, I have decided to go ahead and end my life. Doctor Kevorkian has counselled me not to do this until I was absolutely sure this was what I wanted. I am happy to have his assistance to help me since I am unable to do this myself.

I intend to pull a lever to activate the release of carbon monoxide and nitrogen and I pray Doctor Kevorkian will be exonerated of any wrongdoing in this case. I am so thankful he was able to help me.

Sue Williams's 29-year-old son, Dan, told *Free Press* reporter Lori Mathews that his mother first suggested ending her life four years earlier. He said she was happy at the end, knowing she had a way out, and her death was dignified and peaceful.

"I understood her pain and supported her from the beginning," Dan Williams said. "She loved us, sure, but she wanted it to be over with. It was her wish and I wasn't going to stand in her way. It was up to her, and her alone."

Williams said he hoped good would come from his mother's death: "Maybe we can help someone else. Maybe someone else in the world will ask Doctor Kevorkian for help if they're living a life like my mom did. If they're having problems, there is a humane way."

That prospect enraged Kevorkian's critics. Michigan's governor, Republican John Engler, said he would push for the House to pass Fred Dillingham's ban on assisted suicide. Dillingham begged: "I implore the House to act quickly before more lives are snuffed out."

Medical examiner Dragovic ruled Williams's death a homicide. Fieger said Dragovic was "indulging in the fantasy that an invisible man snuck in there and took Susan Williams by the arm and killed her."

Rita Marker, head of an Ohio-based outfit called the International Anti-Euthanasia Task Force, issued a statement calling Kevorkian a "medical serial killer" of helpless women.

Columnist Arthur Caplan seemed to agree with Marker:

> All his clients were women, ages 54, 43, 58 and 52. None was terminally ill; all were despondent about facing a life of disability and impairment.
>
> The women who have died with Kevorkian's help apparently believed their lives had lost all value. What are others who have disabilities to think when these women, their families, Kevorkian, his legal team and his defenders constantly assert that life in a wheelchair, life without sight and life with pain is life without value? ...
>
> Euthanasia soon will replace abortion as the major source of moral contention on the American social agenda. Issues of the management of death will displace those of the management of birth in a society in which the ranks of the elderly already are exploding, more and more people are kept alive by medical technology and more and more people survive with devastating chronic illnesses ...
>
> Kevorkian's assisted killing of the vulnerable and the frail, his belief that women who see their lives as lacking in value deserve immediate assistance when they say they wish to die, illustrates what is morally wrong with the movement to make active euthanasia and suicide legal. ...
>
> The poor, the disabled and women have the most to lose from Kevorkian's campaign of "mercy." ...

In the United States, women attempt suicide three times more often than men. But each year about 24,000 men kill themselves, compared with 6,000 women, according to the National Center for Health Statistics. These explanations are offered: Women are less willing or able to die by violent means. They use methods that are more likely to fail. And women's suicide attempts are more often cries for help.

In 1990 in Michigan, 862 men and 206 women took their own lives. Nearly half the women used drugs or gas. But 87 percent of the men died by more violent methods, mostly using guns.

The first eight of Kevorkian's suicide patients would be women. That alone provided fertile ground for critics. Some said that vulnerable women were looking for a paternal figure to tell them it was OK to stop looking after others and make the "selfish" choice to die.

"It could be that Kevorkian leads the way and they think 'Oh, good, at last I can rest,'" said Judy Hewitt of the Women's Survival Center in Pontiac.

One researcher, Minneapolis physician Steven Miles, suggested Kevorkian "was acting as a mirror for the hatred of disability—the idea that our bodies must be perfect. . . . women may be more susceptible to that type of reflection."

Asked why his patients were all women, Kevorkian said he didn't really know. He had counseled men, he said, but all had chosen to go on and die a natural death. Maybe women were stronger and less afraid of dying, said Doctor Death:

"Women are far more aware of the quality of life and what's at stake than men."

CHAPTER TWENTY
"I'LL NEVER SEE GOD"

*In the painting, a bearded, long-haired man with
arms folded in a prayerful posture is standing in
a large, cracked, brightly colored egg, as if
hatched from it. Three large rabbits surround the
man. One wears a fur hat and holds a gold
circular hoop or halo above the man's head;
strings extend down from the hoop to the man's
shoulders. Another rabbit holds a gold cross above
and inside the hoop, with strings that go down to
the man's head. The two rabbits are obviously
puppeteers and the man a marionette. The third
rabbit's hand is helping to pry open the egg.
The painting with the Easter theme is
another Kevorkian original.* ❒

Of the five Weaver girls, all raised good Catholics, number four, Sue,
was the sick one: Rheumatic fever. Impetigo. Allergies. Eczema all
over, so bad she would scratch herself with a brush all night. A
malignant tumor on her forehead at age 12, and more than 10 surgeries to rebuild her face.

"The doctor said she was just born with a screwed-up immune
system," said Joanne, the eldest girl.

At 18, Sue started dating the man who ran the local bowling alley,
Les Williams. Williams, 48, was a year older than Sue's father.
Defying her mother, Sue married Les the day she turned 21. In 1962
they had a son, Dan, and moved to Clawson.

Sue sold Avon products door to door, plying her route on a
motorized scooter, since she was legally blind and could not drive a
car. Then her legs went numb. In 1982, when she was 44, she was
diagnosed as having multiple sclerosis. She couldn't play Bingo any
more, or hook rugs, or go to the mall for her morning coffee klatch,
or sell Avon. She couldn't afford a full-time nurse or an electric
wheelchair, and no agency would cover those expenses.

Eventually, she became incontinent. Nurses came to bathe her. Cellulitis attacked her skin, which peeled and stank. Her husband suffered a slight stroke and had a bad heart.

One day in February 1992, she asked her sister Joanne to write a letter for her to Dr. Kevorkian.

Soon, the famous suicide doctor was at Sue's house on South Marias. His sister Margo was running the video camera, in her customary behind-the-scenes role. And Sue, her husband, her son and her four sisters were talking matter-of-factly about the details of her death and her prospects in the after-life.

The tapes of the Sue Williams counseling sessions don't fit the format of a newspaper report. The issues they hint at can't be summarized in a TV clip or a sound bite.

Viewing the tapes, it is clear that Sue's four sisters were very accustomed to Sue's role as the invalid and had no qualms about speaking for her—with one sister even suggesting what day Sue should die. But Sue also had no trouble speaking for herself. At one point on the tape, Sue told Kevorkian she wanted to die because "I'm tired of sitting and watching the day go in and out."

"Is that the only reason?" Kevorkian asked.

"No."

"What are some of your other reasons?"

"I'm trying to think now. (Long pause) Oh, I don't know what else it would be."

Sue's routine never varied. Her husband would get her out of bed, put her in the wheelchair, and take her into the dining room. She would listen to the radio and watch TV all day. Les would feed her dinner and, before bed, put salve on her whole body.

"What in life do you enjoy?" Kevorkian asked her at another point in the tapes.

"Nothing," Sue replied.

No one in the family strongly countered Sue's contention that her life was worthless. Most outspoken was her sister Nancy, who volunteered that she would do the same thing if she had to live a life such as Sue's. Yet at another point the sisters agreed that Sue gave her family and friends lots of laughter, love and good times.

Sue's husband and son spoke little. Though sometimes sounding confused, Sue herself was adamant about her wish to die, affirming her choice again and again.

Some of her sisters wondered whether Sue was risking eternal damnation. Polled by Kevorkian, sisters Joanne, Mary and Barbara all said suicide was a sin, though each said she would not stand in Sue's way.

Kevorkian noted that Detroit's Catholic archbishop, Adam Maida, had pronounced assisted suicide sinful.

"What do you think of that?" he asked his patient.

"It's a sin to keep on living," Sue replied.

Kevorkian remarked: "People say you're playing God when you help somebody end their suffering. . . . But doesn't every doctor play God?"

Sue's sister Mary wanted to know: "Sue, if the Catholic Church teaches that you are going to go to hell over this, do you think that you are going to go to hell?"

"No."

"You don't?"

"I think I'll go to heaven, but I'll never see God."

"Why do you think you won't see God?" Kevorkian asked.

"Because I'm committing suicide."

"Oh. So you think it's a sin then?" Kevorkian persisted.

"No, not really."

"Yes, you do. Yes, you do," her sisters chorused. Mary pressed on:

"Where is your soul going to go, Sue? Where do you feel your soul is going to go?"

"To heaven."

"Well, if you go to heaven then you'll see God," Mary said.

"I don't believe that I'll go to hell."

Kevorkian tried another tack: "Would you feel better if you went on awhile longer and went on to a natural death and then see God?"

"No. No. No. I wish it was tomorrow."

"Don't you want to see God? . . . You want to see God, don't you?"

"No. Not really."

"Well, that answers the question," Kevorkian abruptly concluded. "That made it logical."

Kevorkian used Sue Williams to test the procedure he had devised for Wanda Enditall. "In a way you're making history here," he told the family. "Now I'm playing the part of the specialist, which is an obitiatrist, which means 'Doctor of Death,' so that doesn't affect me when people say that to me."

Kevorkian had the family sign and witness Documents A through Z. He examined Sue's medical records and verified that her doctor knew she wanted to die. But, showing no hesitation at bending his own rules, Kevorkian said it didn't matter if her doctor wouldn't meet with him: "Well, that just means that he doesn't verify your clinical data. That's alright. . . . He's already said your case is hopeless, it's irreversible."

Kevorkian wanted an opinion on her mental competency, too, but said "we couldn't get a psychiatrist because none would make a house call."

Kevorkian suggested Sue's parish priest consult with her: "That way Sue will have the benefit of his expertise in religion, and if he does talk her out of it, all the better."

Kevorkian was angry when the priest, in a written report, concluded that "Sue is being asked to go through with something that she had always been taught is wrong," and added: "In my opinion, Doctor Kevorkian is taking advantage of Sue Williams."

Kevorkian objected: "That is deceit. None of us is asking her to do this. . . . I've never asked anybody to do anything. In fact, I try to tell them to go on. I have with every patient."

He turned to the woman in the wheelchair: "Sue, has anyone ever asked you to do what you're doing?"

"No way."

"Has anyone told you not to do it?"

"No. Uh-uh."

"They haven't? Your family didn't say not to do it?"

"Yes, yes," answered her sisters.

"Yeah," said Sue, looking confused.

"We don't want you to go through with this, you know that," Kevorkian said.

"I would not wait," Sue said solemnly. "I want to go."

Kevorkian had one of Sue's sisters read aloud a statement from St. Thomas More that he said supported assisted suicide.

"The saint's word is directly contradictory to the priest's word," Kevorkian maintained, "and to Archbishop Maida. So, you see, the Catholic Church, if they say it's a sin to help someone commit suicide. . . then St. Thomas More lied . . . Can a saint be that flawed?"

After ending the discussion about religion, Kevorkian told Sue Williams and her family: "This'll probably be the last one I can do for a while, because they'll probably throw me in chains."

Then, concluding the session on Saturday, May 9, he inquired:

"So what is the timetable? . . . Sue, you could go on for maybe a year or two more."

"Oh, I don't want to go on that long."

Sister Nancy piped up: "I don't know how Sue feels, but I feel Friday, because we all work and we're going to go into work and there's going to be people at work, there's going to be a lot of flak."

Kevorkian responded: "I wouldn't say a weekend, would you? The kids are out of school. . . . A Friday would be all right. It's quick. You want it that quick?"

Nancy said: "I don't especially mean this Friday. That's up to you two, but I mean when Sue ends her life, I think she should do it like on a Friday."

Kevorkian explained that the final consent must be signed within 24 hours before the procedure.

"I was thinking of Wednesday," Sue said quietly. No one seemed to notice what she said.

Kevorkian suggested: "I thought Sunday, everybody's sorta free, aren't they? Alright, we could sign it Sunday afternoon late, then do it Monday morning. That bad? Bad?"

"Sign it tomorrow?" one sister asked.

"No, not tomorrow!" Kevorkian said, sounding shocked. "Tomorrow's Mother's Day, you couldn't then. . . But a week from tomorrow sign it, then you'll have 24 hours."

Changing the subject, Sue asked whether authorities would execute a search warrant after she died.

"No, they haven't even searched my place," Kevorkian said. "Everything's going to be in the open. . . . I don't think they'll go to trial on this, because it's going to be different from the other one. I'm going to first call the attorney. We're going to wait for the attorney. Then we're pretty well protected. We don't say a word to anybody. One of you has got to call. I can't call this time. . . . Just call and say there's been a suicide, that's all. And then we wait. Nobody touches anything."

"What happens if your attorney is not available when you call?" a sister asked.

"There'll be somebody available. He has a pretty big staff. . . . If Fieger's not available, Schwartz will be here. They're both very competent attorneys."

(In fact, when Williams's death occurred, Fieger was in the middle of a big trial. From then on, Fieger seemed always to be available on days Kevorkian helped someone die, though Fieger repeatedly insisted he never had advance knowledge of an assisted suicide.)

"I think this time the prosecutor may have doubts," Kevorkian continued on the tape. "I don't think he'll be quick to jump in. . . . He has nowhere to turn because there's no law. . . . So I think this time he'll just gnash his teeth and tear his hair out, but he won't be able to do anything. I may be wrong, because he's crazy, he'll try to do anything."

Kevorkian said they would finish setting the date off camera. In fact, he said, most of the discussion about the date could have been left off the tape. From behind the camera, Margo Janus asked Kevorkian if he wanted her to edit that part out.

"Let it go," Kevorkian said. "It's just an honest, frank discussion, and we haven't said anything that's bad."

Finally, Sue Williams asked: "When the coroner comes to take my body out, what door will they go out?"

Her wish, her son explained, was for her body to be taken out the back door—not the front where the neighbors would see.

In the end, Sue Williams did die on a Friday—six days after her sister Nancy suggested that would be most convenient for her because she could avoid the flak at work.

Watching the tape, I got the impression that Sue Williams didn't want to inconvenience anyone. And I wondered why her sisters were so ready both to agree that her life wasn't worth living and to question whether God would damn her for ending that life.

A year after Sue's death, her husband Les died. And her sister Joanne told *Time* magazine that Sue in fact had agreed when her priest told her suicide was a mortal sin.

"I don't know if she said that in the tapes," Joanne said. "I think it's because she was afraid Doctor Kevorkian wouldn't help her, that if she had said, 'Yes, it's a sin and I think I'm going to go to hell and be eternally damned,' he wouldn't help her. She didn't care, I guess. She was just so determined."

CHAPTER TWENTY-ONE
IN THE CLEAR

"The act of a physician assisting a suicide
is not a criminal act."
—Oakland County Circuit Judge David Breck ❐

If Judge Alice Gilbert's decision was a "vile harangue" against Jack Kevorkian, Oakland County Circuit Judge David Breck's opinion in July 1992 might be characterized as a fan letter to Doctor Death. In dismissing Richard Thompson's murder charges in the cases of Sherry Miller and Marjorie Wantz, Breck sounded like he had borrowed Geoffrey Fieger as a ghost writer.

Breck ruled that the 1920 *Roberts* opinion making assisted suicide tantamount to murder was of limited scope. He said that the *Campbell* court, ruling six decades later on a case involving incitement to suicide, had correctly determined that assisted suicide was no crime in Michigan.

Breck went much further, crossing out the moral line previous courts and many ethicists had drawn between pulling the plug and active assistance in dying. Breck wrote: "If a person can refuse life-sustaining treatment, then that person should have the right to insist on treatment which will cause death, providing the physician is willing to assist and the patient is lucid and meets rational criteria. . . . The distinction between assisted suicide and the withdrawal of life support is a distinction without merit. But for the doctor's act of disconnecting the life support system, or the act of inserting the IV needle, death would not have occurred."

Because Judge Sheehy had erred in ignoring Sharon Welsh's testimony that Sherry Miller pulled the screwdriver to activate the flow of gas, Breck said Kevorkian should not have been bound over for trial in the first place.

For the future, Breck suggested: "This Court is uncertain whether legislation is the answer. Perhaps it is best to leave the solution to the Michigan Medical Society and the State Bar of Michigan."

His startling opinion ended in an unusual plea:

"These final comments are addressed to Doctor Jack Kevorkian: you have brought to the world's attention the need to give this topic paramount concern. This judge, however, respectfully requests that you forego any other activities in this field, including counseling, for the time being. To continue I fear hurts your cause, because you may force the Legislature to take hasty, and perhaps improvident, action. Give the Michigan Medical Society and the Michigan Bar Association more time to do right."

In a sun-drenched parking lot behind his office, Fieger held a press conference. Fieger said Thompson should stop wasting taxpayers' money on his "persecution" of Kevorkian.

"The people of Michigan have an inalienable right to decide for themselves when and how they want to die," Fieger declared.

Out to face the cameras walked a grinning Jack Kevorkian.

Kevorkian said Breck's suggestion that he take a hiatus from his work was inappropriate.

"You're going to watch a person suffer in agony while somebody's debating? I will wait, but not if the case is extreme."

Then he issued his customary invitation to Michigan doctors to work with him.

"It's the responsibility of organized medicine. This is a medical service. It always was. . . . You cannot legislate this. You don't need a law, and no law can address every situation."

Unmuzzled, Kevorkian soon turned the discussion to organ harvesting. It was needed, he said, "so that something positive can come out of death, which is a negative." But he said such a program was "way in the future because society isn't ready."

Fieger regained the microphone and hustled his client away.

There were the usual responses from critics. I got a call from Ron Seigel, who identified himself as head of the Handicapper Caucus of the Michigan Democratic Party.

"Euthanasia and physician-assisted suicide are a nice bunch of code words for getting rid of people with handicaps," he insisted. It was a line I would hear him repeat time and again.

I called Senator Dillingham.

"Kevorkian is going to take this as a clear mandate to assist anybody, anywhere, anytime," the senator said. "I think Kevorkian is going to act decisively and basically open the floodgates."

Dillingham said he hoped Representative Lynn Jondahl's House subcommittee would release the assisted suicide bill. Jondahl, a

Democrat, said he wanted more time.

A *Free Press* editorial insisted it was way past time for the Legislature to regulate, but not outlaw, assisted suicide:

"Only the Legislature ... can set legal standards governing assisted suicide. That duty cannot be palmed off on anyone else—including voters. Cautioning lawmakers against a rush to judgment is ludicrous; Doctor Kevorkian has been plying his public trade for more than two years without intervention by Lansing, and four people have died as a result.

"How many more such deaths will occur, without regulation, while legislators 'study' the issue? When will lawmakers decide to do the jobs they were elected to do?"

Richard Thompson appealed Breck's verdict, but rejected the option of hauling in Kevorkian for violating Gilbert's civil injunction, which was still in force. Michael Modelski filed a voluminous, caustic appeal on November 6, 1992. His brief, more than 100 pages long, tried to string up Kevorkian with his own public and written comments, including the "rosy corpse" reference. Modelski argued that Breck "impermissibly imposed his moral judgments upon the State of Michigan."

"Judge Breck's decision simply creates anarchy in this area," Modelski wrote. "One should think long and hard about whether Oakland County should be converted into a Transylvania, where Kevorkian or any other person, a doctor or a layman, is allowed to prey upon depressed women who are abandoned to their despair. ... Kevorkian's vision of making Michigan a model killing zone for the country and the world must be rejected. One cannot simply shrug and pretend that it cannot happen here."

Rita Marker's International Anti-Euthanasia Task Force and a sister organization called the Nursing Home Action Group filed a brief supporting Thompson's appeal.

The brief said:

> The "right" of disabled people to be killed or "assisted" to die by a doctor is not a right. It is, instead, a message to disabled people which says: Your life has little value. . . . Society encourages you to "choose" death. . . .
>
> In its opinion, the Circuit Court legitimized the depraved ambitions of an unemployed pathologist and further devalued the lives of thousands of disabled people. . . .

Kevorkian enlists those who are in great need of affirming the value of their own existence. Using and abusing this vulnerability, he twists it for his own purposes, persuading them that their deaths, not their lives, are meaningful. [Kevorkian] exploited Sherry Miller's lack of self-esteem and personal worth by using her as his poster girl for obitiatry. . . .

Filled with passion, prejudice and an arrogant medical paternalism, defendant Kevorkian's words and actions make it clear that he will continue on his quest to reduce vulnerable human beings to objects of his own bizarre and deadly decrees. . . .

To accept physician-assisted suicide and euthanasia is to encourage those who despair.

On January 11, 1993, Fieger asked the state court of appeals to dismiss Thompson's appeal. Fieger characterized Modelski's brief as "gobbledygook that may as well have been presented by a preacher on the pulpit."

Observers predicted it would take years for the appeals court to rule.

◻ ◻ ◻

Judge Breck's decision finally brought tears to Sharon Welsh.

There had been no service for her friend Sherry Miller. Sherry had insisted her body be cremated and no funeral held.

For many months after Sherry's death, Sharon Welsh's life remained unsettled. First reporters badgered her, then sheriff's deputies. Then she testified before the grand jury. Next, she took the stand before Judge Sheehy.

"I kept thinking this would end and I would get my life back together," Welsh said.

"Finally, when Breck threw it out in July, I figured it was over. Instead, I got worse. I cried a lot. My whole life had been consumed with Sherry. I had spent so much energy just dealing with the legal hassle and the media that I didn't have time to grieve. Finally it was time to grieve for Sherry and say goodbye."

III

BARGAINING

"One of the Uncles was teaching the boys some wrestling tricks. He said, 'Look, when you're up against an enemy, you've only got two choices: fight, or run away. So it's good to know how to fight, so you won't have to run away.' Another Uncle spoke up and said, 'Sure, and it's also good to know when to run away.'

"Then one of the Elders going by stopped and said, 'There is a third way.'

" 'Oh,' said the first Uncle. 'What's that?'

" 'You can dance with him.' "

—Native American teaching

CHAPTER TWENTY–TWO
COWARDS AND PHONIES

"You know who's scared? The intelligentsia at the
top, because their empire is crumbling. Medicine
and the editorial writers and the judiciary,
all are in cahoots."
—*Jack Kevorkian (1990)* ❏

I visited Jack Kevorkian's apartment a few days after Judge Breck exonerated him. His windows overlooked the hippest stretch of storefronts in Michigan. It was totally incongruous. Kevorkian seemed a person who had not yet gotten with the '60s—much less the '90s.

The decor in his flat was early Salvation Army. His kitchen was cramped, utilitarian. His old couch was uncomfortable. The walls mostly were bare. The place appeared inhabited by a man who either had few visitors or didn't care what kind of impression he created. Fame clearly had not brought him fortune; after all, he provided his suicide services free.

It became clear as I got to know Jack Kevorkian that appearances didn't matter to him. He was not out to create a favorable impression. He didn't seem to care what you thought of him. He didn't varnish his opinions. It was take him or leave him.

Yet I didn't find Doctor Death to be an ogre. He wasn't creepy or sinister like his press clippings. Quite the contrary: Kevorkian was someone who clearly delighted in wit and wordplay. He liked to laugh—and could even laugh at himself.

In fact, his friend and admirer Janet Good told me, Kevorkian was such a jokester that it frequently got him into trouble.

"His joking doesn't fit into the serious business that he should be about," Good told me. "He thinks he can get away with joking about everything, but he can't."

Indisputably, Kevorkian was entertaining. Throughout my visit to his apartment, the invective flowed non-stop, and it was sprinkled with plenty of humor. For more than an hour, Kevorkian railed against the government, the medical profession and organized religion. To him, all were dens of idiots and thieves.

Leaders of the medical profession were "arrogant, greedy, deceitful, hypocritical wimps." As for politicians, he said he hadn't voted in years because it would be "choosing one crook over another." And, of course, he had no use for religious dogma.

"What I'm doing may be theologically immoral and unethical," he said. "But medically it is absolutely moral."

At one point, he half-apologized for his tirades, saying he had long suffered in silence under Fieger's muzzle.

"So much has been heaped on me," he said, referring to all the personal attacks. "Now I get to call people what I like."

Was he alone in his crusade? Kevorkian said he was sure some doctors would join him in admitting they helped patients die, if they weren't so afraid of the consequences of speaking out. He said he personally knew several who were sympathetic.

Public opinion didn't matter much to him, he said: "If everybody was against me and there was one patient who needed my help and you would throw me in jail for doing it, I would still do it."

Kevorkian repeated his vow to starve himself to death if jailed. And, in a new twist, he invited his opponents to watch him conduct his next case every step of the way.

"Let me try it under your auspices," he said. "Watch me like a hawk. Put a group together—a judge, a philosopher, a garbage collector, a housewife—and have the whole group be with me right there to the end."

If Richard Thompson would grant such a group immunity from prosecution, Kevorkian said he would be happy to open his procedure to scrutiny. If anyone suggested a better procedure, he would be glad to change his methods, he said. Trial-and-error was better than sitting around talking about ethics, he insisted.

"Let me run it for a year or two and see if there's any abuse. Then kick me off and let somebody else do it. I've got other things to do with my life."

What other things, I wondered, would occupy such a zealot? Then, as I was leaving his apartment, I saw an easel. I asked him about it. He said he was taking up painting again. His earlier works, he said, had all been lost when he tried to have them shipped from California. People who had seen his past paintings had urged him to take up the brush again. (I never found out whether he produced any new paintings.)

Later, I would learn about the magnitude of the lost shipment. At the time, I didn't fully grasp how much of his other life Jack Kevorkian had left behind in California. I didn't know the famous suicide doctor had been a serious but failed artist, filmmaker, writer and inventor.

Sound bites don't reveal all that.

□ □ □

As soon as I told him about Kevorkian's proposal for a panel of observers, Richard Thompson flatly rejected it.

"It's preposterous," he said. "It's an attempt to grab more headlines. This issue is too serious and will have such a profound effect on our society one way or the other that we should not make this into a sideshow."

□ □ □

In the months to come, I would have many more conversations with Jack Kevorkian. One thing I learned was that bringing up Dr. Timothy Quill's name made Jack Kevorkian apoplectic.

Quill's action in helping "Diane" die—and then writing about it—had brought him widespread acclaim, much to Kevorkian's consternation.

The *New England Journal of Medicine* published Quill's "Proposed Clinical Criteria for Physician-Assisted Suicide" in 1992. Quill argued that in cases where the best comfort care failed to alleviate pain, physicians should make lethal drugs available to competent patients who requested help in dying. Instead of suicide specialists, Quill said primary care doctors in long-term relationships with patients were best equipped to aid in deaths. Not only terminally ill patients, but also some people with chronic debilitating diseases might qualify for such a service, Quill wrote.

Though Quill seemed to be proposing a system of assisted suicide that differed from Kevorkian's mainly in the details of method, commentators in prestigious journals drew sharp ethical distinctions between the Rochester physician and the Royal Oak pathologist.

In a column, Arthur Caplan wrote:

I am convinced that what Kevorkian did in helping Janet Adkins die is completely immoral. Yet I do not believe that Quill acted unethically. . . .

Kevorkian did not know Adkins prior to attaching her to his homemade suicide device; Quill had known Diane as a patient and as a friend for many years before her death. Kevorkian scoured the country looking for someone upon whom he could use his machine. Quill did all that he could to get his patient to choose life, not death.

Kevorkian helped to her death a woman who was questionably competent, was in no pain and who was not terminally ill; Quill wrote a prescription for sleeping pills for a terminally ill, competent woman who was in a great deal of pain. Kevorkian personally hitched Janet Adkins to a machine that he himself had built, promoted and fervently hoped someone would use; Quill fervently hoped he could help manage Diane's suffering so that she never would choose to end her life.

In the *Journal of the American Geriatric Society*, doctors David Watts and Timothy Howell expressed support for Quill-type, passive physician-assisted suicide but found that Kevorkian's "supervising or directly aiding" someone's death "carries significant potential for physician influence or control of the process, and from it there is only a relative short step to physician initiation (i.e., active euthanasia)." Syracuse University law professor Leslie Bender, in "A Feminist Analysis of Physician-Assisted Dying and Voluntary Active Euthanasia," wrote: "The apparent publicity-seeking nature of Doctor Kevorkian and the strange conditions of Adkins' death—that is, the use of this jury-rigged machine in the back of a 1968 Volkswagen van—had skewed the debate about physician-assisted suicide. . . . when Doctor Quill's article was published, his presentation of the issues recaptured the public debate and returned it to a seemingly more medicalized model."

Kevorkian sneered at Quill's "respectable" methods and denounced him for the way he treated "Diane."

"Nobody saw her die. Anybody could have done that—a pharmacist could have done that!" he told me. "You've got to control for complications. You have to be there. You don't just give something to someone. He didn't act like a real doctor. And to top it off, he lied on the death certificate!"

"So for being a coward and a liar, he becomes the front man for the AMA. They love him! He broke the law in New York and nothing happened, he didn't lose his medical license, he didn't get prosecuted.

"The *New England Journal of Medicine* has never even mentioned my name!

"I don't act out of fear, I act out of conviction. Any doctor who does this quietly and secretly is acting out of fear and that's unethical.

"Caplan says he did it the right way! He broke the law, he lied on the death certificate, and he can walk away from that!

"They like Quill because they can control him. That's why they hate me and throw me in jail and take away my license, because they have no power over me.

"Has he done any other patients? Who knows? His case was not documented. Mine are all well-documented and they ignore them."

Quill went on to write a widely acclaimed book in 1993. As his book was hitting the stores, I called him to get his comments on Kevorkian's criticisms of him. Quill said Kevorkian was right: It would have been much better if he had been by Diane's side until the end. His absence, he said, probably kept him from being indicted. Quill admitted: "He's had more courage in being present."

But Quill also said a doctor who gave a patient pills to take home left that patient more autonomy than a doctor who made a house call with a suicide machine. And a doctor who knew a patient well and would be there afterwards if that patient had a change of heart was better equipped to help someone die than an itinerant "obitiatrist," Quill insisted.

I asked Quill about Kevorkian's impact. Quill said: "I think he's certainly put the issue more in the public awareness. He's also scared the hell out of people. He's made people very worried that there would not be enough safeguards, that idiosyncratic doctors would be doing their own thing.

"I don't see this as a right to die. I don't know that we have a right to die. I see this as a path of last resort, trying to respond to extraordinary circumstances that a relatively few people find themselves in, because we can't turn our backs on these people. It's not so much a right to die, as a right not to be humiliated before death."

I also asked Dr. Howard Brody of Michigan State University, longtime chair of the state medical society's bioethics committee, about the distinctions between Kevorkian and Quill—and the difference in the way doctors responded to them.

"I find it very interesting that what Timothy Quill has done has been as well accepted as it has been by so many of his professional colleagues," Brody said. "Even doctors who are strongly opposed to assisted suicide have a hard time getting anti-Quill."

Brody ticked off some reasons:

Quill had a rational patient with a clearly fatal disease. Pain wasn't the issue, so Quill couldn't be criticized for poor pain management. Quill and "Diane" had a long-standing relationship. Quill was a general practitioner with a lot of hospice skills, "exactly the kind of physician who is best trained to deal with a patient like that, not an out-of-work pathologist."

But personality and presentation might have been the key distinctions, Brody admitted:

"Kevorkian, even when he's at his best, comes across as something of a zealot. And he has a hard time when he talks keeping some of his other causes out of it"—such as organ harvesting and death-row experiments. "Quill comes across both in writing and in person as a very compassionate, caring, sensitive person."

Though Kevorkian argued that his self-activated suicide devices gave patients more autonomy and doctors less culpability, Brody agreed with Quill that Kevorkian's suicide house calls put too much pressure on patients.

"The fact that the patient at one point pushes a button or pulls a lever is kind of morally immaterial," Brody said. "The process is set in motion by Kevorkian showing up with this equipment. He hooks up the patients, he sets the standards, the guidelines on how this is to be done, how that is to be done. In theory the patient could say, 'Stop! I changed my mind.' In actual practice Kevorkian himself has said if you say 'Stop, I change my mind' I'm not coming back again.

"Diane, Quill's patient, can take a bottle of barbiturates and look at it and say 'I think I'm going to die tonight, I'm just too bad' and then she can say, 'Oh, gosh, maybe I should sleep on this, maybe I'll see what I feel like in the morning.' So she can struggle with her ambivalence and she can decide to die or not to die. And she is not under direct pressure from Quill standing there staring at her saying 'Are you ready to go now?' and to think 'OK, if the doctor's going to take me seriously I have to go through with it now.' She has the freedom to think about it a bit.

"She can own up to her own ambivalence, which I think is the human response to facing one's death."

□ □ □

I asked Kevorkian again about Timothy Quill.

"Quill's an irrelevancy to me. He's a fraud."

And what about Howard Brody?

"Brody?! He's a phony, too. He used to be against me, but he's come around on the issue since he saw the public's behind me."

CHAPTER TWENTY-THREE
THE JACK AND GEOFF SHOW

*The artist/pathologist portrays the back sides of
two men—or two halves of two bodies—joined at
the spine like Siamese twins. One man has a
beard and wears a suit and bow tie. The other
man, looking to the right, is clean-shaven with a
string tie. In the joined back of the figure is a
large oval-shaped opening, as if the back had
been split open. There is a dim, ghostly white face
inside the split-open back. Atop the split, in the
back of the conjoined neck, is a red, bloody mass.
At the bottom of the split is an iron or steel lock
and another red mass.* ❐

On August 21, 1992, Dr. John Ingold, assigned by the state Board of
Medicine to rule on the matter, denied Kevorkian's appeal of the suspension of his medical license.

In response, Kevorkian called medicine in Michigan "an ethically
dead profession." But in the next breath he pleaded to members of
that collective corpse. If other caring doctors only would step forward, Kevorkian said, "we'll set the guidelines ... we'll be giving the
lead to this benighted society."

A few weeks later, on September 16, Kevorkian and Fieger drove
to Lansing to meet with the Michigan State Medical Society's board
of directors and bioethics committee.

Fieger had called the medical society to request that Kevorkian
speak, ostensibly to comply with Breck's request that Kevorkian give
the medical profession a chance to work with him.

Before he left Royal Oak, Kevorkian told me over the phone that
he planned a wide-ranging talk including his views on his place in
medical history. But he insisted the time had come for doctors to
stop debating abstractions and start focusing on real, suffering
human beings.

"While you're blabbing and flapping your gums, people are dying," he said.

The meeting in Lansing was closed to reporters. When it ended, Fieger and Kevorkian waded into a sea of microphones. Fieger declared he was outraged because the chairman of the meeting had told him to "sit down and shut up" and because the group had refused to view two tapes of sick people asking for Kevorkian's help.

"We were censored," Fieger boomed.

In one tape, played for reporters, a 69-year-old woman described her 22-year battle with rheumatoid arthritis, which included one amputated leg, one lost eye, and hand and foot surgery. She said she had tried three times to take her life.

"I have lost all dignity," the woman's voice said. "If you could put me on your list I would appreciate it."

The medical society should appoint a panel of doctors to examine the woman and try to help her, Fieger said: "You shouldn't ignore her and then castigate Doctor Kevorkian for acting as a responsible physician."

Kevorkian called the committee's refusal to hear the tapes "barbarism."

"Where's the compassion of the medical society to say this is a business meeting?" he asked. "Is business more important than a suffering patient?"

People were swamping him with letters, Kevorkian said. He needed help.

"It is absolutely essential that the medical profession act in some way, shape or form to alleviate suffering," he said.

Kevorkian said he was being treated like the doctors who pioneered vaccination, birth control and heart transplants.

"They didn't learn," Kevorkian said of medical leaders. "They're basically dumb. They don't know history."

Having complied with Breck's request by coming to Lansing, Kevorkian vowed to resume his practice.

"I've held off with a couple of cases," he said. "I can't hold off much longer. I'm going to proceed. . . . Nothing's going to stop me. If you pass a law, it's an immoral law."

Fieger announced: "We've done everything that Judge Breck asked him to do. Now if you don't want or like what Kevorkian's doing, you do something about it. No one can say he's acting alone now."

Fieger said the medical society had a week to respond to Kevorkian's request for help.

Fieger whisked Kevorkian away. Dr. Thomas Payne, head of the medical society, emerged to face the reporters. He passed out a statement calling for "a self-imposed moratorium on any physician-assisted suicide in Michigan" until there was a public consensus on the issue.

"We hope he adheres to this," Payne said. "I hope he doesn't do anything rash."

Payne explained that Fieger was asked to be quiet because he had not been invited to speak. He said the meeting was not the proper forum for the patients' tapes.

Payne said the bioethics committee needed more time.

"We're at least a year from any resolution," Payne said. When asked what Kevorkian's patients should do in the meantime, Payne recommended they find doctors who were skilled at pain management.

❏ ❏ ❏

In a later interview, I asked Howard Brody, who had been inside the meeting, for his account of the day.

"There were really two appearances. Jack Kevorkian spoke for about an hour to the assembled group in a thoughtful and very scholarly way, about how physician-assisted suicide is in fact a long-standing noble tradition. He seemed to be saying: 'If you folks are willing to work with me, I'd like to try to work with you. If you think there's something wrong about what I'm saying, tell me what it is. I'm interested in dialogue. I'm here to share ideas, and I don't claim to have a corner on the truth market.'" Kevorkian deftly and politely fielded questions, and Brody noticed past critics responding favorably.

"If a vote could have been taken in that room at the end of his presentation, I would have thought that his stock just had gone up very high in the state medical society based on that one appearance. He succeeded in putting himself forward in a very different light than what most people thought of him from what they'd seen in the media."

Then came the second presentation: Kevorkian and Fieger talking to the media.

"They described a meeting which did not occur, in which they laid down an ultimatum that said: If the state medical society wants to work with us, they have such and such a period of time to do the following. They went on as if there had been some kind of major negotiation."

Brody said attorneys had advised the committee not to view the patient tapes so no one later could say Kevorkian had consulted with the board. Showing the tapes would have left Kevorkian no time to talk, Brody noted.

"He said in the meeting something to the effect of: 'I don't mind if you don't watch the videos, because you are doctors, you know what it's like to sit down and talk with patients with terminal illnesses.'

"So Fieger in the news conference lambastes the MSMS for refusing to watch these videos. It was a totally different thing being presented outside in the news conference from what was being presented inside. What some of us concluded was that the only purpose of that meeting was to have the news conference outside and what went on inside was irrelevant, basically just used as a stage prop for the Kevorkian and Fieger show."

Chapter Twenty-Four
"Give Me the Gas"

*"It's a universal law that you should not kill
somebody, an unbreakable law. Lots of my dying
patients say they grow in bounds and leaps, and
finish all the unfinished business." Assisted suicide is "cheating them of these lessons, like taking a
student out of school before final exams. That's not
love, it's projecting your own unfinished business."*
—Death expert Elisabeth Kubler-Ross ❏

The first time he saw Neal Nicol, Geoffrey Fieger told me, Nicol and
Jack Kevorkian were trying to figure out how to help people choke
themselves to death.

Thirty years earlier, Nicol had lain down next to a corpse at Pontiac
General and let Kevorkian put the cadaver's blood in his veins. The
two old colleagues had not been in touch for some time when Nicol
called after Susan Williams died to volunteer his services in
Kevorkian's latest crusade.

Soon after, Fieger found the can-do duo in his office trying to
work out a back-up suicide plan. Kevorkian already had lost his
medical license, so he could no longer buy lethal drugs for the
Mercitron. And companies that sold Kevorkian carbon monoxide
were buckling under pressure from the authorities. Kevorkian told
Nicol he wanted to find another way to help people die in case he
couldn't get the gas.

The two old friends explained to Fieger that they were working
on a device that would provide enough pressure on the carotid arter-
ies in the neck to deprive the brain of oxygen.

"It was so ridiculous," Fieger recalled. "I said, 'Jack, you do this,
they'll kill you for this. . . . You can't start choking people to death.'
He says, 'No, no. We're not talking about choking people. We're talking about putting pressure on the carotid artery.' I said, 'Jack, it
won't be a good way to do it.' "

Nicol and Kevorkian scrapped that plan. But Nicol, who now was in the medical supply business, would prove very helpful in other ways. He used his connections to make sure Kevorkian kept getting the gas he needed to assist in suicides. And he started moonlighting as Kevorkian's chief assistant.

For years, Nicol had lived unobtrusively on Paulsen Street in Waterford Township, west of Pontiac. Neighbors said he was a friendly fix-it type who could repair kids' bikes in a jiffy.

In September 1992, Nicol asked his next-door neighbor, 79-year-old Richard Van Huizen, if he would mind if Jack Kevorkian used Nicol's house for a suicide. Van Huizen didn't blink.

"He said the woman was in extremely bad shape," Van Huizen said. "I have seen such pain, five weeks at a time. If I had to continually endure it, I would want the same thing."

Lois Hawes came to Nicol's house on Saturday morning, September 26, about 8 a.m.

By 11 a.m. police had cordoned off the house. Reporters gathered. Through the front window, they could see the sofa bed where Hawes had died by inhaling carbon monoxide gas. Nicol wasn't present—but he would be the next 10 times Kevorkian helped someone die.

No one could dispute that Hawes, 52, was terminally ill. Her lung cancer had spread to her brain, and doctors in April had given her three months to live. Fieger said she basically had lost the use of her hands and was living on a diet of painkillers.

Hawes, who ran programs for disabled children at public schools, had four children; one had suffered severe brain damage after a car accident in 1987. She was an avid reader and organic gardener, always scratching in the dirt in her yard. She lived in the Macomb County suburb of Warren, but, Fieger told reporters, she didn't want to die at home because it was too small and she feared a media crunch.

Fieger doled out extensive information about Hawes within hours after her death. The attorney, who always insisted he knew nothing in advance about Kevorkian's plans, always knew a lot shortly after the patients' suicides. Fieger said "all of Hawes's doctors knew of her wishes and none interfered with her wishes." He said Kevorkian had counseled her for about two weeks. A family practitioner, cancer specialist, internist and several radiologists were consulted and provided medical records. At Kevorkian's insistence, she saw a psychiatrist the day before she died; he attested to her mental competence.

Fieger would not give any of the doctors' names. But he predicted more doctors soon would step forward when they saw that the authorities no longer had any way to stop Doctor Death.

By Hawes's side when she died were two sons, two sisters and a niece. Her last words, Fieger said, were: "Give me the gas."

Reaction to Hawes's death was swift and predictable. State Right to Life leader Barbara Listing said Kevorkian "has become a law unto himself." State Representative Joe Palamara commented: "It's a sad day for Michigan to be in the news again with 'Doctor Death strikes again'. This is just terribly frustrating. We're long overdue in making assisted suicide against the law."

Lynn Jondahl, who had been keeping the assisted suicide legislation bottled up, said: "My great frustration with Kevorkian is that there are no checks and balances to what he is doing. It's clear that whatever the law says is not going to be persuasive to him. He doesn't sound persuadable."

At a national conference on euthanasia in Long Beach, California—not far from Kevorkian's old Termino Avenue apartment—Derek Humphry wasn't thanking Kevorkian for generating the publicity that helped make a best-seller of Humphry's how-to book *Final Exit* (which was basically a well-timed rewrite of *Let Me Die Before I Wake*). Instead, Humphry, who recently had left the Hemlock Society to start a new right-to-die group, told reporters that he wished Kevorkian would stop "muddying the waters."

"The way he goes about it is dangerous and open to abuse," Humphry said. "But we do think there should be a law which permits doctors to do this in a safe and careful way."

□ □ □

In October, Doctor Death tangled with Elisabeth Kubler-Ross, psychiatrist and author of the best-seller *On Death and Dying* and 10 other books. Kubler-Ross, the world's most famous researcher on the dying process, identified the well-known five stages of response to imminent death: denial, anger, bargaining, depression and acceptance. Kubler-Ross told *Free Press* reporter Lori Brasier that she would invite Kevorkian to attend one of her workshops—waiving the usual $600 fee for the six-day session—in the hope she could stop him from assisting in more suicides.

"I would not preach to him," Kubler-Ross said. "I would show him how unconditional love can make any life worthwhile. What he is doing is wrong. He is committing horrible mistakes."

With enough emotional support and pain medication, Kubler-Ross insisted, all terminally ill people can live out their days in peace and comfort. Kevorkian, she contended, was robbing his patients of the most important days of their lives.

"Pain can no longer be used as a valid case for euthanasia," she told Brasier. "Patients are not dopey. They are comfortable, and if we can learn to listen to what they have to say, they can teach us very valuable lessons. With physician-assisted suicide, you don't give the family and the patient the chance to learn some enormous lessons. It's like taking a child out of school two weeks before graduation.

"At the end of people's lives, they become honest again. The only honest people in the world are the psychotic, the very young and the dying, when you throw all of the baloney overboard and get back to basic values."

Kevorkian made a counter-offer: He would go to a Kubler-Ross workshop if she would come to observe one of his suicides.

"Maybe she can learn something," Kevorkian said. "I think if she came along with me, visiting patients and going from start to finish, her perceptions would change."

Kubler-Ross said she had worked with thousands of dying patients and their families over 35 years. Few wanted to commit suicide, she said.

Kevorkian was not impressed by her credentials.

"She's either crazy or somewhat ignorant of ethical medical practices. Every one of my patients would have cursed her. She's healthy, she's not in pain, so it's easy for her to oppose it. So what if she's well-respected? So was Hitler."

The summer in Texas had been good to Martie Ruwart. She had gained a little weight before flying back to San Diego. She took a self-help course her sister Mary recommended to create a greater belief in her own healing powers. By the fall she was back to work part-time at the software company.

In October, Martie felt some lumps in her abdomen. A doctor told her it was just adhesions from the surgery. She sought a second opinion, then a third. Finally a very experienced oncologist told her she likely had tumors in both her ovaries.

At just that time, the CAT scan report she had requested before leaving the Sacramento hospital finally came in the mail. The radiologist reported that he had found two cyst-like protrusions on her ovaries and recommended they be checked out. Five months had gone by without anyone acting on that report.

Mary Ruwart asked Martie to have the operation in Michigan and recuperate at her home in Kalamazoo. That way Martie could be closer to her family.

"I knew if it had spread, it was probably terminal," Mary said.

◻ ◻ ◻

Geoffrey Fieger said Jack Kevorkian needed a media makeover, and that's why the world's most famous out-of-work pathologist was going to Washington to speak to the National Press Club. "He's been portrayed as morose and a killer," Fieger said, "and so it's important that the national press does not see him as a lone wolf helping people commit suicide."

On October 27, Kevorkian told the Washington press corps he was glad to get a chance "to prove that I'm really not the *bête noire* like I was made to feel for awhile."

He also said: "When they call me a pioneer, they're wrong. I'm a person at the right time when the mores are changing."

Kevorkian said he opposed the upcoming ballot proposal in California that set guidelines under which doctors and nurses could help terminally ill people die. Passage of that measure wouldn't lure him back to California, Kevorkian said.

"There, I could help only terminal cancer cases who are going to die within six months. Believe me, that's about 10 percent of the people who need it. I know from experience. . . . I know where the need is. No. Why leave Michigan where I can do all kinds of patients?

"We don't need a law. There's no law in Michigan. It's being done ethically, believe me. Where is the need for a law?"

Once again, Kevorkian hurt his chance to spread goodwill by focusing attention on one of his other preoccupations. At length, he expounded on his latest idea: An auction market for organs. Such a system, he said, "would eliminate the scarcity of organs. . . . The rich would buy them and the list would get shorter. The free donated ones would go to the poor. Have you heard of a better deal than that?"

Earlier in 1992, the obscure *International Journal of Medicine and Law* had published Kevorkian's article on the subject, "A Controlled Auction Market Is a Practical Solution to the Shortage of Transplantable Organs."

In it, Kevorkian wrote that since altruism had failed to meet the demand for implantable organs, "the incentive of commercialization of an organ market would seem to be the only practical solution." Under his system, he predicted, the organ shortage would be replaced by a surplus.

Kevorkian railed against "the foolishness of so-called intellectuals"—with "their emotionally overwrought imaginations" and "bizarre mental contortions"—who would criticize his plan: "Tragically, such sophistry today is costing many thousands of salvageable lives and untold pointless suffering."

Kevorkian pointed out that organ sales were legal in India and common worldwide on the black market. As for price, he proposed letting the market decide. Bidding would be worldwide, in person, by mail, phone or fax. Condemned prisoners would have "priority of choice to donate organs" because "they owe the greatest social debt, and many want to recompensate through an almost miraculous transfer of life and death." And people "who opt for medically justified euthanasia or physician-assisted suicide would also qualify."

Kevorkian even mustered a roundabout economic rationale: An auction market would increase the incomes of transplant surgeons, who would pay more taxes, thus reducing the federal budget deficit.

"For a rational society the choice is obvious," Kevorkian concluded with a flourish. "Let otherwise idle money of the advantaged who are in dire need circulate through new and natural channels among the diverse strata of a coincidentally wanting society—flow freely like the nourishing and revitalizing social lymph it was meant to be.

"Let money maximize altruism."

Syndicated ethicist Arthur Caplan said Kevorkian had gone off his rocker.

"This is a little more macabre than his ideas in the past," Caplan wrote. Caplan contended Kevorkian's proposal would lead to cases where people were killed for their organs.

Weeks later, Kevorkian told me he had modified his proposal: Anyone buying an organ would also have to buy another at the same price for a poor person on the waiting list. And, he said, "Let women run it. I think they're generally more honest than men."

"I refine my ideas as I go along," he explained.

He said he couldn't understand why people opposed his plan.

"I'm just flabbergasted at this insanity around me," he said.

❏ ❏ ❏

In May 1993, the *New York Times* reported there were 23,533 people waiting for kidney transplants, 2,843 waiting for hearts and 2,654 waiting for livers. One out of three people on the waiting lists died before they could get the organs. And only 10 to 30 percent of brain-dead patients who qualified as donors gave organs. The *Times* said transplant surgeons were lobbying in many states for "presumed consent" laws like those in Europe, which would allow doctors to take organs from brain-dead patients unless the family specified otherwise.

CHAPTER TWENTY-FIVE
"HIT THE ROAD, JACK"

"I ask you to make it a felony in the great state of Michigan for Jack Kevorkian or any like-minded physician to prey on another sick, scared, single woman who reaches out for help and is granted only one choice, only one, final, definite and irreversible option. . . . Please stop your great state from becoming the new killing fields of America."
—Diane Collins ❐

Three mornings before Thanksgiving, Diane Collins went to Catherine Andreyev's house in suburban Pittsburgh. Her longtime friend was gone. A neighbor handed Collins a note written in a shaky scrawl on lined yellow paper.

"Thank you for all your love and care," the note read. "I know you would disagree with this decision. Please forgive this and understand this."

Two nights earlier, Collins had visited Andreyev and shared a spaghetti dinner. Andreyev's cancer shackled her with pain, but she was up and walking. The friends laughed and sang songs.

Now Catherine Andreyev, 45, was lying on Neal Nicol's sofa, 350 miles away, with a gas mask over her face.

It was her way of avoiding the fate of her mother, who had suffered an excruciating death from amyloidosis, a rare disease that causes a protein overload. At the end, her mother's tongue was so swollen that she breathed through a tube inserted in her trachea.

Catherine Andreyev had vowed she would not suffer like that. Then, in 1986, she got cancer. It took a breast, then a lung. Andreyev gave up singing in her church choir. She stopped playing her flute, harp and piano. She quit making pottery. She could no longer hike or watch birds in the hills around her home. She quit selling real estate and tutoring children in English. She broke off a promising romance with a pilot.

Andreyev considered a drug overdose but feared she would botch

161

it. As her final summer waned, she called the local Hemlock Society, which put her in touch with Janet Good in Michigan. As she had done for so many others, Good gave Andreyev Jack Kevorkian's phone number. Andreyev could have gotten it herself had she called directory assistance for Royal Oak, Michigan. Despite his notoriety, Kevorkian still had a listed number.

Good later recalled: "I remember the tears. She was so obviously in pain, even on the phone. I remember the lump in my throat. I felt so sorry for her, so empathetic. She told me she was in daily, constant pain. She was really, really at the end of her rope."

Andreyev's friends tried to talk her out of suicide. But she wouldn't be budged.

Panic, an essential element in many suicides, set in as Andreyev weakened. She had planned to meet Kevorkian on December 1, but the day after she ate dinner with Collins she became obsessed with the fear that she would be too weak to make the six-hour drive from Pittsburgh to Detroit. She decided to leave right away. Her friend Betty Ouzts picked her up on Sunday afternoon, November 22. They picked up another friend, Dorothy Shorsher, in Tiffin, Ohio. That night, Andreyev met Kevorkian for the first time. Andreyev was in "great spirits," Shorsher said.

That same weekend, Martie Ruwart came to Michigan on her final trip. She brought her cat Tigre to her sister Mary's mobile home in Kalamazoo. Martie had just spent a week at the Gerson Clinic in Tijuana, Mexico, learning about the strict regimen of vegetable juices, coffee enemas and thyroid supplements that she hoped would turn back her cancer. She remained optimistic, her sister Mary recalled:

"She told me she thought she was going to come here, have her surgery, get well, and go back to San Diego. I don't think she really realized the implications of having more tumors."

Catherine Andreyev sat on the sofa bed in Neal Nicol's house. Her three friends drew close. Leslie DiPietro, who had met Andreyev 30 years earlier, had come from Ann Arbor to join Ouzts and Shorsher. The women played classical music and recited the 23rd

Psalm, the same Bible verses that Flora Holzheimer had read to Janet Adkins before Adkins stepped into Kevorkian's van.

Andreyev hugged and kissed her friends.

"I'm ready," she said.

Kevorkian, Margo Janus and Neal Nicol were ready, too. Andreyev pressed a lever that released the carbon monoxide.

Shorsher later said: "She told me this isn't what she wanted, but this is what was left for her and she was not going to suffer any more. It was her decision, no one else's. I hope people will understand there is a need for people to have a choice when there is no other way out."

Early that afternoon, my editor at the *Free Press* wondered aloud if a Kevorkian-aided suicide was now too commonplace to rate the front page. After all, Kevorkian already had helped five people die, and the paper had carried those on Page One. Wasn't his tale becoming routine enough to move it inside the paper?

Then Diane Collins hit the airwaves, and any thought of downplaying the story vanished.

Collins, calling herself Andreyev's closest friend, went on TV and denounced Kevorkian. The image of a helpless victim seduced by Doctor Death was a characterization authorities, critics and many in the media had made of other Kevorkian patients. Collins's anger buttressed that characterization. Collins made all the newscasts, and the front page, in Michigan and most of the nation.

"Doctor Kevorkian preys on people who are depressed. He was with her less than 24 hours, then handed her a mask.

"She was not in maximum pain. She was not incontinent. She was not bedridden. She was ambulatory. She had good days and bad days, and she was depressed on some of the bad days. Is this the way Doctor Kevorkian would have us answer someone's depression? I don't think any physician has the right to do anything but care— always to care, never to kill.

"She was nowhere near maxed out on what they could have done for her pain."

Collins scolded the entire state: "Shame on you, Michigan, for being the suicide death capital of the nation."

Norma Corwin, a cousin of Andreyev, tried to rebut Collins's characterization: "This was not the act of a hysterical young woman who was afraid to face anything. She probably thought this out carefully and knew exactly what she wanted to do."

Late Monday afternoon, Detroit Archbishop Adam Maida issued a rare press statement calling Kevorkian's actions "inhumane, dangerous and tragic" and promising that lobbyists for the Catholic Church would press harder for a law to ban assisted suicides.

"For Michigan to be known as the suicide state—well, we have enough trouble with our image," Maida said.

Some residents of Paulsen Street said Kevorkian and Nicol were ruining the neighborhood.

"This is going to get the reputation as the place to come to die," Carolyn Keel told reporters.

Dr. Ljubisa Dragovic ruled Andreyev's death a homicide, but Richard Thompson said he couldn't press charges without a law.

"Again, I have to say shame on the Legislature," Thompson said.

Meeting the press at his attorneys' office, Kevorkian said authorities had no business meddling in his business.

"Dick Thompson is irrelevant to this, as he would be to a brain surgery or a kidney transplant or any other medical procedure," Kevorkian said. "I consider this a well-tested, well-thought-out, well-controlled medical procedure. And I consider myself a specialist in this area."

Kevorkian said he had first talked to Andreyev in September.

"Imagine in her condition, in the kind of pain she was in, traveling by car. It shows how much she wanted this."

Michael Schwartz, representing Kevorkian because Geoffrey Fieger was out of town, said he was researching whether Kevorkian still had to call police to report assisted suicides.

"The hospital doesn't call the police when somebody dies from a routine medical procedure," Schwartz said. "What Doctor Kevorkian is saying is that he shouldn't have to do so either."

❏ ❏ ❏

For months, Marguerite Tate had been begging Kevorkian to help her die. In January 1992, she had appeared on *Donahue* with Kevorkian and Fieger. Kevorkian told her she wasn't ready.

Tate, who lived in Auburn Hills near Pontiac, had amyotrophic lateral sclerosis, Lou Gehrig's disease. Its victims gradually lose their ability to move or speak because brain impulses can't reach the muscles. They die gasping for air when diaphragm muscles quit working.

Tate was divorced and estranged from her only daughter. She and her ex-husband had run a cab company together. After their separation in 1963, she worked in the accounting department of a local utility until she retired in 1987.

In May 1992, Tate still hadn't gotten the green light from Doctor Death. Tate told a reporter she was upset because she had lost her gun. The gun was insurance in case Kevorkian didn't come through, she said.

"I don't like being robbed of my ability to make my own decisions," Tate said. "It's really closing in on me now. . . . it's terrible being trapped in this body."

"I used to have very strong muscles," she said. "I gardened. I cut my own grass. I did volunteer work, too. Now I can only lift one arm over my head."

She used her own voice the first time she asked Kevorkian for help. But her speech had become garbled. She started typing her words on an electronic voice synthesizer. Every day, she called Janet Good and used her computer voice to speak.

Good and others from the Hemlock Society visited Tate regularly to talk and pray. Mostly they prayed Tate's suffering would end.

The day Andreyev died, Tate spoke to a reporter through her computerized voice: "I wish he would help me. I wonder what she had that I didn't. I don't think Doctor Kevorkian knows how bad I am. I can't even wash my face. I'm like a baby.

"I want to go as soon as possible."

◻ ◻ ◻

The day following Catherine Andreyev's last act was the closing day of the 1992 House session in Lansing. For 20 months, Richard Thompson, Right to Life, the Catholic Church, newspaper editors and others had been clamoring for the Legislature to stop Kevorkian in his tracks.

On November 24, they would finally get satisfaction. House Judiciary Committee chair Perry Bullard had made a tactical error. He had sent to the floor a bill amending the same section of the Michigan penal code that Fred Dillingham and his House colleague, Nick Ciaramitaro, wanted amended to outlaw assisted suicide. The misstep allowed Dillingham and Ciaramitaro to attach their legislation to Bullard's bill, making an end run around Lynn Jondahl, who had kept Dillingham's measure bottled up in his committee.

With no way to keep the matter from a vote now, Jondahl backed a bill that would set up a commission to study the issue for 15 months. Representative Ted Wallace of Detroit proposed language that would permit doctor-assisted suicide for the terminally ill under strict guidelines.

Kevorkian appeared to be thumbing his nose at Lansing by timing a suicide the day before the floor debate. Andreyev had come from out of state, lending credence to fears that Michigan could become the nation's death-on-demand capital. In the shadow of Doctor Death's sixth suicide, Wallace could muster only 35 of the 56 votes needed to pass his measure.

Lawmaker after lawmaker took to the floor to harangue Doctor Death.

"The public clearly doesn't want the current situation in Michigan to continue where Michigan has become the mecca for assisted suicide," said Representative Ken Sikkema, ignoring polls that indicated Michigan residents favored assisted suicide.

"Hit the road, Jack, and don't you come back no more," taunted Representative Joe Palamara.

Representative Bill Bobier temporarily quieted the chambers by telling how he had watched his father die slowly from cancer. Then he offered an amendment to exempt doctors who withheld food and water from a dying patient.

"I have a very difficult time dealing with a piece of legislation that would make a doctor who withdrew a feeding tube a criminal," Bobier said. But his amendment failed by five votes as the bill's sponsors argued that its language would protect such doctors anyway.

After three hours of debate, the House voted 72-29 to pass a hybrid bill that would set up a 15-month blue-ribbon study of assisted suicide, but meanwhile would make it a four-year felony until six months after the panel reported. Another vote with 75 assents would be needed to give the measure immediate effect, but nobody called for one. Therefore the ban would take effect March 30, 90 days after the official close of the session.

The long stalemate in Lansing over Jack Kevorkian was suddenly over. Approval by the Senate, and Governor Engler's signature, were foregone conclusions.

Thompson sounded relieved.

"I'm pleased that we've decided to join the rest of civilized society on this issue," he said. "It's an important victory for life and the vulnerable in our society. We are sending the message to the handicapped, the elderly, the infirm, that we think you're important."

Representative Shirley Johnson said House members were afraid to vote against the bill lest they lose Right to Life's endorsement in the next election.

"They weren't voting their conscience," she said. "They were voting the way Right to Life told them to."

Minutes after the bill passed the House, I called Kevorkian. "The stage is set for fun," he said. "They don't realize the dumb mistake they've made."

Kevorkian said he had gotten seven phone calls that day from people asking for his help, five from out of state.

"I knew it would come to this," he said. "This is legislation that is directed primarily against one person. That doesn't happen very often. Nobody else is threatening to do anything. The law is barbaric.

"This law can do nothing but hurt patients and perpetuate human misery. This is a step backwards and proves that Michigan is in the Dark Ages. No other state will do this. No other state is run by a benighted governor like Engler and religious idiots like Dillingham."

Kevorkian said he didn't time Andreyev's death to antagonize Lansing.

"I never take an action to affect or not to affect legislation. I never time things for anyone but the patient."

When reporters arrived at Fieger's office for a late afternoon briefing, they discovered he was on a Caribbean cruise and would miss a chance to pitch some of the bitter sound bites the media loved to snap up. Schwartz, the Barracuda, pinch-hit.

"This act represents one giant step toward barbarism and unenlightenment in the state of Michigan," droned Schwartz, whose speaking style was as narcotic as Fieger's was hyperkinetic. "There are numerous persons in our state and elsewhere who are victims of diseases and who every day are living in desperation, people who are worried there will come a day when they can't control their own destiny. To these people Doctor Jack Kevorkian has come to represent hope.

"What the Michigan House of Representatives has done today is to rob these people and others of the hope that they will not die in horrible pain and misery, to rob from the victims of ravaging disease the hope that they can die in peace, to rob from every one of us the right to control our own destiny.

"The Michigan House has acted without compassion, has acted in vengeance against Doctor Kevorkian. Many representatives made it clear that this act was aimed specifically at Doctor Kevorkian. This is a personal vendetta."

Schwartz turned his attention to Diane Collins.

"If she was such a close friend, how come Ms. Andreyev didn't tell her about her consultations with Doctor Kevorkian, which had been going on for months? She was not a confidant. . . . She is ignorant to be making the charges she's making. Diane Collins is a lady with a political agenda."

After the press conference, a newspaper reporter pulled Schwartz aside to complain about lack of access to the three friends who were at Andreyev's side when she died.

"You know, these people come in from out of town and they are walking right into an international news event," said the reporter. "Then they think it's OK to just disappear."

"They don't come for the purpose of being a part of an international news event," bristled Schwartz. "They come because they want to be near someone they love."

"Well, if I were your PR adviser, I'd tell you this," the reporter persisted. "After the next time, just bring a couple of these people here for a press conference for 10 minutes and we'll all be happy."

◻ ◻ ◻

Weeks before Andreyev's death, California voters had thumbed down Proposition 161. As in Washington in 1991, the proposal to legalize assisted suicide under strict controls had led handsomely in polls only to sink in voting booths. In both states, the opposition spent millions on ads to defeat the proposals. But many supporters blamed Kevorkian's ill-timed actions—the double suicide at Bald Mountain in 1991, the death of Lois Hawes and the unvarnished remarks at the National Press Club in 1992. Right-to-die organizations' attempts to make doctor-aided death look respectable paled before the TV images of a smirking Kevorkian leaving death scenes. Even supporters of assisted suicide were dismayed.

"Kevorkian thinks he's God, but he's not God," said State Representative Maxine Berman, who voted against the House bill. "The Legislature thinks it's God, but it's not God either. And these poor people, they don't want God, they just want somebody to help them."

Some doctors feared the new law exposed them to potential prosecution for practicing comfort care for the terminally ill. When dying patients developed resistance to painkillers, it was becoming more accepted to raise dosages to levels that could cause death. Many doctors already were uncomfortable about dishing out morphine, mostly out of the nonsensical fear of making an addict of a dying patient. Now doctors might be looking over their shoulders for a Right to Life nurse or a publicity-seeking prosecutor who might charge that their pain control regimen constituted an intent to kill. Even frivolous charges could ruin a physician's career.

"The irony is that patients are going to Doctor Kevorkian because they can't get adequate pain relief," said Dr. Howard Brody of Michigan State University. "Now more could be going because their doctors will be afraid to provide them that relief."

Even Thomas Payne, the medical society president and staunch critic of Kevorkian, expressed strong doubts about the law.

"We're afraid that some physicians will be reluctant to treat, and others will be reluctant to stop treating," Payne said.

Some critics accused lawmakers of letting Kevorkian push them into passing a bill that couldn't hold up in court.

The law "would overturn centuries of legal doctrine, deter doctors from providing patients with sufficient pain medication, and could actually increase Michigan's suicide rate," warned Representative Perry Bullard. "The first court that hears a challenge to this law will invalidate it."

Using the carrot of the study commission to entice Democrats and the stick of the temporary ban to lure Republicans was a marvelous vote-getting tactic but created a strange mixed-breed offspring. No one in Lansing could recall any other bill that outlawed an act while setting up a commission to study whether the act should be outlawed. What would the courts think of it?

Schwartz said he and Fieger would challenge the law on grounds it invaded privacy and usurped constitutional rights to life and liberty, and that it was a bill of attainder—a piece of legislation illegally aimed at a single individual.

The Michigan chapter of the American Civil Liberties Union said it also planned to sue.

"This is not a bill that would affect just Doctor Kevorkian, but it would criminalize the actions of a loving spouse," said Howard Simon, the state's ACLU director.

For his part, Kevorkian called the law a puny weapon.

"They were going to shoot off this big cannon at me, and all they could fire was this pea-shooter," he crowed. "This isn't going to stop me."

Even his staunchest opponents agreed with that assessment.

"I think the only thing that's going to stop him is prison or somebody wiping him out," said Senator Jack Welborn. "I honestly believe he enjoys it. That's how he gets his jollies."

The local press reacted to the new legislation with glee and grief. There was little soul-searching in the editorial offices of the *Detroit News*, a paper famous for its right-wing editorials.

"Mrs. Andreyev could have died exactly the same way by locking herself in a garage with the motor running," the *News* noted. "Why involve a physician at all?"

While some said the new law constituted government interference with personal choice, the *News* found a way to turn that argument on its head:

"As government picks up more and more of the tab for caring for sick and elderly people, there would inevitably be pressure for such folks to 'get out of the way.' . . . It's hard to see how death would not become a cottage industry among the elderly. Physician-assisted suicide would bring Big Government into what ought to be an intensely private and personal decision."

Contrarily, *Free Press* political columnist Hugh McDiarmid scorned "an unholy alliance, including a large, feckless majority in the state House of Representatives, zealots from Right to Life of Michigan, and, implausibly, the grim reaper himself, Doctor Jack Kevorkian" that produced a law "to insure that Michigan would avoid being tagged as constructive, progressive, sympathetic or even thoughtful in the manner of allowing terminally ill, mostly elderly people, to die gracefully and with dignity, if they so chose." Lansing's action, McDiarmid wrote, "means that Michigan clearly has blown a chance to escape its Kevorkian-inspired reputation for clumsy, even ghoulish experimentation and to become, instead, a responsible leader in the challenging new field of medical ethics and morality."

News editorial cartoonist Draper Hill saw a way to rescue the state's image.

"Perhaps we're not selling the Kevorkian thing with sufficient imagination," he kidded, and drew hypothetical billboards such as "Welcome to Michigan—Mecca for the Moribund" and "When Death Takes a Holiday—He Goes to Michigan."

On December 2, a local minister and gerontologist, Dr. Jack Duty, revealed the results of his poll of 385 Oakland County residents. Three out of four people said they would support terminally ill loved ones who wanted a doctor to help them die. Nearly 60 percent said the Legislature should not decide the issue of physician-assisted suicide.

"That's terrific," Kevorkian told me on the phone. "You think it's going to have any effect on those dodos in Lansing? They're acting against common sense, the changing of the times, against rationality, against compassion. They're decerebrated humanoids—do you know what 'decerebrated' means? They're the vestiges of the Dark Ages, the Inquisition. They're just automatons, like cigar store Indians.

"History will tell them what their law's worth. It will be struck down in the future. You can't fight changing mores. It isn't Kevorkian that's doing anything, it's changing mores.

"If there's going to be blame put on anyone, it's on the medical profession. These political hacks who call themselves doctors, like Payne and Brody. All they have to say is this is a medical service. Now it's up to the profession to lay down guidelines. Now Kevorkian will stop.

"Why do you need a law? Get these undertakers like Dillingham out of this. We don't need these guys passing bad laws.

"They ought to pass this law in Lansing and then about 500 doctors in this state should do this all at once. What are they going to do, throw 500 doctors in jail?"

Senator Dillingham dismissed Dr. Duty's survey even before I had finished explaining to him how it had been conducted.

"Those polls aren't worth the powder to blow them up with," he said.

The next day, meeting in special session to tidy up year-end business left by the House, state senators fell over one another jumping on the anti-Kevorkian express. Even Democratic Senator John Kelly—an abortion rights supporter, political maverick and Right to Life opponent—scrambled aboard. On the Senate floor, he denounced Kevorkian as a "psychopath" and a "sicko."

"He takes women in their fifties, not just with terminal illnesses, but with chronical illnesses, and terminates their lives," Kelly boomed.

Welborn called Kevorkian "Jack the Ripper." (Other wags sometimes called him "Jack the Dripper.") John Schwartz, the Legislature's only physician, said assisted suicides were "no more than murders" and blasted "everyone who has written about this" for "hyper-philosophizing" and putting Kevorkian "on a pedestal."

There were only a few whispers of dissent. Senator Jack Faxon said his colleagues were being "bamboozled."

"It's absurd," he said. "You don't write legislation for one person."

The Senate passed the bill 24-6, beating back all attempts to amend it. Engler soon would sign the law to put Doctor Death out of business as of March 30, 1993.

Columnist McDiarmid mused sarcastically: "Now, thanks to those brave public servants, we are all safe again—safe from Doctor Jack Kevorkian, the *bête noire* of pathology, the mad monster of medicine, the vile, body-snatching, bloodthirsty, evil genius who had threatened to turn Michigan into the SUICIDE CAPITAL OF AMERICA!"

❏ ❏ ❏

An hour after the Senate vote, the media returned to Fieger, Fieger & Schwartz to face Michael Schwartz again. Fieger was still in the Caribbean, missing the camera time he relished.

Two women entered the small law library. One was in a wheelchair. The other walked with the support of a nurse.

The woman in the wheelchair, wearing a black shawl, was Marguerite Tate. At 70, she was toothless and disheveled. The cameras could record how far downhill she had gone.

The other woman was breathing heavily as she fell back in a chair. She wore a light green pant suit and looked weary but alert. Her name was Marcella Lawrence. She said she had emphysema, osteoporosis, arthritis, cirrhosis of the liver, heart problems and ulcers.

Schwartz appeared with Kevorkian and the pair issued their expected denunciations of the Senate.

"The real victim of this bill is not Doctor Kevorkian," Schwartz intoned. "The real victims are the people of Michigan—your grand-parents, uncles, aunts, God forbid, your sons and daughters and eventually you. In its lack of compassion, the Michigan state Senate has robbed you of the right to decide when you have had enough, when you can't bear the pain and suffering any longer."

Kevorkian blamed the medical society for not acting.

"The doctors in Nazi Germany by obeying immoral laws caused untold human misery. The doctors in Michigan are going to perpet-uate the same human misery.

"As a physician, I am not bound to obey immoral laws. The suf-fering patient comes first.

"Everyone paints me as a monster. What have I done wrong? I have not done anything unethical. Is this high-powered group going to come up with anything better?"

Kevorkian discussed the cases of Tate and Lawrence. He said he had insisted for months that both women see more doctors. If he truly was luring victims, Kevorkian said, Tate and Lawrence would have been gone by now.

"They were ready months ago," he said. "These two patients have suffered a lot for my sake because I've insisted they do things they didn't want to do."

Kevorkian showed the reporters a videotape of Tate that had been made several months earlier. She held her head up and could talk intelligibly but at one point said "my mind is cracking" and started to cry. When the video ended, reporters asked her questions, but her speech was too slurred to comprehend and she could hardly gather the strength to press the buttons on the keyboard of her voice syn-thesizer.

"Marguerite Tate has no quality of life," Kevorkian said. "Everyone can see that. Look at her. What good is pain control for a quadri-plegic?"

Lawrence, a divorced former nurse, spoke clearly and matter-of-factly of her desire to die. Her various ailments had worn her out, she said. Her life was dreary, meaningless and full of unending agony.

"I wish those legislators could have my pain for just one night," she said. "I can't go shopping in a supermarket. I haven't played Bingo in a year. I'm losing my sight. If I was up on the 23rd floor, I think I'd jump."

She had plenty of drugs to kill herself, but she said she feared botching it. She did not want to wind up a vegetable and be a terrible burden for her only daughter, who lived in Ohio. Her son had died two years earlier of cancer.

Lawrence said the legislation was merciless.

"People who feel like their life is not worth living any more should have the right to die," she said. "I feel like the Legislature should walk in my shoes or walk in her shoes before they make these laws."

"Are you ready to die?" a reporter asked.

"Absolutely. It's my body. I have no fear. I feel like I've led a good life and I'm ready to meet my maker."

Kevorkian thanked the women for coming to the press conference. Then, at the request of photographers, Kevorkian stood between the women, put a hand on each of their shoulders, and smiled for the cameras.

On December 7, Martie Ruwart underwent surgery in a Grand Rapids hospital. The surgeon came out of the operating room and told her sister Mary that he had removed two grapefruit-sized tumors from Martie's ovaries. He had taken her uterus and appendix. And he had felt, all along the inside wall of her surgical cavity, little bumps that were like beads of wax on a wet surface. The surgeon confirmed Martie likely had only months to live.

When she woke, Martie turned to her sister and said:

"What's the bad news?"

Mary told her: "Well, Martie, it was cancer. They took two grapefruit-sized tumors out of your ovaries and you've got lots of little ones on your peritoneal cavity." She asked how many, and Mary told her the doctor said there were too many to count.

Martie insisted on talking to the surgeon the next day.

"Well, how many of them are there?" she asked him. "Give me a number."

"About 50 to 100," the doctor replied.

On December 12, Marguerite Tate called Janet Good and typed these words into her voice synthesizer:

"Thank God. I am so happy. Our friend is finally here and it's going to happen."

□ □ □

On the morning of December 15, Marguerite Tate, in a blue nightgown, lay down in her brown lounge chair, looked at photos of her parents and tried to cheer up her friend Garvin Mosser, whom she had dated in the 1930s.

"She was trying to keep up my spirits," Mosser recalled, "so she started talking about the good times, the old times we had together. I held her hand until they were all set to go. She waved at me and smiled and that was it. I walked out. I couldn't take it any more."

When police arrived at Tate's home, they found her body in her living room. On a bed in a rear bedroom was the body of Marcella Lawrence. Each woman wore a gas mask attached to a canister of carbon monoxide. In the house were Mosser, a neighbor of Tate, Lawrence's daughter and friend, plus Jack Kevorkian, Neal Nicol and Margo Janus.

Mosser later told a reporter:

"You have to understand how it was for her. It just wasn't working. If she wanted to take a pill, she'd have to use her finger to shove it down her throat. She couldn't go to the bathroom by herself. None of her muscles was working. It wasn't any kind of life for her.

"I'm tore up inside. Just tore up. I can't believe she's gone."

A few hours after the deaths, Governor Engler signed the bill that would make what Kevorkian did for Tate and Lawrence a criminal act.

Fieger, back from vacation, was raring to go. "I'm tanned and rested," he told me on the phone.

At a press conference, Fieger said the deaths were planned weeks earlier, and the timing had nothing to do with Governor Engler's action. He also said the law wouldn't faze Kevorkian:

"Doctor Kevorkian has informed me that he is held to a higher standard. Doctor Kevorkian intends to disobey any immoral laws."

He denied that Kevorkian encouraged people to die.

"Doctor Kevorkian's main counsel is to allow these people to go on to the end, to seek treatment. But available to them is this option."

Fieger said any criticism of Kevorkian was the work of "a right-wing, fanatical religious minority" who want to "tell us what we can and can't do."

Fieger said Lawrence, who lived in Clinton Township in Macomb County, had come to Tate's house in Oakland County to die partly because "I don't want to put [Macomb County Prosecutor] Carl Marlinga through these murder charges. I don't want to get them involved in this."

Fieger released a letter Lawrence had written a week before her death. It was addressed to "The Residents of The State of Michigan" and said, complete with misspellings:

> I was ready to give up a long time ago, but Dr. Kevorkian keeps telling me that I am not ready to die. He has had me go to this specialist and that specialist to see if they could help to alleviate some of my pain. My regular doctor has also asked me to go to other doctors and has sent me to a pain clinic. If my pain was in one place in my body they might be able to help me by giving me a nerve block. But the pain is in too many places to be of any help.
>
> I *refuse* to go to anymore doctors. All of the doctors seem to think I should continue to try this and try that and I should go here and go there. I can't and I refuse to force myself anymore! I suffer too much!
>
> I am appalled at some of the things I have heard on television! Rush Limbaugh said that he doesn't tell lies on his program and yet all he did was lie! He made it sound as if Dr. Kevorkian grabs people off the street. The truth is, it's very difficult to get the doctor to help you. ...
>
> The specialist who performed my Thoracotomy said that he would only give me one to two years to live and that was seven years ago. I've gotten alot worse yet I am still here and I can't take this any longer!
>
> In taking one's own life there is always the risk that even after you swallow a lethal dose of pills that your stomach could make you vomit even though your body has absorbed enough of the medication to leave you in a vegitative state indefinately, merely existing in a nursing home. There you will be repositioned every two hours and your family can come and visit never knowing if you realize they are there.

The Michigan legislature is making a big mistake. I certainly hope that they never have to watch a member of their family suffer in severe excrutiating pain!

It is doctors like Dr. Kevorkian who can help a person die with dignity which is every persons right! Before this becomes a law the people of Michigan who support Dr. Kevorkian need to march in protest of this law and make their voices heard!

Just remember always—But for the Grace of God—YOU could be walking in my shoes!

Hours after the suicides, a neighbor told a reporter that death had been Marcella Lawrence's Christmas wish.

"She said, 'I'll have a great Christmas with my son. We'll be together.' "

CHAPTER TWENTY–SIX
DEVIL OR ANGEL

*We can see the legs of Santa Claus coming down
a chimney. His boot is crushing a baby lying in
the fireplace. A pale nude figure standing in the
living room is wearing a dunce cap and is
wrapped in red wire and holiday strands. Two
presents with pink wrapping are
on the floor nearby.
The painting is a Jack Kevorkian illustration
of Christmas.* ❐

"Army of opponents rises up against Kevorkian," the *Detroit News*
headlined its Page One story the day after Marguerite Tate and
Marcella Lawrence died. On the jump page, the headline was:
"Kevorkian's sanity is questioned."

Ed Rivet, legislative director of Right to Life of Michigan, told the
News: "He continues to exploit people who are emotionally and
physically vulnerable and now has got to the ghoulish point of
parading people out in front of television cameras before killing
them."

Ned McGrath, a former TV newsman who now worked for the
Catholic Archdiocese of Detroit, said: "Not only are these vulnerable
people being coached to kill themselves, they are being exploited by
Kevorkian and his attorney for their own publicity purposes."

To back the assertion of mental illness, the *News* quoted no less
an authority than Oakland County Medical Examiner Dragovic,
who said: "I'm very suspicious that a psychiatric disorder may be a
motivating factor in these deaths. It's a question of insanity. This is
not normal behavior."

Howard Brody, the MSU ethicist, characterized Kevorkian as a
publicity hound: "It's obviously pretty sad that he feels driven by his
own agenda to continue. I think it's a sincere desire to help patients,
but the forum is so strange to many of us that we're dumbfounded.
We can't relate to it. We don't know how to play that game.

"He's doing this in the public eye. It's a political-social agenda, the way he's going about it. He's made the media the center of this. Many died in hospices and hospitals today, but you're calling me about two deaths."

Sally Baker, a neighbor of Tate who was also stricken with terminal cancer, was quoted saying: "Doctor Kevorkian is doing the work of the devil."

Former marathon runner Gary Nussbaum of Los Angeles saw Kevorkian as an angel. Nussbaum, left paralyzed by a freeway sniper in 1987, told *Time* magazine that he hoped to see Kevorkian before the March 30 deadline.

"I'm going to be one of the lifeboats off the Titanic," he said.

Fieger at first responded churlishly to the article, saying Nussbaum might no longer be a candidate for his client's services: "We would seriously reconsider him since he's popping up in a magazine like that."

Fieger said Nussbaum was among many patients who were getting panicky.

"The patients have become more desperate," Fieger said. "They feel they have a window of opportunity in which to act. But Doctor Kevorkian says he will not hasten their desire to die, nor will he hold off" just because of the law.

A day after criticizing Nussbaum, Fieger released a card Nussbaum's mother had sent to Kevorkian. It read: "You have given my son the comfort which a sense of control over one's life offers—this is the first time in over five years he has had this experience. I can see how this has reassured and relaxed him and I am grateful to you."

The mother's words were inscribed inside a store-bought "Christmas Card for a Special Doctor" that read:

> "You're the kind of doctor/ who has a special flair/
> for making people feel better/ and for showing/
> that you care."

Fieger also released a letter Nussbaum had sent Kevorkian in July. Nussbaum had written: "Nothing is normal. Every day, I live with humiliation, complete dependency on others, the chronic turnover of personal care attendants and the loss of my freedom.

"Death is an enviable option."

Fieger characterized Nussbaum, 34, as "a mentally competent

quadriplegic with no quality in his life. He has a right to make the decision. Some day, Gary may change his mind, but we can't decide that.

"You have a man who is likely to suffer horribly for another 40 to 50 years. We are not talking about somebody having a bad day."

❏ ❏ ❏

"Kevorkian has talked more people out of committing suicide than he's helped," Alan Marsh of Grand Rapids told me. "The papers never print that."

Marsh was healthy in 1970 when doctors injected into his spine a drug called Panoque prior to an X-ray. Fifteen years later, he developed arachnoiditis, a paralyzing disease of the spinal cord. The pain started in his arms and legs and spread to his stomach.

After Janet Adkins died, Marsh wrote Kevorkian. Kevorkian invited him to appear on *Donahue* with Marguerite Tate in January 1992. Before going on the air, Marsh told Kevorkian he planned to start a support group for arachnoiditis sufferers.

"He said, 'You ain't ready for death, Al, you're doing too much good for other people. Just hang in there. Maybe in a few years they'll find something to help you deal better with the pain.' "

Tate and Marsh became friends. She called him every night for almost a year. Her last words, Marsh said, were: "Tell Al goodbye."

"I cried all night" after she died, Marsh said. "She suffered as bad as I do."

Marsh said he wouldn't use Dr. Kevorkian "until the time comes when I'm kept alive by machinery so hospitals can make money off me."

"The politicians don't know a damn thing about medicine," Marsh railed. "They ought to take that Thompson and hang him by the heels in downtown Detroit. I wish he could have the kind of pain I have."

Marsh said Kevorkian called him on Christmas Day in 1992 and asked him to contact Nussbaum—"because he's a lot like you." Marsh said he wrote Nussbaum and got a call back. Nussbaum told him he was back with his girlfriend and getting his life turned around and no longer wanted to die.

❏ ❏ ❏

On January 4, 1993, Fieger spoke at a Macomb County Bar

Association meeting. Fieger allowed that he might run for governor.

"I've got to run against Engler just on his looks," he quipped. "He is so ugly I can't stand looking at him anymore."

Fieger also threw a bouquet to Richard Thompson: "He's a real cold fish. A nice little swastika would warm up his office considerably."

Fieger wondered aloud what Macomb County Prosecutor Carl Marlinga might do if Kevorkian assisted a suicide in his county.

"I hope Carl wouldn't do what Thompson did, because then we'd have to kick him around the block a few times," Fieger said.

If jailed, Kevorkian would go on a hunger strike, Fieger again vowed, and "either it will shame us all when he dies and society is revulsed by his killing . . . or there will be a period of unenlightenment and we will fall back into a Dark Age to be reborn in another time."

Fieger blamed the media for sensationalizing Doctor Death.

"To a certain extent, we use the media," he admitted. "They want to dramatize his image, not the reality. But when you're in Disneyland, you have to play by Disneyland rules."

Fieger said that Kevorkian kept turning down chances to go on a speaking tour, where Fieger estimated he could get $10,000 a talk. (Fieger's own speaking fee reportedly rose from $700 to $2,500 in the first part of 1993.)

"He has no desire to be rich," Fieger explained. "He's in his own little prison in his apartment. He has no car. He lives on Social Security and slight savings. He buys clothes from the Salvation Army. He doesn't eat much. I've asked him to go on a speaking tour and he won't do it.

"But long after we're gone, this man will be remembered for trying to remove this monolith in society."

The Fieger statement that caused the most waves was an off-the-cuff remark that Kevorkian was "itching to get across the state line" to help patients in Ohio. "I hope he doesn't go," Fieger added, "because they have the death penalty in Ohio."

When I called Kevorkian to ask him about that, I learned that Fieger had spilled the beans without his client's permission.

Kevorkian said he only recently had learned Ohio had no law against assisted suicide. If he had known that before, he said, he would have "gone farther" with other Ohio patients.

I also learned that Doctor Death didn't like to travel far because he was afraid of flying. "If the plane crashes, that's an awfully rough way to go," he told me.

But Ohio was only 60 miles away.

"I could even walk," Kevorkian told me. "I'd hitchhike, but nobody'd pick me up."

Assisting a suicide in Ohio, Kevorkian said, would be "a test to see if their Legislature is as stupid as the Michigan Legislature."

By Kevorkian's standards, Ohio passed the test. Within hours after Fieger's leak hit the news wires, legislators in Columbus were making "Jack the Ripper" speeches and editorial writers were viewing with alarm the Slippery Slope of assisted suicide.

"It's almost like a contest to see who will be first" to introduce an anti-Kevorkian bill, said Tim Pond, a lobbyist for the Catholic Archdiocese of Columbus.

"We don't want Ohioans added to his body count," said Janet Foler, a leader of Right to Life of Ohio.

Spurned, Kevorkian canceled his Ohio plans. Within months not only Ohio, but also neighboring Indiana and Illinois had passed new laws against assisted suicide.

Fieger thought the flap amusing. An office worker heard him singing a line from the old Crosby, Stills, Nash & Young anthem about the 1970 killings of Vietnam War protesters at Kent State University.

"Four dead in O-hi-o," Fieger reportedly crooned.

◻ ◻ ◻

In a month's time, from January 20 through February 18, Kevorkian assisted in seven suicides, nearly doubling the total he had performed in the 2 1/2 years before the Legislature voted to outlaw his practice.

To his opponents, it was a macabre spree buttressing their warnings that Michigan would become a magnet for suicide-seekers if Kevorkian were allowed to operate unchecked.

To his supporters, the deaths were proof of the doctor's continuing compassion and courage in the face of persecution.

To the media, which suffer from short attention spans even on the most compelling stories, the deaths were becoming routine. Each patient used the same method: carbon monoxide delivered through a gas mask, activated by the patient releasing a clip on a tube. Each died in the morning, at a private home. Unlike most of Kevorkian's early patients, many had terminal cancer. Kevorkian, Neal Nicol and Margo Janus were always present and refused to answer questions from police or reporters. Fieger controlled all the information. Each death was followed by a news conference at which Fieger spewed familiar invective in well-honed performances. Even Fieger seemed a little jaded. His voice started to lose a little of its edge. His slams at Thompson and the Right-to-Lifers sounded trite.

"The bizarre has become almost banal," the *New York Times* observed about the suicides.

Kevorkian told the *Times* that panicked patients were flooding him with requests and the pace was wearing him down: "We can only do so much and then we're saturated. You really couldn't do one a day of these; it just takes too much work. If we had three or four in a row we'd be bushed."

Kevorkian told the *Times* he had mixed emotions about the impending law: "pleasure that they're making fools of themselves, disgust, even contempt, that they would even think of perpetuating human misery by law. . . . I don't call it a 'law.' It's the arbitrary codification of an edict, for the sole benefit of a barbaric religious clique."

One day, when I asked Kevorkian about his cause, he told me: "It's not a cause. I've given up on that. I just want them to get off my back. All I care about is my patients."

For local journalists, the challenge was to decipher ways in which each suicide broke new ground.

Patient number nine, Jack Miller, was Kevorkian's first male. His was also the first death to take place outside Richard Thompson's turf. On January 20, in the mobile home in Huron Township that he shared with his friend Cynthia Coffey, Miller, 53, once a rugged lumberjack, put on a mask to end his battle with bone cancer. Wayne County Prosecutor John O'Hair did not act, citing the confused state of the former law and the impending new law.

Fieger said Miller had been a patient at the Hospice of Southeastern Michigan under the care of Dr. Jack Finn, but Finn "was totally unable to relieve this man's suffering." Near the end, Miller joked he didn't have to eat because he was taking two pounds of painkillers a day, Fieger said. The hospice refused to comment, and Finn never returned my calls.

Fieger also revealed that Kevorkian had instructed him not to challenge the new law before it took effect.

Miller's death was the first Kevorkian "assist" that failed to make the front page of Detroit's two major dailies. Searching hard for an angle, the *News* ran a tasteless profile in which Miller's ex-wife and estranged children complained about his drinking problem, his bad temper and his "Jekyll and Hyde" personality. Weeks later, the ex-wife and children contended that Miller had been too weak to pull the clip to release the gas. But police closed the case and the county medical examiner, Bader Cassin, stuck to his ruling that the death was a suicide. Fieger said the family and police were "just trying to create a story where none exists" and that Miller was perfectly capable of pulling the clip.

Bubbling just under the surface was a bitter feud between Coffey and Miller's estranged family members, who were angry that Miller did not get their consent to his suicide.

I met Coffey at a meeting of the Hemlock Society weeks after Miller's death. She said people were still driving by her home, stopping and gawking and sometimes yelling. She declined to give her side of the dispute with Miller's family.

After Miller's death, the *Free Press* editorialized:

"Doctor Kevorkian's supporters applaud him for forcing assisted suicide to public attention. That distinction, such as it is, was conferred with the first suicide in which he took part. Since then, he simply has made up his own rules as he has gone along. . . .

"Doctor Kevorkian recently hinted he might like to ply his lethal trade in Ohio. A bus ticket from Detroit to Toledo costs $11. We'll pay his fare—one-way."

❏ ❏ ❏

The Michigan State Medical Society wanted to quell doctors' fears about the new assisted suicide law. In the February 1993 issue of *Michigan Medicine*, a monthly magazine for the state's 11,000 doctors, Howard Brody urged doctors to increase their knowledge of good pain management and ignore any potential threat of prosecution. The society's attorney said doctors shouldn't let the new law change how they practiced medicine. Even Richard Thompson contributed an article to reassure respectable doctors he wouldn't go after them.

"Physicians can give as much medication as they see fit to alleviate pain, even if the consequences of that medication contribute to the death of the patient," Thompson wrote.

Brody wrote in the magazine that Kevorkian's campaign had convinced medical society leaders that "the public has to a large extent lost faith in us, and fears that we will ignore their pain and suffering and keep them alive with medical technology in opposition to their stated wishes."

Brody also predicted that doctors who quietly assisted patients in dying would continue to do so despite the new law.

❏ ❏ ❏

On February 3, Kevorkian addressed the annual meeting of the International College of Surgeons at Sinai Hospital in Detroit. It was a rare chance for Doctor Death to speak at a respectable medical forum. Kevorkian gave no hint of any travel plans.

The next morning, he was 250 miles away, assisting a double suicide in Leland, a small resort town in northern Michigan. The patients were an 82-year-old former agricultural official, Stanley Ball, and a 73-year-old Indiana woman, Mary Biernat. Both had terminal cancer. They died in Ball's lakeside home, becoming the first Kevorkian-assisted suicides outside the Detroit area. Each patient had two children nearby at the end.

Ball, a retired cherry and peach grower, was the cooperative extension agent for picturesque Leelanau County from the mid-1940s to the early 1970s, when his wife died and he retired. Until shortly before he died, he would walk or ski the mile to the center of town almost daily, and he was still downhill skiing in his late 70s.

Ten days before his death, Ball's doctor gave him a prescription for a powerful painkiller. Ball never filled it. In a suicide note dictated to his daughter, Ball said:

"I'm 82 years old, I'm blind and I have cancer of the pancreas. I've lived a great life and done most of the good things people get to do. But now my health has deteriorated to where I'm in pain. I'm itching, I've lost my appetite and life is not worth living. I want to end my life at the earliest opportunity."

Biernat, who had breast cancer that had invaded her bones, lived in a resort community called Lakes of the Four Seasons, outside Gary, Indiana.

Her sister-in-law Julie Bryja said Biernat had been diagnosed with cancer 15 years earlier and in recent months it had spread to her spine.

"I went to visit her on Monday and she could hardly stand the pain," Bryja said. "She had lesions all over her body." But, Bryja said, Biernat "was in very good spirits. I told her to hang in there and I would pray for her. She said: 'Don't pray for me. I can't live with the pain. It's impossible.' "

Her oncologist, Ray Drasga, said Biernat did not mention pain as her major symptom.

The two deaths caused a tremendous sensation in Leland, a sleepy town that is almost comatose in the dead of winter. Reporters flew in from all over the world to hoist beers at the local inn and squeeze drops of information from the locals.

The Leelanau County prosecutor, Thomas Aylsworth, at first thought the news was a joke. Aylsworth often chewed the fat with Leland townspeople, and one of the favorite topics was Kevorkian. But no one expected Doctor Death to show up in town and provide flesh to the bones of their debates.

"When I got the call that there were two bodies and that Doctor Kevorkian was involved, I said: 'Oh, come on,' " Aylsworth told reporters. Aylsworth questioned Kevorkian, Nicol and Janus for a few hours, then released them. The county medical examiner swiftly ruled the deaths suicides. But Alysworth said: "If Doctor Kevorkian had committed this crime after March 30, I would have done everything in my power to see that he was jailed."

At a press conference that afternoon, Fieger said "several very prominent physicians" had approached Kevorkian after the Sinai Hospital speech and offered to work with him privately. Fieger issued a public plea for those doctors to come forward and back Kevorkian.

No doctor did.

Fieger said Kevorkian would no longer talk to the media because "I finally convinced him that the only sound bites they use are when he's acting strident. That gives the wrong impression. He's really a nice, calm person most of the time. But if you argue with him, he is like a bantam rooster. I know that doesn't come across well on TV."

After the press conference, Fieger again insisted he knew nothing in advance about Kevorkian's patients. Then he said that the only major religious group not yet represented among the suicide patients was Judaism.

The next morning, Kevorkian sounded feisty on the phone. He said he was glad the stories about Ball and Biernat were not on the front page.

"It isn't even newsworthy what I do now," he said. "It's finally accepted practice. That's great. That's what I've wanted all the time. Jesus, it's about time!"

Kevorkian told me that the Sinai talk had gone well, and that "several doctors are willing to help me analyze cases in private" but not help him assist patients in dying.

"You think they're going to risk their reputations?" Kevorkian asked, but added: "I think the pendulum is swinging." Some doctors and hospitals were changing policies toward very ill patients, even giving them barbiturates to help them die, he said.

"These guys do the actual killing! And their licenses aren't suspended.

"They hate me because I am so open and blatant about it. But that hatred they showed me is fatal. They played right into my hands with that law. I needed that law.

"Eventually these guys are all going to use my device, because that way the patient can do it. But they're probably going to hate it because they hate me. It's irrational."

On February 8, Elaine Goldbaum, 47, died in her apartment in Southfield with a friend and her 17-year-old daughter at her side. She became Kevorkian's 12th assisted suicide patient—and the first Jew. In Detroit, the news of her death was overshadowed by the dispute between General Motors Corporation and NBC-TV over the network's staged crash studies of GM truck safety.

Fieger opened his press conference by saying:

"If Jack Kevorkian lives to be a thousand, he won't kill as many people as GM trucks do."

Fieger released a letter, dated December 21, from Goldbaum's doctor, which said he had been treating her for several years for progressive multiple sclerosis.

"She has been confined to a wheelchair for several years, and has severe disease with marked decreased mobility, marked ataxia, and paraparesis. The patient is totally disabled because of these disabilities and will be so indefinitely with no chance of recovery."

Fieger also distributed Goldbaum's letter of December 28 requesting Kevorkian's help:

"I have given this much thought and after trying to convince me of other alternatives, my family understands my suffering and respects my right to decide what is best for me. It is my decision alone to make."

Goldbaum wrote that she was diagnosed with MS in 1978, but was able to work full-time and raise her daughter until 1988, when she became permanently disabled. Her teenaged daughter took care of her for three years until she could no longer "physically or emotionally continue." Her daughter then moved in with her father and his wife.

Goldbaum continued:

> I can no longer financially stay in my home. The alternatives are demeaning to me. I am not able to take care of my bodily needs. Feeding myself is getting harder and harder. . . . The loss of dignity is atrocious. I have no control over my urination and need to wear diapers 24 hours a day. I cannot do anything for myself. I am very uncomfortable sleeping at night, I cannot even turn myself.
>
> I am totally confined to my wheelchair and there is no hope that I will get better, just worse. I can no longer continue living like this. The quality of my life is totally diminished. Living for me is so stressful, I do not want to go on. I am just tired of needing assistance and taking medication. I just want to end the constant suffering I experience every day with no hope of getting better. I have nothing to look forward to but continued pain and loss of dignity.
>
> I am Jewish and have been raised to believe that suicide is a mortal sin. Doctor Jack Kevorkian, your assistance in medicide will get me into heaven.

In that final cryptic remark, Goldbaum seemed to be saying that Kevorkian's device transformed her act from suicide into something God would accept.

Fieger noted that Jewish custom is to bury the body within 24 hours, but he said: "I expect the medical examiner, Dragovic, to be as disrespectful to this family as he's been to others" and keep the body several days for a thorough autopsy.

"He is a shill for Richard Thompson," Fieger charged. "A suicide is a homicide when Jack Kevorkian is involved."

□ □ □

Michael Modelski, who left Dick Thompson's employ at the end of April 1993 in a dispute over Thompson's strict work rules, told me his boss should have done more to stop Kevorkian from going on a spree.

When he didn't appeal Judge McNally's ruling on Adkins, Modelski said, "a lot of people took it to mean that Thompson wasn't serious about it, that he milked the issue and walked away from it."

After Thompson appealed Judge Breck's ruling on Miller and Wantz, he took no action on Kevorkian's cases in 1992 and 1993.

"Ultimately it destroys the credibility of our office if we continue to bring these charges and have the cases dismissed," Thompson explained to me.

Modelski said Thompson should have gotten a contempt citation against Kevorkian for violating Judge Gilbert's injunction. But the penalty for contempt was only 30 days in jail and a $250 fine. Thompson said that would have been "almost an extravagance of form over substance." Thompson also said charging Kevorkian for violating the injunction likely would have ruined any chance of a later murder charge because of double jeopardy.

"That made sense up to a point," Modelski said. "But by the time they got up to 10 bodies we probably could have wasted one or two cases to go with the injunction."

Modelski said he believed Thompson was watching the polls.

"We were taking so much flak for going after Kevorkian that Dick just chickened out," Modelski said. "Then other prosecutors said if Thompson's not following up any more of these, why should we put ourselves out?"

With Thompson's inaction, "all of a sudden the assembly line started going," Modelski said.

□ □ □

On February 9, the Dutch parliament passed the world's most liberal law on euthanasia. It did not legalize mercy killings, but guaranteed doctors immunity from prosecution if they followed guidelines. The practice had been tolerated by Dutch courts for at least 20 years, and a 1991 government report estimated that physician-assisted suicide accounted for at least one in 50 deaths. But some said that physician assistance in most such deaths went unreported, and the real number might be closer to one in 10.

□ □ □

On February 11, Archbishop Adam Maida aired his views on the value of suffering in a *Free Press* opinion column:

> Persons with terminal illness or those born with severe physical or mental limitations are needed by all of us, because they help us to see the full range of gifts within the human person. ...
>
> Every moment of life is precious, from the first moment of conception until the last natural breath. In that process, even suffering—yes, even terminal suffering—has value and meaning. ...
>
> ... we all know that suffering cannot be eliminated from our lives. In a strange sort of way, as the saying goes, suffering is good for the soul.
>
> Why? Because it draws us out of ourselves and helps us to be more sensitive to others and to our need for them. When we come face to face with people who are suffering, we learn to see the real value of a person—the gift of life itself.
>
> There is yet a deeper perspective on suffering: When it is accepted with patience and love, it can be a source of healing for the individual and for those who are part of the extended family.
>
> Understanding and accepting our human limits—whatever they may be, especially the ultimate limit of death—can be a kind of threshold experience by which we move from one level of life to something much deeper.

Maida's column brought a stinging response from Pastor Thomas Eggebeen of St. Paul's Presbyterian Church in suburban Livonia.

"Maida," he wrote, "offers some wonderfully warm platitudes about suffering as it might have been experienced in other ages, when it was intense but short-lived ..."

But today, things are much different, Eggebeen argued:

The course of life and death is interrupted by a vast array of technologies, catching patients at the threshold of death and pulling them back, again and again, until their suffering is transformed into a hideous torture of body and soul. . . .

It is an act of gross irresponsibility to forestall death by every means possible, and then, when recovery is no longer likely, simply to abandon patients, with our prayers and best wishes for the interminable suffering they must bear.

The archbishop's . . . recalcitrance on this matter, and that of the Roman Catholic Church and the various right-to-life groups aligned with it, reveal an unbalanced, if not neurotic, regard for suffering.

Kevorkian is on the right track . . .

❏ ❏ ❏

On Monday morning, February 15, police were summoned to a small house in the Detroit suburb of Roseville. They found 70-year-old Hugh Gale dead, a canister of carbon monoxide attached to a gas mask over his face. His wife Cheryl Gale was present along with Kevorkian, Neal Nicol and Margo Janus.

Gale, a retired merchant marine sailor and former security guard, died in the same chair where he had spent the last three years struggling to breathe because of his emphysema.

"He couldn't lie down or he would drown in his own mucus," Fieger said.

Gale was suicide number 13. His death took place in Macomb County. Fieger had warned Macomb Prosecutor Carl Marlinga to expect an ass-kicking if he interfered. Marlinga, a Democrat who had announced he would run for the U.S. Senate in 1994, sounded miffed that Kevorkian and Fieger hadn't notified him of Gale's death in advance.

"I find it distasteful the way in which Doctor Kevorkian self-righteously feels he is the only one who knows the truth on this issue," Marlinga said. "There was no reason his attorneys couldn't have given our office a call in advance."

Michael Schwartz replied that Kevorkian didn't seek publicity nor give advance notice of suicides. He accused Marlinga of pandering for votes.

In Lansing, momentum was gathering for a new attack on Kevorkian. The recent spate of deaths had convinced Right to Life that it could make a deal to secure enough votes for an immediate ban, moving up the date from March 30.

Ed Rivet of Right to Life said he feared a string of deaths if the Legislature didn't act quickly.

"My greatest fear is the week before the effective date, he'll be killing someone every single day. We could have multiple bodies going down every day."

Representative Joe Palamara, who had told Kevorkian in December to "Hit the road, Jack," now said:

"This is one self-appointed death guru who obviously has no respect for human life. The only thing that's going to stop him is to have a jury of Michigan citizens determine he violated the law that was passed by the Legislature."

Fieger said Kevorkian's opponents were "Nazis" and "religious nuts."

"They enjoy human suffering. They believe human suffering is the way you get into heaven. And yet these are the same people who support the death penalty. They are the worst sort of hypocrites who periodically inveigle themselves into government."

Kevorkian told the *New York Times*:

"I'd like to see them move it up. Let's get the charade under way faster. Let the world see what cruel fools they are."

CHAPTER TWENTY–SEVEN
"I WANT DOCTOR KEVORKIAN!"

"Just getting in contact with me relieves people. Sometimes just talking to me on the phone, they say they feel better. It's like insurance. You feel good if you have it. If you don't, you feel a little edgy. Insurance is the option that relieves panic. The insurance I offer is that you don't have to die in pain. That relieves them, and many go on to die from the disease."
— Jack Kevorkian (1993) ❐

Martie Ruwart left the hospital in Grand Rapids with the 50 to 100 tiny bumps inside her abdominal cavity and returned to her sister Mary's mobile home in Kalamazoo.

Again Martie refused chemotherapy, because her doctors told her it would give her only a 30 percent chance of reduction in tumor size. She also rejected the option of another operation to flush her abdominal cavity with chemotherapy drugs. Martie felt too weak for more surgery.

Instead, Martie tried to stay on the Gerson diet. Her sisters hired several women to make juices and care for Martie while Mary was at work. But Martie felt too full to drink a glass of juice every hour.

She began taking enemas of shark cartilage, thought to be effective in preventing blood vessel growth in tumors. She drank Essiac herbal tea, an American Indian remedy for cancer. The tea relieved her full feeling and allowed her to eat more.

But juggling the coffee enemas required by the Gerson diet with the shark cartilage enemas was too much. Martie gave up on Gerson.

She was losing weight. Her sisters Mary and Teresa, who lived nearby, tried to fatten her up with homemade cream soups and trips to restaurants for pasta. But Martie couldn't sit up for long. Her back was giving out and her stomach hurt all the time.

In the middle of January, Martie enrolled in a local hospice—the home comfort care program that is limited to the terminally ill.

Mary and Martie asked hospice personnel if they had Doctor Kevorkian's phone number. The reply was: "Sorry, we don't get involved in that."

Martie's pain medication was making her drowsy and constipated, so her sisters weaned her off the opiates. She was going through withdrawal the day a hospice social worker came to interview her. The social worker noticed Martie seemed depressed and asked:

"Do you ever think about suicide?"

"I think about Doctor Kevorkian a lot," Martie replied.

The next day, the hospice doctor put Martie on an anti-depressant and upped her pain medication. In response, Martie's stomach bloated like a balloon and her gut shut down.

Martie next went to a gastrointestinal physician who told her that the dosage of anti-depressants was five times what he normally prescribed. He did a CAT scan. It showed no large tumors. But the doctor said her symptoms signaled that her bowels were being strangled by multiple small tumors. He tapped her stomach to drain the fluids, but she had a large pocket of fluid behind her liver, too dangerous a spot to drain.

It took days for Martie to recover from each medical procedure. She was taking so many medications that Mary had to keep a log. The pressure of the fluid on her stomach made her feel full. She would vomit if she ate too much. She woke up every few hours at night.

Martie found some relief in her sister's hot tub. She soaked in the tub three or four times a day to relieve her pain.

Soon, Martie began vomiting a lot. A bulge on her left side below her breast bone grew larger; likely it was a tumor. Her rectal channel was partially blocked by what was probably another tumor.

By late January, she could no longer hold down water. She was down to 80 pounds.

The doctors indicated that trying to feed her would only prolong her suffering. The best course, they said, was to keep her on as much pain medication as she needed to feel comfortable.

Facing the end of her life, Martie began to try to gain some control. At Martie's request, her sister Teresa called directory assistance in Royal Oak. On January 31, Teresa dialed Jack Kevorkian's phone number. She told him about Martie. Kevorkian said he wanted to see Martie's medical and psychiatric records. The sisters sent him the records by overnight mail.

On the night of February 9, Martie got out of bed three times to vomit. She cried out from the bathroom:

"Nobody listens to me! I want Doctor Kevorkian *now!*"

Mary decided: "Well, I'll call him just to calm her down."

It was 10:30. Mary apologized for the late hour.

"That's OK," Kevorkian said. "I'm a night person."

Kevorkian wanted to meet Martie before committing to helping her die. But after Mary explained her desperate situation, he said he would make an exception to his rules. If the Ruwarts could find a house, Kevorkian said he could schedule her for Saturday the 13th.

Hearing the news, Martie improved noticeably. For the first time in weeks, she could hold down a little food and water. She had been bedridden, but now she was up part of the day.

"It was wonderful," Mary recalled. "She was like a new person. I thought I'd never see the old Martie again."

Making the decision to die wasn't as hard for Martie as coping with the disease had been.

"There's not a lot of fear of dying in our family," Mary said. "There's a fear of suffering."

About what happens after death, Martie told her sister: "I think probably your consciousness goes on in some way, but if it doesn't you don't know about it, so what is there to worry about?"

On Wednesday the 10th, Martie's brother Bill flew in from Texas to be with her in her last days.

The next day, her father came to visit. He said she could use his house in Grosse Pointe Woods to die in.

Martie was in great spirits. At times she felt so good that she started to wonder if she really needed Kevorkian's help.

Late Thursday night, Mary Ruwart called Kevorkian to tell him they had a house. But Kevorkian said his supply of carbon monoxide had been cut off and he needed the weekend to make changes in his apparatus so that he could better ration the gas. It was devastating news.

"Martie was real scared. She kept worrying that he was going to cop out on her," Mary said.

On Saturday morning, February 13, Kevorkian told the Ruwarts that he had a slot open for Martie on Monday. The sisters called their father.

He said he had changed his mind about letting them use the house.

"That's when all hell broke loose," Mary said.

Martie went into a tizzy. Then she told her sisters: "This doubt that I had because I was feeling a little better is gone. I know now how much I want this because I am really bummed out."

Utter panic consumed the Ruwarts for the next 36 hours. If they didn't find a place, Martie's opportunity might be gone. Kevorkian had told the Ruwarts the Legislature was getting ready to ban his practice.

Where to go? Mary's home was out because Kevorkian wouldn't assist a suicide on rental property. Martie's sisters Karen and Teresa asked their spouses, but after talking on the phone to Fieger, their husbands decided there could be too many repercussions.

An old friend of Martie from college told Martie she could use her house in Lansing to die in—even though it could jeopardize her government job. But Kevorkian was nervous about the questions Martie's friend asked.

"I think he initially perceived we had a lot of family support," Mary said. "But now he was really beginning to wonder. He said: 'Martie, look, you've got to get someone where there's no questions. You've got one more chance to find a house.'

"Martie was getting strung out. She was really in a panic."

On Sunday morning, Valentine's Day, Martie told her sister Teresa:

"When I woke up this morning, I knew my decision was the right one. It's exactly what I want to do."

Martie wanted to make backup plans.

"Can I shoot myself in your house?" she asked Mary.

"I said, 'Martie, you know, we'll think of something. Don't feel like this is the only thing that can happen,' " Mary recalled. "So she didn't worry too much. But I did, because I knew I was going to have to think of something else.

"We were terrified. I was thinking: If you shoot yourself in my house, I better be around to make sure you do a good job. I don't want you lying there for hours."

There was one other hope: Gary, an old college friend of Mary and Martie. In a stroke of good fortune, Mary reached him on the road. By Sunday evening, he had gotten back to his home in Lansing and gotten his wife's OK to use their home for Martie's death.

At 6:30 Sunday night, Mary called Kevorkian to tell him they had found a place for Martie to die the next morning. But Kevorkian said he had filled the Monday slot—with Hugh Gale—and could do Martie on Thursday, if she didn't mind sharing a house in Waterford

Township with another patient from out-of-state.

"I felt the commitment in his voice," Mary said. "Up until then, I hadn't been sure."

The sisters were relieved, though they were still worried that Kevorkian's Monday assist might propel the Legislature into immediate action.

The various pressures—the pending legislative action, the short supply of gas, Kevorkian's timetable—may have influenced the timing of Martie's death, Mary said:

"Part of her decision was: I have time pressure here. If I don't do it now I might have to do something I don't like as much."

Martie put her affairs in order down to the minutest detail. On Tuesday the 16th, she had Mary dictate a letter to the hospice saying she was dropping out of the program—to spare hospice officials any embarrassment. She wrote thank-you letters to her co-workers in San Diego. She ordered flowers sent to all her doctors. She settled all her financial business and left instructions for distributing her possessions. She left the bulk of her estate to promote *Healing Our World*, the book she had helped Mary write.

On Wednesday the 17th, her brother Bill parted tearfully from his sister and flew back to Texas. Her brother Michael had decided he would not attend his sister's death. Her sister Karen would meet them at a motel in Waterford Township, where Kevorkian had instructed them to come.

That afternoon, Mary and Teresa put Martie on a foam pad in the back of Mary's 1985 Charger hatchback. Mary stopped at the mobile home park office to pay her rent. The manager asked how Martie was doing.

"She's not doing real good, so we're taking her to Detroit for a change of scenery," was all Mary could think to reply.

The secrecy was difficult.

"The hardest thing about this is that we could not be straightforward with people that we liked and trusted," Mary said.

The Ruwarts were a large family, with many branches. If word got out, someone might try to interfere. And it had to be hush-hush at work as well. "If we blew the chance, then she would be suffering," Mary said.

Wednesday evening, three of Martie's friends met the Ruwarts in Waterford. Kevorkian, Neal Nicol and Margo Janus soon arrived to conduct and videotape a counseling session.

"They were real warm people," Mary said. Martie called Kevorkian "my angel" and hugged him.

"She was a big fan," Mary said.

Margo began rolling the videotape. Martie lay on the motel bed and explained her decision:

"I wish right now to end my suffering. I don't feel it's worth going on. . . . I want to die because this is the only way I can ease my pain."

Martie said she didn't want to wait until she was incoherent and doped up, but wanted to go while she was still lucid.

Kevorkian was light-hearted. He said: "Do you want to see a minister?" Martie said no. He said: "If I insisted that you see a minister, would you see one?" She looked at him quizzically and then said, "Sure, I'll do whatever it takes."

Kevorkian asked if Martie had any anger about her disease.

"I had a good life, that's the way I look at it," she said. "I feel like my life's complete. I got to the stage where I was able to see my whole life and how all the parts fit together. So I feel like I've completed my journey."

Martie signed a consent form. Kevorkian told them about the other person who was scheduled to die. He was also from California and also had cancer. The sisters asked if Martie could go second the next day, because they intended to stay up late talking.

Kevorkian, Nicol and Janus left to have a session with the other patient and his group. They said the two groups could meet later, but everyone ended up too tired for that. The Ruwart sisters and Martie's friends had hoped to have one last pajama party with Martie, but instead she conked out and everybody went to bed.

The next morning, Martie told her sister Mary that she had hoped she would feel good but in fact felt awful. She was sick to her stomach and afraid she was going to vomit.

"She said that maybe that was just as well, because it was pretty obvious to her and to everyone that she had run out of steam and was tired. It was time to go," Mary recalled. "She was very much at peace."

Martie's old college roommate had decided she did not want to be there at the end. She said her goodbye to Martie.

Mary's face fell with fear when Margo Janus entered their hotel room crying shortly after 10 a.m. Had something happened which would interfere with Martie's suicide?

"She said, 'Well, I just witnessed the other one and it's always hard on us. And I feel bad for your sister, too.' "

Margo led them to a house. They didn't know whose house it was and didn't ask.

The man from California had died in a back bedroom. The Ruwarts never saw him or anyone who had been with him.

Neal Nicol pulled out a sofa bed in the living room—the same bed Lois Hawes and Catherine Andreyev had died on. Martie lay down right away. She signed another consent form.

"We all hugged her and we told her we loved her and we said our last goodbyes," Mary recalled.

Kevorkian showed Martie how to pull the string with her finger to detach the clip from the tube leading to the carbon monoxide tank. He told her she could stop any time, that she didn't have to go through with it. He said there was no hurry. But Martie was in a hurry.

"She was anxious to do it, that was quite obvious," Mary said. "She was definitely ready. She had no hesitation. She was ready to go."

Kevorkian and Nicol placed a gas mask over Martie's face. It didn't fit quite right, so they cut a little bit off the bottom. They told her that if she felt any distress or hesitation to say something or to signal.

"It's hard to imagine a more supportive group," Mary recalled. "They watched out for her, made sure she was comfortable."

At about 10:50 a.m., Martha Ruwart said: "OK, guys, I'm going to do it."

Her sisters and friends drew near. She pulled the clip.

She talked to them for a little while.

"Oh, oh, oh, it's kind of hard to breathe," she said. Teresa rubbed her head a little.

Then Martie said: "I feel like I'm going to fall asleep."

Her friend Gary asked if she could still hear them talking.

Martie said: "You're kind of far away. This is probably the last time . . . "

"It was real peaceful, like she was falling asleep," Teresa recalled.

For about 30 seconds, Martie didn't breathe at all. Then she had a few spasms and spit up a little bit.

Then, eight days before her 41st birthday, Martha Ruwart died.

Her angel had taken her away.

Chapter Twenty-Eight
No Chance to Grieve

*The artist Jack Kevorkian put two childlike faces
with bright yellowish hair in the center of a
canvas. Beneath them is a ghostly blue face with
white eyes and pink teeth in an open mouth.
Above them is a huge red open mouth with
bared teeth. ❐*

Kevorkian and Neal Nicol told Mary Ruwart to dial 911. Officers and emergency medical crews quickly arrived. They checked Martie's body for vital signs, but to the relief of her sisters and friends did not try to resuscitate her.

Fieger soon arrived and handled the authorities. Mary just cried, letting go of the accumulated stress of weeks.

"I felt so responsible for everything," she said. "If it went wrong, I was going to have to do something else. I had made that commitment to Martie that I wouldn't let her suffer."

After two hours, police let everyone go. Fieger led the Ruwart sisters outside. Teresa was carrying Martie's coat and thinking about the person who had worn it just a few hours earlier when she looked up and saw a huge crowd of reporters, TV camera crews, neighbors and gawkers.

The sisters had been so preoccupied planning Martie's death that they hardly had thought about what would follow.

❐ ❐ ❐

I was not one of the reporters gathered around Neal Nicol's house. I probably would have been, had I not been on vacation from the *Free Press* that week. After all, Kevorkian was my beat.

I heard Kevorkian had helped two people from California die, but I was too busy with other things that day to keep an ear open for names and details. It wasn't until dinnertime that my sister called and told me what she had just seen on TV—that one of the Californians who died at Neal Nicol's was my first cousin Martie.

As children, Mary Ruwart and I played together a lot. Martie, a year younger than I, played mostly with my younger sister. Our families lived only a few miles apart. At their house, we liked to play a stock market game Mary had invented. At our house, our cousins liked to play "monster under the stairs."

As Martie Ruwart breathed through Jack Kevorkian's gas mask, she didn't know that I was a journalist covering the now substantial list of people who made that choice. Neither did her sisters—they weren't following my career that closely. And I, as was too often the case, was badly out of touch with my mother's family and didn't know Martie was terminally ill, much less that she was in contact with the man who was my prime assignment.

When Martie died, I already had signed a contract to write this book. Now, suddenly, with this million-to-one occurrence, the Jack Kevorkian story became of intense personal as well as professional interest.

Journalists usually are hidden behind the stories they write. But I could no longer leave myself out of this report. There was no way to avoid the first person singular.

Regardless of where the villains might be cast in this sprawling morality play, regardless of how even-handedly I would attempt to report it and write it, my cousin's choice required me to step forward and use the word *I*.

❐ ❐ ❐

As soon as Mary Ruwart walked into her home, the phone rang. It was a local TV reporter.

"Nobody tells the other side of this story," the reporter told her. "Can we send a camera crew out to talk to you?"

Mary needed a few minutes to think. Martie had left money to promote *Healing Our World*—a book which Martie's help made possible. Mary thought: "She left her savings to promote the cause of individual choice, and if I talk about her choice, I am fulfilling her wishes." She called back and agreed to the interview.

"I started talking to reporters, because she would have wanted me to do that," Mary said. "It was almost like another project we had planned together."

In the weeks and months to come, Mary would give interviews to many radio, TV and newspaper reporters. She would speak about her sister's life and death at scores of meetings.

Talking about Martie made Mary feel she was still strongly connected to her.

"It gave her death more meaning that she chose a way that gives me a forum to talk about something connected to individual rights and is helping me promote the book, which is what she wanted to do. It's like we were partners again working on the book. She did her part, now I'm doing my part.

"Martie, I'm sure, is just delighted. If she had to die of cancer this young, at least she went out in a very meaningful way that may eventually help to make other people free from suffering. She would have liked that very much."

▢ ▢ ▢

The Ruwart sisters could not tell in advance their many cousins, aunts and uncles and farflung relatives about Martie's choice. Because of a mix-up in communications, they didn't realize until too late that most relatives weren't getting the full story of her death first-hand.

Like me, most of the clan found out by seeing or hearing a news report or getting a call from another relative who had.

The sensational aspects of Martie's death cast a shadow over her friends and relations. Relatives found themselves, sometimes contrary to their own sense of values and dignity, talking more about the circumstances of her death than mourning her loss. Such is the power of the media to shape perceptions.

The absence of any service for Martie contributed to the aura of unreality about her death. Her sisters, still pressured by media requests and battles with authorities, were too exhausted to take the lead in organizing a memorial. Other relatives felt it was not their place to act.

And so an awkward silence fell over the family. When I went to my aunt's retirement party a few weeks after Martie's suicide, I heard little talk of my dead cousin.

▢ ▢ ▢

The medical examiner's office did an autopsy on Martie the day after her death. The sisters had no say in that.

"That was very upsetting," Mary Ruwart said. "We just felt violated."

The medical examiner put "pending" as the cause of death. Michael Schwartz said officials sometimes did that and might not rule for up to six months. It was "politics," he said. Officials at the examiner's office were curt when Karen Swindell, Martie's youngest sister, called. Weeks later, Dragovic ruled her death was a homicide.

Karen, who was handling arrangements for Martie's cremation, was startled when the man at the funeral home wanted to ask her questions about Kevorkian's personality.

Karen recalled thinking: "My sister just died, leave me alone."

❏ ❏ ❏

The Californian who died in the back room of Neal Nicol's house the same day Martie died was Jonathan Grenz. Grenz, 44, was a real estate agent in Costa Mesa. A year before his death, he had surgery for a fast-moving throat cancer and woke up from the operation without a voice. Then, his mother died from cancer.

Grenz's sister, a doctor who practiced in Florida, was present when he died. Fieger made a big deal of that, claiming that the deaths of Ruwart and Grenz were "different than all other cases" because the medical profession cooperated.

Grenz left a suicide note in which he expressed his grief that he was no longer able to eat, exercise or leave his house.

"I guess there's no reason to prolong any of this," he wrote. "I'm just not going to get any better and time goes by so slowly that it is unbearable.

"Life is not life anymore."

After his death, a work associate, Linda Healey, told reporters Grenz was suffering from depression because of the recent traumas and needed time to regain an appreciation of life.

"They cut his tongue out and, of course, he was shocked. He had no idea the surgery would be that drastic," Healy said. "Then his mom died. He was overwhelmed with grief. . . . They never gave him a chance to grieve over his losses.

"He was in a very depressed period of his life. It takes time to recover. But he wasn't terminal. John wasn't immobile, he wasn't helpless, he wasn't bedridden. He was still walking and driving around. He was going through a time of crisis and looking for options.

"If that option with Doctor Kevorkian wasn't available to him, he would be alive today. He didn't evaluate what John was going through."

Kevorkian dismissed Healy.

"She's not a psychiatrist," he told the *Free Press*.

Michael Schwartz acknowledged that Kevorkian never got any psychiatric reports on Grenz but made a decision to help him after seeing his medical records and talking to Grenz and his family.

"Without question, Mister Grenz was not suffering from an inability to make an informed decision," Schwartz said. "Nobody asked him to come to Michigan. He chose to do that on his own."

☐ ☐ ☐

After Martie's death, Teresa Ruwart's boss tearfully told her how she had watched her father and stepfather suffer through fatal cancers.

"I just wish that what your sister had was available to them," she told Teresa.

The *Kalamazoo Gazette* conducted a phone-in poll. Respondents overwhelmingly backed Kevorkian. But Teresa was irked by the people who said Kevorkian had no right to decide when people should die.

"Doctor Kevorkian had nothing to do with her decision," Teresa said. "Doctor Kevorkian didn't say, 'Here, Martie, it's your time, it's your turn to die, and I'm going to kill you.' He didn't do anything like that. Martie was the one who made the choice to die when she died."

If Doctor Kevorkian had not been able to help, Martie likely would have killed herself anyway, her sisters said. And if not, she probably would have been drugged into unconsciousness. She would have died without choosing the time and place. Her sisters might not have had the chance to say goodbye or be with her at the end.

"We've been real fortunate," Teresa said. "My mom died and Martie died, and with both we knew they were going to die. When you know that somebody's going to die, you can prepare ahead of time."

The way Martie died was best for her and her family, Mary said.

"It was about as good as those things could go. She had people around her, she didn't have to die alone. She was lucky. So many people don't get the opportunity."

On February 26, her sister's 41st birthday, Mary wrote the intro-duction to the Russian and Romanian translations of *Healing Our World*. She wrote this about her sister:

"One of her final requests was that her savings be used to pro-mote the principles of *Healing Our World* throughout the world. Indeed, she provided the seed money for the translation and print-ing of the book you are now holding. Please let her legacy help you and yours to uncover the path of peace and plenty that rests within these pages."

CHAPTER TWENTY-NINE
THE LORD WORKS IN STRANGE WAYS

"If I were Satan and I was helping a suffering
person end his life, would that make a difference?
Any person who does this is going to have
an image problem."
—*Jack Kevorkian (1993)* ❐

In her home across from the Hygrade plant in Livonia, Lynn Mills told me that the hot dog aroma wafting across the street bothered her only during pregnancies. She had three daughters and wanted another.

"I've been praying to God for two years now for another baby girl and he hasn't given me one," Mills said. "Sometimes the answer is no."

When I visited Mills in early March 1993 to get a fuller understanding of her role in the new uproar about Jack Kevorkian, Christmas wreaths still draped the back fence and the front porch. In frames on walls inside the cluttered house, Jesus pulled back his shirt to show his Sacred Heart, Joseph held a crown over the Christ Child, and Our Lady of Guadalupe, "Protectress of the Unborn," watched over a pile of laundry on the dinner table. Above the TV, Rush Limbaugh flashed his teeth. The radio god had scribbled "Happy Birthday, Lynn" on his publicity photo.

Since finding a piece of garbage that had raised new questions about the death of Hugh Gale, Mills had been so busy she hadn't even had time to listen to Rush. Reporters wanted profiles. TV wanted shots of her holding Kevorkian's discarded document. Radio stations wanted her to debate Geoffrey Fieger. Montel Williams wooed her, then stood her up. A *Time* magazine photographer came to take her portrait.

"They never said picture," she said. "They always said portrait."

All the publicity made a try at a state Senate seat—something she'd been mulling for a while—look promising. Name recognition was no problem now. If only she could get rid of those three-times-a-week migraines, and get her husband to agree. He had abided with the anti-abortion marches, even her short stints in jail, because he supported that cause. But his wife's recent mega-notoriety wasn't putting dinner on the table for him.

"He said, 'I suppose I should be happy for you, but I want you'—this is a real sexist remark—'tied to the stove with an apron.' I turned to my daughters and said, 'That's male oppression, darlings, recognize it when you see it.'"

Male oppression?

"I'm not a feminist, but I am a human being with a mind of my own. I just will not go along with the feminist agenda."

She said President Clinton should offer mothers who stay at home a $10,000 annual tax credit.

"I'm not saying pay me for doing housework," she said, waving a hand at the laundry. "Obviously I don't do a lot." Women who don't want a career shouldn't suffer for that choice, she explained.

"The other day I came out in a new suit and asked my husband, 'How do I look?' And he said: 'If you made eighty thousand you'd look great but you don't make anything.' He's entitled. You know, we go without a lot."

Mills's eyes looked always on the verge of overflowing—or flashing in anger. She said she cried for a week after Clinton won the election. But then she slapped some new bumper stickers on her mini-van—"Don't Blame Me, I Voted for Bush" and "If Hillary Doesn't Trust Him Why Should I?"—and started working on the 1994 elections, targeting pro-abortion Senate candidates to stop Clinton from packing the Supreme Court.

But God—or at least the national leaders of Operation Rescue—had other plans. At first, however, Lynn Mills wasn't prepared to carry the banner against Jack Kevorkian.

"God couldn't have chosen a more uneducated person. God couldn't have chosen a more unlikely person. But he chose me."

In December 1992, fellow activists Dawn Stover and Andrew Burnett of Portland, Oregon, publishers of *Life Advocate* magazine, called Mills. In 1991, a jury had imposed punitive damages of $500,000 on each of them for repeatedly blocking entrances and harassing patients at a Portland abortion clinic. Stover told a newspaper in 1990 that she had been arrested 20 to 30 times for abortion protests in the previous four years.

"They said, 'We want to do a story on Kevorkian. We want you to go out and picket him,'" Mills said. "I guess they wanted to expose him. But I just didn't feel the climate here was good."

Mills said she believed "that the whole area loved Kevorkian and that everyone was on his side. I was only gauging by what I'd heard on radio talk shows because I'd never read an article on Kevorkian. I'd turn the TV off, I'd turn the radio off. I didn't want to deal with it. I thought it was bigger than me. I thought it was nothing I could handle. And my focus was the innocent babies in the womb.

"We never mentioned Kevorkian in any of our newsletters except to say that he would be a perfect surgeon general for President Clinton. But I knew what he was doing was wrong. I felt it very deeply. Every time he killed somebody I broke down and cried."

Mills told her friends she didn't want to picket Kevorkian. She made up an excuse. It was Christmas. She was too busy. But the real reason was: "I only do things that will be really effective, and I'm not going to go out there and slaughter myself with the public and possibly do damage to the pro-life cause that I've nurtured along for 11 years."

On January 20, Mills was on the Pennsylvania Turnpike, driving to an anti-abortion rally in Washington, when the radio blared the news of Jack Miller's death—number nine for Kevorkian. Mills said she cried again. At the march, more national leaders of the movement pressured her to do something.

"I skirted the issue," Mills admitted. "But when we came home, he just kept whacking people left and right."

The day Hugh Gale died, Mills got a phone call from an old friend and anti-abortion crusader in the Detroit area.

"She called me up sobbing: 'What are we going to do?' She was just beside herself. She said she had to rush to the hospital to be by her dad's side because what message was this sending to her dad, who had more wrong with him than Hugh Gale? She had to comfort him and tell him he was a worthwhile human being and say 'Please keep on living, Dad.' "

After her friend hung up, the phone rang again. Stover and Burnett said they were coming to Detroit on February 22 to launch a rescue of Kevorkian's patients. Mills agreed to the plan.

On February 18, when Martie Ruwart and Jonathan Grenz died at Neal Nicol's house, Mills didn't turn off the TV set. She saw reports of Nicol's neighbors complaining about Kevorkian.

"I had no idea four people had died at this one location," Mills told me. "A bell went off in my head: I've got to go out there and find out if the neighbors would help us. If they'd let us know when he was going to come out again, we could possibly offer someone an alternative to carbon monoxide—hope, life, mercy, compassion, everything we believe Kevorkian wasn't offering."

February 22 was her husband's birthday. Mills drove to the airport to pick up Stover and Burnett. Coming off the plane, they waved a *USA Today* at her. Next to the headline "House at the end of life's road" were a small picture of Nicol's house and a large photo of Kevorkian. The story began:

> WATERFORD TOWNSHIP, Mich.—People call Paulsen Street here the road of death.
>
> The street, surrounded by elm and birch trees, seems like any other corner of a quiet Detroit suburb.
>
> But when Jack Kevorkian drives up to a two-story brown house here, neighbors know someone will die.
>
> Someone will put on a plastic mask, turn on the "suicide machine" and inhale carbon monoxide.
>
> Four people have done this on Paulsen Street so far.
>
> "People in the area think it's creepy," says neighbor Dawn Lyons. When Kevorkian comes in his white van, the buzz begins: "Uh-oh, it's going to happen again."

Mills drove her friends to Royal Oak to show them where Kevorkian lived. Parked behind the apartment building was the VW van that was the last stop for another visitor from Portland, Janet Adkins.

A man staggering into the pub next door yelled:

"I'm going into Mister B's and have a cool one, then I'm going to go see Jack and do it."

Over dinner at a nearby Greek restaurant, the three activists plotted tactics. Mills would talk to Nicol's neighbors. Stover and Burnett would watch Kevorkian. They were sure he would strike again soon.

Before dawn on Tuesday, Stover and Burnett were camped in a rented car outside Jack's place.

"If they saw him carrying canisters, they were going to try to take them away from him," Mills said.

Mills dropped her daughters at school and drove to Paulsen Street, using a map from a recent *Detroit News*. Mills walked up to a house that had a "Happy Birthday Jesus" sign on it. She was surprised to find the woman who lived there was pro-Kevorkian.

As she drove away from the house, she saw a man carrying a garbage bag down his driveway. She recognized his house from the *USA Today* photos. The man walked to his mailbox, took out the mail and shoved some of it into the trash bag. Then he left the bag at the curb.

Mills had a sudden epiphany.

"I had seen the garbage in the neighborhood, but it didn't even dawn on me until I saw the garage door open and Neal Nicol taking garbage out. . . . There was never any hesitation in my mind that I would take it."

God had led her to garbage before—four times, at abortion "mills." Behind a couple of clinics in Lansing, she had found 38 tiny bodies in formaldehyde. Whenever she found fetuses in the trash, Mills made sure they got buried in a Catholic cemetery.

Mills was now state director for Operation Rescue. No longer did she sift through garbage herself.

"Frankly, somebody else does it for me now," she told me.

In 1990, a Mills deputy trash-picker found a slip with the names of two women and a date. When that date arrived, Mills was outside the abortion clinic with signs bearing the women's names and pleading "DON'T KILL YOUR BABY" and "WE CAN HELP YOU." The American Civil Liberties Union, which once had defended Mills's right to picket abortion clinics, sued her, claiming she had violated the women's privacy rights. The suit still was in the court system in mid-1993.

Driving past Nicol's house, Mills tried to summon Burnett on her car phone, but failed. She was hoping he and Stover would come out and snatch the trash because, Mills said, "I didn't want to ruin my reputation with the neighborhood."

Mills went to Dawn Lyons's house and learned she also backed Kevorkian, contrary to the impression left by *USA Today*. Leaving, Mills noticed fresh tire tracks in the snow in Nicol's driveway. His car was gone. She grabbed the bag and stuck it in her van.

"I had no idea what we were going to find," Mills said. "I just knew that people had died in that house. I couldn't go into the home, but here was part of the house coming out to me.

"I just did what any good cop or reporter would have done. Maybe if more investigative journalists were digging around in garbage instead of putting bombs on GM trucks, we'd all be better off."

❏ ❏ ❏

While Mills drove home with a reeking bag of garbage, Right to Life's Ed Rivet was counting heads in Lansing. There was a move afoot for an immediate ban on assisted suicide. Kevorkian's recent spree had put the fear of God into legislators.

"Who knows how many people he could kill in the last week before March 30?" Rivet told lawmakers.

Rivet had a deal: Clean up the bill's language to give more explicit protection to hospice workers and doctors who practiced standard comfort care, and put the law into effect immediately. Rivet knew he had the votes. So did Fred Dillingham. Jack Kevorkian was about to have his lights really punched out.

❏ ❏ ❏

At dinner Tuesday at Mills's house, Stover and Burnett were tired and discouraged.

"They were up for stopping Jack that day," Mills said.

All they had gotten were photos of Kevorkian crossing the street and walking down a sidewalk. He had done nothing more sinister than go to the store.

"They said they were just being obedient to God by being here," Mills said. "They could be here for a week and nothing might happen."

After dinner, the three donned rubber gloves and went to the basement. Mills, wearing a George Bush sweatshirt, opened the bag she had found at the end of Neal Nicol's drive. Out tumbled rotten grapes, banana peels, cigarette butts, coffee filters, plastic baggies, bits of tubing, rubber gloves, scraps of paper and some mail addressed to a previous resident.

"You're not supposed to throw somebody's mail out and he did that," Mills confided in me. "I haven't even disclosed that to anybody else."

They spied a long, narrow piece of white paper.

"We saw the EKG strip with the beating heart and the heart going to a flat line, and that was like watching somebody die right there," Mills said. It might have been the record of my cousin Martie's last heartbeats.

Then Burnett found an official-looking document. At the top it said "Michigan Obitiatry - Zone 1," "Final Action" and "Confidential."

In each upper corner was a large black H. It was Kevorkian's "Document H" on the death of Hugh Gale. Cheryl Gale, Neal Nicol and Margo Janus all had signed their names at the top of the document to indicate they were present at Gale's death. At the bottom, only Jack Kevorkian's signature was under the section labeled "Procedure."

As Burnett read "Procedure" aloud, "we all kind of sat back, grabbed our hearts a little, took a deep breath and held back the tears," Mills recalled. "Or tried to hold back the tears."

The document looked as if it had been typed on an old portable with keys that needed cleaning and a carriage that produced wavy lines. It read:

> Patient placed plastic mask over nose and mouth, elastic band around head. A plastic tent was put over his head and shoulders, lid at top open. The patient then pulled a string tied to his left index finger, other end attached to a clip, which was pulled off a crimped plastic tube, opening it from the outlet valve of a canister of CO gas to the mask. In about 45 seconds the patient became flushed, agitated, breathing deeply, saying "Take it off!" The tent was removed immediately, the mask removed, and nasal oxygen started. He remained conscious and oriented, and within a minute calmed down to his normal breathing pattern. He was more relaxed and a bit somnolent, but awake and oriented. The patient wanted to continue. After about 20 minutes, with nasal oxygen continuing, the mask was replaced over his nose and mouth and he again pulled the clip off the crimped tubing. In about 30-35 seconds he again flushed, became agitated with moderate hyperpnea; and immediately after saying "Take it off!" once again, he fell into unconsciousness. The mask was then left in place. Hyperpnea continued for about 35-40 seconds, after which a slower and calmer breathing pattern ensued, lasting about 8 minutes, gradually diminishing in rate and intensity. Heartbeat was undetectable about 3 minutes after last breath.

Document H clearly was a godsend.

Mills and her cohorts took the document to a copy center and made huge blow-ups. They debated what to do next. If they took it to the Roseville police, would some desk sergeant toss it?

"I'm leery of trusting police departments who might think I'm just a wacko," Mills said. "Ultimately I decided to turn it in to a man I knew wouldn't ignore it."

Mills said she had met Richard Thompson only once—at a GOP dinner the previous summer—though she often had called his office to voice her support for his efforts to get Kevorkian.

It was late at night now, and she didn't know how to reach Thompson. There were 15 Richard Thompsons in the Oakland County phone directory. There was no answer at his office. Finally, a sheriff's department staffer put her through to an assistant prosecutor.

"She said: 'You mean you have physical evidence of a murder?' " Mills said. "That was the word for what it was. She said she would leave a message for his secretary in the morning."

Wednesday morning, Mills called Thompson's secretary.

"At first I thought, 'Oh no, she thinks I'm a nut too,' then finally she said, "Do you have a fax?' "

Burnett always traveled with a fax machine.

"So we faxed it and we just sat back thinking we were excited over nothing; the Oakland County prosecutor thinks we're nothing but a bunch of ding-dongs. Then Dick Thompson called me and said: 'This is incredible. When can you get here?'

"On the way out there Andrew and Dawn are playing it down and I'm saying, 'No, it's murder, it's murder' and so I personally felt very satisfied when Richard Thompson said possibly it was evidence of a homicide."

The three told Thompson they were going to hold a press conference Friday morning to release the document.

"We weren't playing hardball with them or anything, but this was too critical to sit on," Mills said.

Thompson told them not to tell anyone about the find. But Stover had already called several activists around the country.

Stover and Burnett returned to Royal Oak to shadow Kevorkian. That afternoon, Kevorkian told Fieger that two cars occupied by people carrying Bibles were following him.

That evening, the national director for Operation Rescue, the Reverend Patrick Mahoney, flew in from Washington D.C.

The find in the garbage, Mills told him, was providential.

"I was at the right spot at the right time. I think God led me there."

CHAPTER THIRTY
WHITE-OUT

> *Kevorkian's painting "Give Us This Day" features*
> *a nude figure squatting inside a cave. The body is*
> *like a baby's but the face that of an old man. The*
> *eyes are downcast, forlorn. Behind the man is a*
> *yellow face. Yellow forearms and hands that*
> *appear to match this face are in corners of the*
> *canvas. There is a gaping hole in the face. The*
> *squatting man is eating a dripping, yellowish*
> *mass of flesh torn off the face. Tearing away at*
> *the yellow forearm is a large gray, furry, vulture-*
> *like bird with a huge white beak.* ❐

On Thursday, February 25, the proposal to slap an immediate ban on assisted suicide reached the Senate floor. Lawmakers took turns trying to exceed their previous rhetoric. Senator John Kelly made three speeches, calling Kevorkian a "psychopath" and a "serial killer."

"He executes people and then goes on the evening news and says: 'What are you going to do about it?' "

Senator Vern Ehlers of Grand Rapids said Kevorkian had "the moral sensitivity of a moose." Senator Doug Carl of Utica observed: "Fifteen and counting, that's the number of bodies that have assumed room temperature with Doctor Kevorkian's help. This man must be stopped."

The vote was even more lopsided than the first time around. Opponents of the ban figured they had lost anyway, welcomed the clarifying language to protect doctors, and didn't mind putting Kevorkian out of business five weeks sooner. The House passed the immediate ban 92-10 and the Senate 28-6.

"In the history of the Michigan Legislature, this is the depth, the nadir of their existence," Michael Schwartz said.

Over the phone, Fieger told me he was glad he had returned from a short trip out of town. He started singing: "I'm back to let *them* know I can really put it down. *Do you love me ... ?*

"We're going to have the trial of the century," he said. "They're trying to codify the Bible. They're carrying out their precepts of religion and not the desires of the people who elected them."

Outside Kevorkian's apartment, Stover, Burnett, Mills, Mahoney and two local supporters heard the news on the radio as they kept vigil.

"We figured there was going to be a search," Mills said. "We hoped and prayed that something was going to happen. We were out there watching, listening to Rush Limbaugh."

In mid-afternoon, Gwen Voletti, a courier for Fieger, drove to pick up Kevorkian for a previously scheduled interview with *Newsweek*. When Kevorkian stepped onto the street, protesters came out of nowhere and surrounded him.

"It was like *Night of the Living Dead*," Voletti told me.

Kevorkian and the protesters started to argue. Voletti told him to get in the car.

Burnett and Stover tailed them to Fieger's office and parked in an adjacent lot. When Voletti told Fieger about the protesters, he charged out of the office and leaped over mounds of snow toward the car, yelling and waving his arms wildly.

"He charged at my vehicle with a baseball bat, running, screaming, cussing and yelling," Stover later told the press.

Other witnesses said Fieger, though menacing enough, didn't have a bat. Stover and Burnett took off.

Fieger told the media:

"If they come back I'll take the biggest bat I can find to them. Or I'll get a gun and shoot them. I'm not going to be intimidated by these religious loonies. It's a joke."

After finishing the interview with *Newsweek*, Fieger was ubiquitous on the evening news.

"This law is an outrage and it's contrary to the wishes of the people of the state of Michigan," Fieger told Rich Fisher, the Channel 2 anchor.

When Fisher asked whether Kevorkian would abide by the law, Fieger replied:

"He's indicated that any law which makes people suffer, that makes criminals of dying patients and of their family who cares because they would assist them out of this world and reject the religious dogma that says suicide is a sin, any law that makes them criminals and that criminalizes that activity is immoral."

Fieger said he was confident the law would be struck down.

"The people of the state of Michigan and a jury of Jack Kevorkian's peers don't believe that religious fanatics should have control of our lives and our deaths."

Fisher asked whether Kevorkian would assist in a suicide that night or the next day.

"I don't know," Fieger said. "He really doesn't talk to me about that."

Fisher surmised: "I have a feeling you want this issue to go to court to have it resolved once and for all."

Fieger smiled.

"Sure, I want to kick their butts."

Just after 5 p.m., TV cameras rolled at the Capitol as Governor Engler signed the bill making Jack Kevorkian's practice a felony from that moment forward.

"I think that most of the people of Michigan are uncomfortable with the power that he has assumed for himself," Engler said. "No one wants to see a loved one suffer, but Jack Kevorkian doing his thing is simply too much."

On Channel 4, anchor Mort Crim noted that "it isn't often that the governor goes on live television to sign a bill into law." Then he introduced Fieger and Kelly, the Legislature's foremost maverick cast in the unlikely role of a moderate.

Fieger threw the first punch.

"What the governor just did would have sentenced the people who ended their lives with dignity last week—Jonathan Grenz and Martha Ruwart—to a few more months of unagonizing, er, agonizing and unending pain, and he did it gleefully with applause. Believe me, the people he named are supporters of the religious organization known as Right to Life."

"Senator Kelly, are you a shill for the religious right?" Crim asked.

"Absolutely not, I've never voted with Right to Life in my entire 15 years in the Legislature before this particular bill," Kelly replied.

For three minutes, Kelly never stopped talking—about how the Legislature was trying to reach a reasoned decision on euthanasia and how *Mister* Kevorkian was out of control—and Fieger kept shouting over his words:

"Who's qualified? Name a doctor who's qualified. . . . You keep calling him Mister Kevorkian. When did you revoke his medical degree from the University of Michigan? . . . Have you ever spoken to one family member of the people Doctor Kevorkian has helped? What family member came to you and indicated they wanted Doctor Kevorkian to be criminalized? The only people who have come to you are the leaders of the religious right."

Kelly, uncowed, smirked as he got in the last word:

"It's too bad that Mister Kevorkian has a lightweight like you defending him."

A minute later, Kelly and Fieger resumed their mud-wrestling match on Channel 7 with Bill Bonds. Bonds, Detroit's highest-paid, most popular and most volatile anchor, this night seemed calm compared with Kelly and Fieger, who did little but shout at each other.

On the same newscasts, tape rolled of Richard Thompson saying that the new law wouldn't be enough to get Kevorkian convicted if other witnesses refused to talk. Thompson was using the opportunity to pitch for a favorite plum—investigative subpoena power so that prosecutors wouldn't have to impanel a grand jury to compel testimony from reluctant witnesses, as he had been forced to do in the Wantz and Miller cases.

"What a ruse," Justin Ravitz, a former Recorder's Court judge, commented to reporters. "It sounds to me like Richard Thompson is trying to exploit a frenzied situation to gain powers he will utilize in other cases that may be a danger to someone's constitutional protections."

Off the air, Thompson and Macomb County Prosecutor Carl Marlinga met behind closed doors with Oakland County Circuit Judge Richard Kuhn after court had closed for the day. They emerged with a signed search warrant.

Reporters joined the swarm outside Kevorkian's apartment. Fieger's protests about right-wing nuts stalking Kevorkian had given the Operation Rescue team some welcome publicity.

"We didn't have to lift a finger," Lynn Mills said. "The media just kept coming"—and in time for the evening newscasts.

To pique interest, Reverend Patrick Mahoney's Washington office put out a release announcing a press conference Friday morning. The release was headed "KEVORKIAN'S THIRTEENTH VICTIM HUGH GALE KILLED AFTER HE BEGS KEVORKIAN TO STOP" and claimed "Hugh Gale's death was a painful and agonizing one over an extended period of time as he cried out for Kevorkian to stop."

By 6:30 p.m., all the reporters had left. Mills told a lone remaining

TV cameraman he had an exclusive. Police from Roseville, where Hugh Gale had lived and died, were entering Kevorkian's back door in Royal Oak. At the same time, other police officers were kicking down Neal Nicol's door in Waterford Township.

Kevorkian was still at Fieger's office. Fieger was on a radio talk show.

On the street, Mahoney told Channel 7: "We are here to take a stand for human life and to expose this man for what he is, which is basically an assassin. I don't think there's another word for it."

Prosecutors Thompson and Marlinga called a press conference to drop a bombshell. Police had found a different version of Document H in Kevorkian's apartment.

This version contained a different account of what happened after the gas flowed into Hugh Gale's lungs a second time. The first nine sentences and the 13th and last sentence under "Procedure" were identical. The three sentences in between had been altered. There was now no mention of a second request by Gale to "Take it off!"

The last four sentences of the version Mills had found read:

> In about 30-35 seconds he again flushed, became agitated with moderate hyperpnea; and immediately after saying "Take it off!" once again, he fell into unconsciousness. The mask was then left in place. Hyperpnea continued for about 35-40 seconds, after which a slower and calmer breathing pattern ensued, lasting about 8 minutes, gradually diminishing in rate and intensity. Heartbeat was undetectable about 3 minutes after last breath.

The last part of the version police found was much different. I have added italics to indicate the new language:

> In about 30-35 seconds he again flushed, became agitated with moderate*ly increased rate and depth of respiration, and muscular tension without overt action (an exaggerated response seen in cases of marked loss of pulmonary reserve). Agitation abated in 10-15 secs. with unconsciousness, calmer gasping breaths for* about 8 minutes, gradually diminishing in rate and intensity. Heartbeat was undetectable about 3 minutes after last breath.

Someone had applied typewriter erasing fluid to the 37 words that no longer appeared. Traces of those words could be identified beneath the new typing. With what appeared to be the same manual typewriter, someone had typed over the new words to construct an account which made sense grammatically and fit the exact space available.

Jack Kevorkian's signature still appeared, unaltered, below the "Procedure" section. Nothing else was different on the other sections of the document. At the top, in both versions, the date was listed erroneously as "Feb. 12." (I would later learn that was the originally scheduled date for Gale's suicide.)

Marlinga said Gale's death would be investigated as a homicide. The prosecutors said it was perfectly legal for Mills to search Nicol's trash—courts had ruled garbage at the curb was not private. Thompson insisted the execution of the search warrant had not been timed to follow Engler's signing of the stop-Kevorkian law.

As Kevorkian sat sequestered in Fieger's office, Fieger called a counter-press-conference at the unusual hour of 10:30 p.m. He put Cheryl Gale before the cameras to answer his questions. He asked her if her husband had wanted to die. She said "yes." He asked if he ever changed his mind. She said "no."

On WXYT radio, Thompson and Marlinga spoke with talk-show host Ronna Romney, a Republican activist and former daughter-in-law of former GOP governor George Romney, who found national fame as a presidential contender when he said he had been "brain-washed" into supporting the Vietnam War. Ronna Romney already had reached her conclusion about the documents:

"Of course this is the danger that people have been talking about. What happens if you hook up a machine and you change your mind and they don't believe you and they just keep going? Do they know better than you when you should end your life?"

On Channel 7, Bill Bonds solemnly led off his 11 o'clock news-cast: "The prosecutors are talking homicide." After 10 minutes of breathless reports from all quarters, Bonds introduced Fieger and Marlinga.

His face aflame, his voice rising, Fieger looked ready to leap out of his chair and start punching.

Bonds tried to ask a question, but Fieger jumped right in:

"Bill, Bill, you didn't show your viewers Mrs. Gale, who just came to your studios live and told you that what the prosecutors were saying was a lie. You just made it seem to your viewers as if there's some facts in this. This is a lie. I would say to you frankly that Mister Marlinga and Mister Thompson better turn over their law licenses because this is an outrage."

Bonds looked offended.

"Mister Fieger, I was just going to say that I talked a few moments ago with both Mrs. Gale, the widow of the patient of Doctor Kevorkian, and I talked to Mister Nicol, and they both said they would take an oath and swear that he only said 'Take off the mask' once."

"Right," Fieger shot back. "Doctor Kevorkian makes a typo on a document which he corrects himself—he doesn't have to alter his own document, he's keeping them in his own house—and they're making it seem like this is Watergate. That's ridiculous. And this is all at the behest of a radical religious organization. This sounds to me like fascism in the middle of the night."

Marlinga tried to discuss the document: "As far as whether it's reliable, that's going to be subject to whether we get the handwriting authentication, whether Doctor Kevorkian or somebody else will admit to the authenticity of the document."

Fieger cut him off: "Or the other thing, Mister Marlinga, is you're going to have to show how Mister Gale, who had full use of his hands, wasn't able to take off a mask that you claim Doctor Kevorkian wouldn't take off. . . . Now how could Mister, uh, Doctor Kevorkian murder anybody with a man who put on a mask on himself and then could take it off? You just made it up!

"Instead of getting a phony document, why didn't you call my office and I would have given you every document? . . ."

Bonds tried to referee: "Geoff, if you're going to ask the prosecutor a question, let him answer it."

Fieger seemed hysterical: "It's a shame, Bill, it's a shame what happened tonight."

Bonds sounded put out: "Well, this is freedom of the press. This is a controversial issue. There are two sides to it."

"No, there aren't two sides to this."

Marlinga said: "The important thing over here is that this isn't just one typo. There are a number of lines which would be incriminating that are blanked out and changed to something else."

"Oh, so Doctor Kevorkian sat at home and wrote out a confession of how he killed people?" Fieger exploded, drenching each word with sarcasm. "Mister Marlinga, are you nuts? Are you nuts?" Fieger was shrieking now.

"We consider this a possible homicide. Certainly anybody who was there is a possible suspect..."

"Who held him down?" Fieger screamed.

"But mere presence at the scene of a crime is not necessarily a crime in itself."

"Who held him down?"

"We're going to have to determine whether he did have the use of his faculties, whether he could have taken off the mask. Certainly according to this report, if you read it, it appears that at some point he became incapable of taking it off."

"Oh, when did that happen, Mister Marlinga?"

"All I'm saying is that we have one document. It's a beginning."

"Shame on you. Shame on you."

Bonds interjected: "Are they suspects? Are they suspects?"

Fieger jumped in, shouting: *"What? One document and you went and got a search warrant and kicked in doors in the middle of the night ... You're going to run for the Senate. That shows the people of the state of Michigan what kind of man you are!"*

"Mister Fieger, Mister Fieger, his political decisions regarding the future do not seem this evening to be germane to what happened."

"Hey, listen, this is a politically elected prosecutor who without one iota of proof suggested that Jack Kevorkian when five people were present held a man down."

"Can you, Mister Marlinga, have a final statement? And then we'll get back to Mister Fieger."

Marlinga: "Yes ... the reason that the search warrant had to be executed is that we see here from these documents that there was a willingness to change the words. If there was a willingness to change the words, if there were advance notice, there is also a possibility based on that willingness that the evidence could be destroyed altogether, and we would not have had the original had we given advance notice."

Bonds: "How soon will you make your decision? Then, I'd like to have Mister Fieger..."

Fieger: "I beg you, charge him with murder tonight."

Marlinga: "... we'll have to have all of these people in to give a statement and Doctor Kevorkian of course does not have to give a statement..."

Fieger: "No, no, they're not talking to you at all. Charge him with murder!"

Marlinga: "... under the Fifth Amendment he has that right. But if he wants to, he's welcome to. If he wants to offer an explanation we'll be happy to listen to it."

Fieger: "Bill, I asked him to charge him tonight so that his political career can be effectively ended. All he had to do was call me. Why would Doctor Kevorkian throw away a document if he needed to change it? He changed it on his own document? That's ridiculous!"

Bonds: "All right, Geoffrey Fieger, thank you very much, and Prosecutor Marlinga, thank...."

Fieger: "Show the tape of Mrs. Gale!"

Bonds: "And—uh—we're in the process of editing and it's our hope that we get it on in time. This ran rather extensively and it got rather heated and we thought that this was the well, this was the heart of tonight's debate, controversy. We have to make decisions as we go and we try to be fair to each of you."

The tape of Cheryl Gale was not shown on that newscast.

Chapter Thirty–One
Much Ado About a Typo

"I might very well have been in jail without his pugnacity, his obstinance. You can't bulldoze over Fieger. Everyone knows that."
—Jack Kevorkian (1993) ❑

The next morning, Fieger was up early and all over the electronic place. He was also back in total control of himself.

Local TV reported that Fieger had challenged Marlinga: "Either arrest Doctor Kevorkian today, or shut up."

On *Today*, Fieger irritated Bryant Gumbel by interrupting and avoiding his questions. Gumbel tried to pin down Fieger: "He did not white out the words 'Take it off' from that report?"

"The original report was a mistake," Fieger said, "He only said 'Take it off' once and Mister Gale took off the mask himself—once."

Minutes later, on *Good Morning America*, Fieger appeared on a split screen with Ed Rivet of Right to Life. Joan Lunden asked a question about the documents, but Fieger started right in: "I'm surprised Mister Rivet is not wearing a hood on his head because he's a member of an organization that bombs abortion clinics."

Fieger insisted: "This is all much ado about nothing. The prosecutors are making this up and they raided his home in the middle of the night like the Kristallnacht.

"It's an outrage. Try him again if you want to. What's going on here in Michigan is the radical terrorists like Mister Rivet are hysterical, they're taking over our Legislature and they're going to impose their religion on us."

❑ ❑ ❑

I called Fieger's office and requested an interview. He told me to come right over.

Looking fit and feisty, Fieger read aloud a fax from someone who objected to his use of the Kristallnacht comparison.

Smirking, Fieger dictated a reply to his secretary:

"Dear Mr. Whoever-You-Are: I disagree, paren, as I'm sure you, comma, apparently, comma, disagree with me, paren."

Then he paused and chortled:

"Did Alice Gilbert ask you to write this letter?"

Fieger reviewed his media schedule. He was already booked for Rich Fisher and Bill Bonds that afternoon. Everybody else in radio and TV wanted him, too. It was a great day to be Jack Kevorkian's attorney. It was a great day to see your rhetoric come alive, in the flesh.

"They're nuts. They're the people I told you always were doing this," Fieger smirked. "I don't think, frankly, I could ask for a confluence of events which more appropriately underscores what I've been trying to tell everyone. I couldn't have written the script better."

Fieger said Margo Janus and Neal Nicol had prompted Kevorkian to change the document.

"He had written it, he had copied it, he had given it to everybody, and apparently they had all talked about, you know, the notes and everything, and they said, 'Wait a second, you got a mistake here,' and he said 'Yeah, there's a mistake' and he corrected his original and kept it. . . .

"I don't need to explain this. Listen, you got headlines 'Kevorkian May Be Guilty of Murder' and somewhere down in the body of the thing you got the wife of 22 years saying that's ridiculous. It seems to me this is a continuation of the bullshit.

"I'm tired of this, man, I'm serious. I don't have to make up stories for the fucking goofball loonies. OK, that's the facts of life, and if somebody thinks that suddenly Jack is killing people, that's fine."

The police and the press, Fieger screamed, had never been interested in any of the documents Kevorkian assiduously kept.

"We got 'em for every case since Susan Williams. We handed 'em out to all you guys, you didn't give a shit about 'em.

"*You guys don't even like the fucking videos. The fucking videos—go look at them! Their own words don't mean anything to you.* I remember Janet Adkins. She says 'I want to die.' Oh no, she didn't really mean she wanted to die. We can tell she was blinking her eyes in a secret SOS code."

Fieger said Kevorkian placed a plastic tent over Gale's head to hold more gas in. Gale wanted it removed because it made his face hot and he felt like he was suffocating, Fieger said. Gale's emphysema accounted for the agitation, he said.

"He has spasms of the lungs so bad they thought he was almost dying during some of the interviews," Fieger said.

But why did Kevorkian originally write "Take it off" twice?

"Because it's the same language as the—he's just repeating it. He sometimes types, talks on the phone. Don't you ever talk to Jack? He picks up the phone, he's typing, he's doing everything.

"Jack Kevorkian's the most honest man I've ever known. He's honest to a fault. He never, ever does anything dishonest."

Fieger's voice rose to righteous indignation.

"I can't get fucking anybody from your fucking paper to investigate the fact that Maida conspired with Sheehy . . . that charges were brought illegally by Thompson . . . I mean I can't get you guys to look at any of this bullshit. And you want me to dissect a fucking piece of paper that was thrown away! I ain't gonna do it anymore.

"The fact of the matter is, he's not going to be charged, OK? And if he was, I get to look like Clarence Darrow again, because the case will be dismissed immediately. So it's a win-win situation for me. And in the interim, Mister Marlinga's Senate campaign will be ruined because the people of the state of Michigan will recognize, will realize that the Right to Life lunatic fanatics are actually, really in charge. And I'll be able to say that in the press every day a thousand times. So if they want to say that, that's fine. If it was up to me I would want them to bring the charges, OK?"

Fieger then spun out his theory of the previous day's events: Thompson and Mills had conspired to time the search after the Legislature's vote. Thompson went into Kuhn's chambers after hours so there would be no public record. Thompson tipped off Mills and the press that the cops were coming to Kevorkian's door.

"The whole scene was orchestrated by Thompson," Fieger charged.

"Thompson's a sick man. I say to you on the record that Mister Thompson is mentally ill. He has what's called a Napoleon complex. I'm not kidding you. It's because he's a little guy."

While I was interviewing Fieger, the Reverend Patrick Mahoney was thundering at his press conference.

"Hugh Gale did not die with dignity. He pleaded that the mask be taken off. It was clearly a murder taking place. Mister Gale did not want to die.

"It seems Mister Fieger has taken the legal profession down the same path as Mister Kevorkian has the medical profession—to the pits of hell. He's not even an ambulance chaser, he's a hearse chaser. He's a disgrace to the profession."

Back at the *Free Press* office, I talked to medical and legal experts about the hurdles prosecutors faced. Medical experts told me that Gale's agitation fit with symptoms of oxygen deprivation. Normally, carbon monoxide would induce unconsciousness before it interfered with breathing. But Gale's emphysema left him gasping for breath before he was knocked out. His "Take it off!" could have been caused by the unexpected sensation of suffocation.

Legal experts told me that even if Gale had requested that the mask be removed and Kevorkian had ignored him, Kevorkian probably had not done anything illegal. The law doesn't compel anyone to rescue a person in peril. In fact, had Kevorkian interfered, Gale could have been left with brain damage and Kevorkian could have been held liable for that.

As I was finishing the interviews for my story, about 3 p.m., I got a call from my assignment editor. Could I help another reporter find which friends and relatives of former Kevorkian patients were having second thoughts about him? I didn't know that any were, I told him. It seems the editors, in their morning story meeting, had budgeted a 20-inch story based on the premise that Kevorkian supporters were defecting. And now it was necessary, three hours before deadline, to find someone who fit the hypothesis.

In fact, Kevorkian's supporters were holding firm—despite the media's premature conclusions, despite the headlines that blared "Suicide may be a murder."

In the end, that's the way the story was written.

Interviewed by another *Free Press* reporter about the new law on assisted suicide, Mary Ruwart commented:

"When legislators feel that they can tell people who are suffering that they must live, then they are becoming masters and the people slaves."

CHAPTER THIRTY-TWO
"JACK 15, THOMPSON 0"

"Kevorkian has polarized the issue long before it has to be polarized."
—Patrick Hill of Choice in Dying, an advocacy group for the terminally ill ❐

At 1 p.m. Saturday, February 27, Lynn Mills, Dawn Stover, Patrick Mahoney and their Right to Life cohorts arrived on Main Street in Royal Oak to march and preach and pray. They were shocked to find, in front of Kevorkian's apartment, dozens of raucous marchers holding signs:

"WE LOVE KEVORKIAN"
"DIE WITH DIGNITY"
"DOCTOR LIFE"
"I BACK JACK"

Quickly, the police worked out an arrangement: The opposing groups would alternate half-hour stints picketing beneath Kevorkian's second-story windows.

Kevorkian was not at home. His van was still parked in back, but he was staying at his sister Margo's apartment in Troy.

The pro-Kevorkian group was a motley assortment of 50 to 75 people. Several sources fed the stream: Janet Good and the Hemlock Society stalwarts, members of the fledgling organization Friends of Kevorkian, and people who came just to annoy the right-to-lifers.

Dawn Haselhuhn told me she had formed Friends of Kevorkian in December, after reading newspaper accounts of Marcella Lawrence's plea for citizens to march in support of assisted suicide.

"I decided she was talking to me," said Haselhuhn, who had met Kevorkian a year before. As a diabetic, she supported his crusades for organ harvesting and assisted suicide. "My kidneys are failing. One day I may need it. If I need it, I want it available."

When she heard on Friday about Operation Rescue's plans for a rally, Haselhuhn moved quickly. She called radio and TV stations

228 | Appointment with Doctor Death

and stayed up all night making signs. It was her idea to show up at noon and beat Right to Life to the punch.

Ignoring the rabble, Stover, wearing a fluffy white coat and white gloves, waded into the mikes on the sidewalk. Lynn Mills took up a position nearby and told news crews every last detail of her garbage haul. Each woman held a huge blowup of Document H, the disputed Hugh Gale exit paper. Some marchers taunted them:

"Isn't there enough trash in Oregon? Go home!"

"There's some garbage out back—why don't you go look in it?"

They waved Haselhuhn's signs. The sentiments were clearer than the spelling:

"IMPEACH ENGLER"
"DOCTOR K IS OK"
"HUGH GALE WAS NOT MURDERED"
"RELIGOUS FREAKS GO HOME"

They started chanting: "Jack and Geoff in '96."

Police said time was up and ushered them down the street. Mahoney, wearing a University of Michigan baseball cap, took up the pulpit in front of Kevorkian's door.

"If you believe in justice and mercy come up here," he said, scanning the crowd for supporters.

"I believe in justice and mercy," said a woman carrying a pro-Kevorkian sign. She pushed closer. Police shooed her away.

"We are here because this is the Roe-vee-Wade of assisted suicide," Mahoney said. "We will not be silent any longer. We have come from all over the country to stop Jack Kevorkian, and in the week we have been here he has not killed anyone.

"The state of Michigan took a courageous stand this week, but if the state ban is overturned by the courts, we are going to come back to Detroit and issue a call to activists all over the country to see that Jack Kevorkian will not kill again."

Mahoney introduced another minister, Joseph Slovenic of Cleveland. He said softly: "We as Christians need to offer something of hope to people who are upset and depressed, to give them an alternative to dying."

"Ever been hooked up to a machine?" someone yelled.

Mahoney said his followers would use "non-violent physical intervention" to stop Kevorkian. "We're not going to break any law."

Why, a reporter asked, had it taken them nearly three years to start this protest?

"We were self-centered and apathetic and indifferent," Mahoney said. "And we were wrong to be that way. But we're waking up now."

The group of about 20 formed a line and began marching, softly singing "Blessed be the rock of my salvation."

Peter Thomason and his 12-year-old daughter Elsa had come from Washtenaw County's Operation Rescue group.

"A lot of our efforts were focused on abortion, but we know this is going to be the next issue and we will focus on it," Peter Thomason said. "We work for the beginning of life till the end of life."

Mills courted the cameras again.

"Obviously Fieger and Kevorkian are quaking in their boots," she said. "Hugh Gale obviously asked not to die."

Mahoney spotted Mills alone with reporters and yanked on Stover's coat. "You have to stay by her," he whispered.

Stover sidled over to Mills. Mills asked me if I had ever investigated how Kevorkian fit the psychological profile of serial killers.

"He really enjoys killing, you can see that," she said.

Stover steered the conversation her way.

"The eyes of the nation are on this man," Stover said. "We came here because there was no outcry. We need to mobilize the local community and stop Kevorkian.

"The issues are the same as with abortion. There are the same people on both sides. These people"—she glanced at the ragtag opposition—"are the same people. Life taken unjustly on any end of the spectrum—it doesn't matter."

How exactly would they try to stop Kevorkian?

"To save a pre-born child you put your body between the intended victim and the person who plans to do the killing. We will do the same here. I don't think a confrontation can really be avoided."

The marchers started a new hymn: "Holy, holy, holy Lord, Heaven and Earth are filled with your glory." One wore a hat that proclaimed "Jesus Is My Lord." Some carried Bibles. A few toted signs:

"CHOOSE LIFE."
"LIFE IS GOD'S CHOICE."

In a third-floor window above the procession was a huge golden monstrance—the sacred vessel used in the Catholic Church to hold the consecrated host in processions. Kevorkian later told me the monstrance belonged to his neighbor, who collected religious art objects.

Down the street the pro-Kevorkian forces were singing a parody of the Army marching song "Sound Off": "I back Jack and so should you. If you don't they'll choose for you."

Passersby gathered in the middle of Main Street.

"Who are those people?" said a bystander to a woman friend. He was wearing a studded leather collar and had a ring through his nose. She was in whiteface and her shaved head was topped with multicolored spikes of hair.

As the Christians and the lions switched places by police decree, Kevorkian supporters chanted at their opponents: "Pray, you'll need it, your cause has been defeated."

The Friends of Dr. K brandished more signs:

"MY LIFE AND MY DEATH ARE MY BUSINESS—NOT RIGHT TO LIFE OR THE STATE'S"
"GARBAGE PICKERS GO HOME"
"RIGHT TO LIFE BELIEVES IN SLOW, PAINFUL HORRIBLE DEATH—SO DID THE SPANISH INQUISITION"
"IF YOU CHOOSE LIFE, YOU CAN CHOOSE DEATH"
"LYNN MILLS—GO HOME, GET A JOB, GET A CLUE"
"JACK 15, THOMPSON 0"

One marcher yelled, "Operation Rescue just overpopulates the planet with people we don't need."

Bumper stickers sprouted: "BACK JACK—GAS ENGLER."

Taped to the front door of 223 Main was a scrawled note signed in the name of Jack Kevorkian's landlord:

"DEAR HERD MAKING THIS A CIRCUS I WILL DO MY BIT I WILL LET YOU *ONE AT A TIME* FOR $1000 CASH TO COME IN AND TOUCH HIS DOOR & HAVE YOUR PICTURE TAKEN THAT'S *CASH* ONLY
— BILL RASMUSSEN"

Down the block, I caught Mahoney and asked about the turnout. "It's a little bit disheartening," he admitted. "Jack Kevorkian is very popular in this town. This issue divides people in the Christian churches. It's been a little bit dispiriting not to see more of an active effort locally."

Maybe, Mahoney theorized, people in Michigan were too close to the situation to see what Kevorkian meant. Maybe local people had become inured to the deaths.

What did Mahoney make of his side's successes of the week —the passage of the law, the find by Lynn Mills, the hiatus in Kevorkian's work?

"God desires to move in our lives in our situations and waits for us to react. When we were obedient to Christ and took a stand this week, look what's happened. More has happened for our cause in this one week than in the past three years."

In front of Jack's place, Franklin Dickerson of Farmington Hills lugged a verbose sign:

> Operation Rescue philosophies provide:
> ● No choice—imposing their moral principles and attempting to chill our rights
> ● No compassion for the sick
> ● Prolonging and even contributing to others' suffering and misery
> ● Adding to problems of overpopulation and burdening the world economy . . .
> ● BESIDES—THEY YELL TOO LOUD

"Operation Rescue is just picking a fight," Dickerson said. "They're the ones taking it to this level."

What would Dickerson do if Operation Rescue were to return?

"I'll be back here too," Dickerson said. "I think Kevorkian's a good man. If he tells me he doesn't want me here, then I'll leave. Otherwise I'll do the best I can to support what he's doing."

At about 2:30 p.m., Dawn Haselhuhn scaled a concrete sidewalk planter and shouted hoarsely to her forces:

"We won!"

CHAPTER THIRTY–THREE
THE CIRCUS

"These are knee-jerk reactions by unthinking people. The Michigan Legislature is like a bunch of retarded children lashing out in spite. Hemlock should disband too—they're an obstacle for doctors."
—Jack Kevorkian (1993)❐

Kevorkian was in an upbeat mood when I called him March 2. Things finally had cooled down and he was back home after hiding out for five days with his sister and with Fieger.

"Now it's time to relax a bit, weather the storm and see what happens," Kevorkian said.

He said he'd watched TV reports on the demonstrations.

"What a circus! It was a big circus. Who would have thought that would have happened out in front of my apartment?"

Kevorkian said the events of the last week had made him more of a celebrity.

"People are stopping me on the street now, shaking my hand. What they did, those people, was galvanize the public."

Did he fear a return of the protesters?

"The lunatics are irrelevant. They've shot themselves in the foot, if not the belly. The opposition to them is so crystallized now and they are in such a minority. This is counter-productive for them. They just scream names at everybody.

"They have a divine mission all right: It's frightening other citizens."

Assisted suicide was not comparable to abortion, Kevorkian insisted: "We're talking about sick, mentally competent adults. The fetus is not sick, not mentally competent, and it's unclear whether it's even a person."

Asked about Fieger's TV performances, Kevorkian stirred.

"Only he can get away with that. He's got that natural talent. If anybody else spoke like that, it would offend people. When he screamed at Marlinga 'Are you nuts?' I thought that was the best approach."

Kevorkian said he also enjoyed how Fieger reacted to the people who had been stalking him:

"He said 'I'm going to take a bat and smash you like a melon.' I love that."

We got talking obliquely about the Gale case; Kevorkian refused to answer direct questions. I told him what legal experts had said about the difficulty of conviction.

"Both Thompson and Marlinga know that technically and legally there's no obligation to intervene in a suicide," Kevorkian said.

Then I told Kevorkian what Fieger had said about his honesty.

"That's true," Kevorkian said. "If there was a situation where I had to lie, I would squirm and squirm, if it was a lie on which life or death depends."

CHAPTER THIRTY-FOUR
THE DOWNFALL OF THE NAZIS

A crowd gathers beneath a man on a window ledge. A voice in the crowd yells: "JUMP." One cop tells another: "Get Kevorkian outta here."
—*Editorial cartoonist Chip Bok in the* Akron Beacon-Journal ❐

A week after Lynn Mills fished Document H out of Neal Nicol's trash, a reporter dredged up something embarrassing from Mills's past.

At 16, Mills had downed a bottle of sleeping pills in a rest room at a mall, the *Detroit News* revealed. A store co-worker found her, and a pharmacist gave her an antidote.

"I didn't offer that to the media," Mills told me. She said a reporter found out about it from her fellow activist Andrew Burnett. "I guess it coming out is OK, but I'm not happy with it. I feel like a woman who aborted admitting I aborted a child.

"It plays into the story well. I wish it didn't. I wish nobody knew about it."

Mills said she would not discuss why she attempted to end her life.

"There are a lot of teenagers out there who attempt suicide. I am not alone. I'm just very glad Jack Kevorkian wasn't there.

"I understand how people feel when they do it and then they change their minds and then somebody gives them hope to be a worthwhile person. If I had done it, I wouldn't have my children. My husband wouldn't be blessed with a wonderful wife. I'm sure he's glad I wasn't successful."

Her own past, Mills said, made her determined to offer an alternative to people who might seek out Kevorkian. But exactly what that might be, Mills wasn't sure: "Maybe it's just getting them to a proper hospice."

What if their pain couldn't be managed?

"I don't think we should make laws for a few hard cases. I don't know enough about it. If your doctor can't control your pain, are you going to just turn everything over to him and let him kill you? We shouldn't give the medical profession a new industry. Are we going to have abortion mills and suicide mills side by side?"

The document she found, Mills said, "shows that you can't control assisted suicide. Kevorkian violated his own code of ethics. He says that if anybody shows any ambivalence towards the medicide process, he will no longer be eligible to continue. Right there when Hugh Gale said 'Take it off!' that should have been the end of it.

"People change their minds every day. Ask any hospital how many people have slashed their wrists. Should we take those people and let them bleed to death?

"We think all life is precious. We can't be the judge and jury of who is to live and who is to die. I'm a pro-life activist dealing with the babies, the children who are innocent. They are helpless, but on the other hand these people are hopeless who deal with Jack Kevorkian."

But what would she do if her migraine headaches were constant?

"Survive the best I can. That's what I do now. I wouldn't go see Jack."

Mills said she didn't intend to go searching through refuse again in the Kevorkian cause.

"I think they all bought shredders," she laughed. "I don't know that there's anything I can glean from the garbage anymore."

She said she didn't mind her reputation as a trash-picker.

"I have a tough skin. . . . People go out and garbage-pick all the time. I would be guilty of a crime in aiding and abetting a homicide if I hadn't turned it in. I did my duty and I'm not going to apologize for it."

Mills believed the document was a sign of Kevorkian's false pride.

"Why is Kevorkian writing things like that down? What was the downfall of the Nazis? The paper trail they left. What was Nixon's downfall? He taped every phone call. Kevorkian has no legacy to leave, he's got no children, no wife, no family. His legacy and his ego is what he's doing here and how he feels he's changing history. And his stupidity of wanting a legacy is going to be his downfall."

The day after I interviewed Mills, I phoned Kevorkian again.

I told him that Lynn Mills didn't believe that he would starve himself in jail, as he had threatened to do.

"It doesn't really matter what she thinks," Kevorkian said. "I don't think she thinks at all. Most of the critics don't know anything about what I do. They're just spouting their emotions."

Kevorkian said he would be vindicated eventually—but probably too late for him to appreciate it.

"Luckily I'm not going to be around to read all these histories," he said. I told him I hoped he would be around to read my book.

"I don't know," he said. "I'm kind of old. I'm the oldest guy in the whole scenario."

I couldn't tell from his voice whether he was serious or kidding.

"So what?" I asked.

"That means you're closer to croaking," replied Doctor Death.

IV

DEPRESSION

"I'm not off my rocker. I am different. But so was Freud.
They're saying the same about me word for word."
                                        —Jack Kevorkian (1990)

CHAPTER THIRTY-FIVE
SHADOWS AND LIGHT

*"Penumbra: 1. a shadow cast (as in an eclipse)
where the light is partly but not wholly cut off by
the intervening body: a space of partial
illumination between the perfect shadow on all
sides and the full light."*
—Webster's Third New International
Dictionary ❐

In the days that followed the revelations about Hugh Gale's death, TV viewers became very familiar with excerpts from a videotape of Kevorkian's February 11 counseling session with Hugh Gale. One clip showed Kevorkian saying: "Now remember, relax and enjoy the time you have left, because that's important. Every minute you can enjoy, enjoy."

Gale replies, in a voice gasping for air: "There's not much joy in life."

"I know that," Kevorkian says.

In another clip, Gale says: "Can't we make this the final session? Because I want to take my life, you know that."

The clips—and the answers Cheryl Gale gave at Fieger's press conference—were Fieger's best evidence that Hugh Gale desperately wanted to end his life. Weren't his own words and his widow more believable than some piece of trash?

The ball was in Carl Marlinga's court. But unlike Richard Thompson, a staunch Right to Life supporter, Marlinga was a moderate Democrat who favored legalizing assisted suicide. Marlinga couldn't dismiss the case, but he also couldn't prove Kevorkian had murdered Gale without corroborating testimony from those at his death. Fieger, who represented everyone at the scene, wouldn't let them talk.

Without their testimony, all Marlinga had were two pieces of paper. Yet those documents, in their deep ambiguity, became talismans for the opposing camps Kevorkian's bold crusade had helped to create. And they illustrated how the unemployed pathologist, in the autumn of his star-crossed and lackluster career, had become a celebrity of the first rank—a person whose every word and action could be closely scrutinized and contrarily interpreted.

To critics of Kevorkian, the changes in Document H were incontrovertible evidence that Gale had changed his mind and Kevorkian had murdered him. That fit into their preconception that Kevorkian, like a Svengali with an IV, seduced patients into dying. The documents were like the Holy Grail for those who argued that legalizing assisted suicide would grease the Slippery Slope into enlightened barbarism.

To the other side, the changes were immaterial and the documents proof that a massive conspiracy of religious "fanatics" and their political lackeys was working against freedom of choice.

Fieger never disputed the authenticity of the documents.

He characterized the changes as a "typo" and explained them either as the perfectionism of a stickler for detail or the immaterial slip of an absent-minded doctor. By Fieger's account, Kevorkian had typed the original on his old $2 manual typewriter. He made copies and gave them to Janus and Nicol. They pointed out the "mistake." Kevorkian then took the original, whited out 37 words and, in a clever word game, concocted a new version that fit the space available and tracked grammatically.

In the age of word processors, which erase mistakes and hide duplicity, the documents were almost charmingly quaint. But they were also opaque, concealing important facts.

What had caused Gale to flush and become agitated—not once, but twice? Claustrophobia caused by the mask? Heat caused by the tent? An emphysema attack? A reaction to the gas? Panic? Ambivalence? A change of heart?

How soon after his second agitation did he fall unconscious? Was his second agitation itself a request for help? Could he have been revived, or was it too late?

In a split-second, perhaps, Jack Kevorkian might have been confronted with a devil of a dilemma, might have come face to face with the opened Pandora's box full of the ambivalence and ambiguity that surrounds the edge of death. And he might have chosen to leave well enough alone.

Or he might just have made a typo.

□ □ □

On March 1, the American Civil Liberties Union filed a lawsuit challenging the state's ban on assisted suicide.

"As much as the public is transfixed on Doctor Kevorkian," said state ACLU director Howard Simon, "the issue is about the delivery of medical care to terminally ill patients and the effort on the part of our state legislators to force suffering people to endure pain and suffering beyond what they want to."

The ACLU, representing two cancer patients, Ken Shapiro and Teresa Hobbins, and seven health care professionals, claimed the law infringed on constitutional protections to privacy and violated technical state lawmaking procedures.

One of the plaintiffs, oncologist Dr. Ken Tucker, said: "There are occasionally patients I see who want to get it over with. A physician should be able to help them make this decision."

Writing in the *Free Press*, Elizabeth Gleicher, an ACLU-affiliated attorney handling the case, argued:

"Government's obligation in this matter is not to coerce us to preserve life at all costs; it is to respect the dignity, privacy and personal freedom of competent adults."

Shapiro said the new law would bring the government into the doctor's office: "It'll be a doctor-prosecutor-patient relationship."

In a later interview, Shapiro, 50, told me he had been living with cancer since his mid-30s. On several occasions, he was told he had mere months to live. Once, he planned his own funeral. Each time, he beat the odds, to the astonishment of all the experts. But, he said, "the odds are overwhelming that eventually I will die of this disease. It's really just a question of when.

"It's such a fear to know that it's possible that I could wind up as a vegetable and in incredible pain so I could die the way society says I have to.

"If we are going to die anyway, why can't we die in a compassionate, dignified manner? If I am terminally ill and I want to preserve a legacy for my family, I don't see why I should be forced to go bankrupt in order to make Right to Life happy.

"Do we have to let ourselves be drugged into oblivion and sit there as a non-functioning human being just to die a politically correct death?"

To the surprise of many, Fieger announced that Kevorkian would not assist in any more suicides until a judge ruled on the ACLU's request for an injunction.

❏ ❏ ❏

Cheryl Gale couldn't stand being muzzled for long. On March 2, readers of the *Detroit News* found her story on the front page. Gale, defying Fieger's orders to stay silent, had unburdened herself to freelance writer Harry Cook.

(Cook, an Episcopal priest and former *Free Press* assistant city editor, in January had written a column for that paper headlined, "Kevorkian's way is better than unmitigated suffering." That opus might have helped squeeze him out of his regular spot on the *Free Press* op-ed page. Cook one day found a note in his mailbox saying his column had been canceled. After hearing from Cheryl Gale, Cook offered to give his dramatic exclusive to the *Free Press* in exchange for getting his column back. *Free Press* editors refused, and Cook went down the street to the longtime rival *News*, which since 1989 has been joined at the wallet to the *Free Press* in a joint operating agreement.)

Gale told Cook it was ridiculous to suppose that her husband was forced to die against his wishes.

"As if I had sat there and let Doctor Kevorkian murder my husband," she said.

Gale said her husband did say "Take it off" twice—but in the same breath. It was just another of his emphysema seizures, when he would gasp for air and panic. She said "Take it off" referred to the tent, not the mask. She said the tent's purpose was to keep the carbon monoxide from escaping into the room.

Gale said Kevorkian told her husband: "I know it was very uncomfortable for you. Let's just stop. I can come back another day if you still want this." Hugh said: "Let's get on with it."

The second time, Cheryl Gale said, the tent was not used. The Gales held hands. Hugh pulled the clip. Again his face flushed and he went unconscious. She insisted: "It was very, very peaceful."

The widow said Kevorkian tried to come up with reasons for her husband to go on living: "Doctor Kevorkian really made Mister Gale talk him into it."

Gale said Marlinga had made the investigation into "a three-ring circus" and owed her an apology. She said recent days had been a nightmare: "My life has been terrifying—having my door banged on at all hours of the day and night, Geoffrey Fieger ordering me not to say anything to anybody.

"I am afraid of the religious fanatics. 'In the name of God,' they say. It does something to my insides when I hear people say it that way.

"I'm afraid to leave my own home."

Gale said she was worried that people might doubt her morality.

"So I decided to tell everything I know," she explained. "Fieger said anything I said could be used against me. But I don't understand how telling the truth can be used against you."

Marlinga said he needed witnesses to shed light on the Gale case "and I do not intend to gather that information by cutting newspaper clippings or gathering videotape from television stations." So Marlinga decided to compel testimony by empaneling a coroner's inquest, a rarely used investigative technique.

California was out to get Kevorkian, too. On March 3, *San Francisco Chronicle* columnist Debra J. Saunders compared him to Frankenstein—a comparison that Kevorkian said he welcomed.

"The fictional death doc also treated corpses and near-corpses as if they were old heaps in a body-parts junkyard," Saunders wrote. "It's no wonder that others in the physician-assisted death movement can't run fast enough from Kevorkian. The death doc's forthright embrace of body-parts harvesting and auctions show [sic] the euthanasia movement for what it very easily could turn into—a cold-blooded death machine that finds expanding reasons and social benefits in suicide."

Authorities in California were trying to take away Kevorkian's license to practice medicine there. In a complaint filed February 23, Dixon Arnett, executive director of the state medical board, wrote: "Doctor Kevorkian is NOT an 'angel of mercy' as he would have you believe. Dying in the back of a Volkswagen van with your blood splattered all over because 'the angel' could not find a vein in which to insert a needle can hardly be characterized as 'Death with Dignity.' "

In an interview with the Associated Press, Kevorkian called the actions "nice Gestapo tactics." California medical officials, he said, were "worse than Nazis. At least the Nazis were honest about what they were doing. These guys are trying to do it under the guise of democracy. These guys are dishonest and corrupt."

Replying to Kevorkian's criticism, Arnett offered: "In my opinion the guy's from the dark side."

□ □ □

Early in March, families and friends of Kevorkian's patients held a reunion at a restaurant in Southfield. They told reporters that Doctor Death was really a warm and compassionate man who acted only at the request of their loved ones.

"Doctor Kevorkian was always caring and gentle" with Sherry Miller, Sharon Welsh said. "That's more than she got from a lot of other people."

Doreen Ackner said her sister Elaine Goldbaum told her that Kevorkian was "doing her a mitzvah"—an act of charity.

"He gave her back the dignity her disease destroyed," Ackner said. "She got control of her life and death, and nobody can take that away."

Sue Williams's sister Nancy Vervaras, who had requested that Sue die on a Friday, told critics to back off: "If Sue was here today, she'd tell them off. I get so mad when I hear these people say they've given up. They haven't given up. People don't give up.

"There's a time to die. I'm going to die one day. You're going to die."

Kevorkian told the group to confront critics with one question:

"Ask them: If they care so much about suffering people, when's the last time they went down to the inner city and brought an impoverished family out to their house for dinner?"

□ □ □

On March 9, the *Daily Tribune* of Royal Oak reported that Kevorkian had sued the City of Clawson to get back from police the tank, regulator, mask and tubing used in Sue Williams's death.

City Attorney Jon Kingsepp said he couldn't understand why Kevorkian wanted the stuff back.

"Maybe it's for sentimental reasons," he quipped.

Even Miss America was against Jack Kevorkian.

On March 11, prominent Catholics—including 1989's Michigan-born Miss America, Kaye Lani Ray Rafko-Wilson—attended a fundraiser in the Detroit suburb of Novi for the Catholic Campaign of America, an organization which had its sights trained on assisted suicide, among other things.

"I totally disagree with euthanasia," said the beauty queen and nurse. "I think we're all given this wonderful gift and I don't believe that one person should help another to be able to end their life."

Also attending were Tom Monaghan, the Domino's Pizza owner who was active in right-wing Catholic circles; Rusty Hills, Governor Engler's prime spokesman, and Mary Ellen Bork, wife of the rejected Reagan Supreme Court nominee.

Thomas Wykes, executive director of the Catholic Campaign of America, said the purpose of the meeting was "to send a clear signal at this point that the Catholics in Michigan and across the country believe that life is worth living. We have to start looking at people as more than just disposable entities."

Lynn Mills showed up for dinner but was given the cold shoulder as a rabble-rouser when she started passing out copies of Document H.

Fieger commented on the gathering: "We need more of these people around us like we need a hole in our heads. These people are religious terrorists."

◻ ◻ ◻

The day after TV's Public Broadcasting System carried a two-hour special on euthanasia in the Netherlands, I called Kevorkian for a review. He told me the forum in Boston that was part of the show was "much too formal, too nicey-nicey. The discussion was bland, tired. . . . There were just these Ph.Ds, these ethicists, and the MDs. Of course they all were against it. Ron Adkins spoke from the audience and he made sense, but that didn't matter to them.

"A priest got up and said life was a gift. That was an astounding revelation! If life is a gift, then why doesn't he go out and give that gift? Why doesn't he go out and create babies if life is a gift?"

Chapter Thirty-Six
Media Savvy

"All the pressure and the attention, it's like a gnat buzzing around you. None of it bothers you, but it buzzes, and it won't go away."
—Jack Kevorkian (1993) ❐

Doctor Death's dilemma was attracting attention worldwide.

There was *Newsweek*, quoting the most famous resident of Royal Oak:

"I make patients suffer. But they do it for me because they trust me and they know the option is there. They know they're not going to die in extreme agony. I keep them going as long as possible.

"It's a strange phenomenon. Not one of them fears death, not one. I've had all kinds of religions, and not one wanted a religious consultation. Religion is totally irrelevant to what they want."

And, Kevorkian admitted, death scenes moved him:

"It's tough on me. You've got to steel yourself. Every doctor does. If a doctor didn't do that, he couldn't function. Medicine is a real tragic profession in most cases. You steel yourself and you cannot empathize too much, although I do. Several times tears have come into my eyes. These are not happy moments. The ending of a human life can never be a good moment."

Asked whether the prospect of going to jail scared him, Kevorkian replied:

"Well, I've been there twice and I wasn't frightened. When you walk down the aisle with holding cells on each side, and someone spots you and then there's suddenly an uproar of cheers, and hands come through the bars to shake your hand, would you worry? That happened both times."

There was *20/20*. On March 12, newspapers across the country ran photos of Kevorkian and Barbara Walters. The famous TV interviewer was wearing a face mask attached to a tube and canister. She was holding a clip and a string in her right hand. *Newsweek* quipped in a caption: "Yes, but she never inhaled."

Kevorkian's appearance with Walters on *20/20* marked the apex of his rehabilitation. Both Kevorkian and Fieger were calm and reasoned. Kevorkian took pains to fend off his image as an eccentric, saying he was just a regular guy who chewed on a cigar while playing cards.

"Just ask my poker buddies," he said.

Kevorkian vowed to defy the law soon and to stop eating if sent to jail: "In effect, the state will assist my suicide."

The acclaimed news show never balanced the interview with as much as one quote from a Kevorkian opponent.

A few days after the show aired, Kevorkian told me that it was "a little more objective and honest than most."

But there was one inaccuracy, one of Kevorkian's poker companions told me: He didn't just chew on cigars, he smoked them. And he drank warm Squirt at the card table.

Actually, Dave Kovl had only played cards twice with Doctor Death. Kovl sent me pictures he had taken of Doctor Death being a regular guy in another regular guy's basement. Kovl said Kevorkian cracked regular guy jokes with an extra wry twist.

Once, when the dealer announced the game as "low card buried," Kevorkian flicked his cigar and deadpanned:

"I'm a pathologist. I like things buried."

George Adams, the *Health Care Weekly Review* publisher who kept in touch with Kevorkian, played cards with Doctor Death on occasion, too. Adams said Kevorkian kept a good poker face and loved to recite off-color jokes and limericks.

Having lunch with Kevorkian was becoming an event, Adams told me. People would constantly come up and shake his hand and say, "God bless you" and "Keep up the good work."

Fame hadn't changed Kevorkian's strange eating habits, Adams said. Doctor Death would eat only very bland, overcooked foods. When ordering a hamburger, he would always instruct: "Burn it."

There was also Simon Kinnersley, a reporter for the London *Daily Mirror* who came to Detroit in March to do that popular paper's first feature story on Kevorkian.

Kinnersley found out I was the *Free Press*'s Kevorkian expert and rang me up. He said he had spoken briefly with Kevorkian on the phone but was making no headway toward a sit-down interview. Could I help?

Unfortunately I couldn't. I was having the same problem.

For many months my relationship with Doctor Death had been

something of a cat-and-mouse affair. I would call him on the phone, ask him a few questions, and we would chat. Usually he would say something noteworthy or provocative. I would take notes. Sooner or later, he would tell me Fieger had forbidden him to give interviews. I would persist in the conversation, and often he would continue.

My cousin's death afforded me—for a time—even firmer common ground. Our conversations got friendlier and looser. Early in March, Kevorkian confided to me that he liked most of the Kevorkian jokes that were a staple of Jay Leno and David Letterman. In fact, Kevorkian said, he had written a limerick for Leno about a year earlier. He had trouble remembering exactly how it started, but it went something like this:

> A new machine I've been trying / to devise could be used for applying / to comics like Jay / when the eggs that they lay/ in their monologues bomb / and they're dying

Our phone relationship started to change after I detached myself from daily reporting and took a leave for full-time book writing. Kevorkian would throw up Fieger's red flag earlier and earlier in our conversations.

Finally, on March 16, Kevorkian abruptly ended a call by declaring: "I can't talk about my work, because you're making notes of everything I say. I know that. And I'm not supposed to give interviews. You're weasling things out of me. If I seem curt, it's because I have to be. I can't give interviews without Fieger's permission."

And Fieger, busy with a high-profile murder trial, wasn't returning my phone calls, though he continued to dole out Kevorkian to the likes of *Newsweek*, *Time*, *20/20* and the *New York Times*.

So all I could tell the British journalist was good luck. Kinnersley arranged an interview with a family member of one of Kevorkian's patients. The night before he flew in to Detroit, Kinnersley phoned and asked if there was anyone else I thought he should visit. I suggested Richard Thompson.

"The prosecutor? Oh, right. That would make for a bit of a balance, wouldn't it?" And he congratulated me on a good idea.

Kinnersley stopped by my house after he flew in from the airport and interviewed me about Kevorkian.

"What kind of a doctor is he?" he asked. I told him he was a pathologist.

A day later, after talking to Thompson, Kinnersley told me he felt much more "torn between the two." Thompson's arguments were well-made, he said, adding: "I didn't realize that Kevorkian never practiced with live patients, only dead tissues."

The British reporter said he felt sorry for Thompson.

"He's sort of frying, isn't he, on this? He doesn't get much chance to get his message across. The other side is pulling the heartstrings. And he says it's wrong and comes off looking like the bad guy.

"Where do you draw the line? Where's the beginning and the end of this sort of thing? Do you include people with disabilities or who are just depressed?

"A lot of these are middle-aged women. They might just happen to be going through some sort of mid-life crisis."

Kinnersley said the home office wasn't sure quite what to make of this Doctor Death chap—and neither, frankly, was he.

"I talked to my editor this morning and she said: 'Well, what kind of a line are we going to take on this?' And I said 'I really think we should have to play it right down the middle and let the reader make up his own mind.' I mean, is he a licensed mass murderer or truly an angel of mercy? One person says one thing and another says the other."

Despite *Newsweek*, *20/20*, the *Daily Mirror*, *USA Today* and all the other national and international media outlets scurrying to get a fix on Doctor Death, Random House was not.

While the quick-hit media of television and daily print journalism were hot for Doctor Death, New York book publishers didn't get it. The *Chicago Tribune* reported, in a Sunday feature titled "Tale of the Terminator," that a noted author-physician commissioned by Fieger to write a book about Kevorkian couldn't get the time of day from the big publishing houses.

Dr. Harold Klawans, author of nine popular books and a foremost maverick neurologist, had penned a provocative book proposal, reported the *Trib*. More than 30 publishers had passed on it.

Klawans and Fieger had become friends after Klawans had testified as an expert witness in Fieger's tardive dyskinesia case in 1980. Klawans and Fieger were going to split the book royalties. Kevorkian would get nothing because he wasn't interested in making money.

Kevorkian never saw the book proposal. But the man who was the object of more media attention than any doctor since Livingstone had no trouble figuring out why it was rejected:

"It's a conspiracy! The authorities that run our society don't like this idea. They will do anything to thwart it. All editors are against it. Owners of newspapers and publishing houses are against it. All the hacks that run the AMA are against it."

Even Miss America was against it.

Chapter Thirty-Seven
The Line Goes Dead

"Penumbra: 2. the shaded region surrounding the dark central portion of a sunspot."
—Webster's Third New International Dictionary ❑

The first coroner's inquest in Macomb County since the late 1950s looked like it would be a battle royal between Kevorkian's feisty attorneys and a new foe, Macomb County Prosecutor Carl Marlinga.

"This is nothing more than an attempt to save Marlinga's political career," Fieger scoffed. And Michael Schwartz said it really didn't matter how many times Hugh Gale had said "Take it off!"

"There is no criminal penalty for not stopping someone in the middle of a suicide," Schwartz said.

Marlinga disagreed, saying "the law imposes a duty to save a drowning man if you pushed him in."

On March 22, Kevorkian, Neal Nicol, Margo Janus and Cheryl Gale sat on folding chairs in Judge Mark Switalski's tiny 39th District courtroom in Roseville.

Asked to testify, Kevorkian told the court: "I refuse to answer because it's shameful for a blameless citizen to submit to an inquisition deceitfully called an inquest."

Asked if he was taking the Fifth Amendment to avoid self-incrimination, Kevorkian bristled: "I will not use the word 'incriminate.' There's no way I can incriminate myself if I've done nothing illegal."

Nicol, Janus and Gale also refused to testify. Instead, the four listened as Roseville cops told what they found at the death scene. They watched a videotape of Gale taken after his death. They heard county medical examiner Werner Spitz say that Gale's lungs were coal-black from tobacco and his blood full of carbon monoxide.

Shortly after lunch, Fieger and Marlinga approached the bench. Switalski then abruptly announced the inquest was over.

Holding separate press conferences outside the courthouse, Fieger and Marlinga explained they had reached an agreement: Nicol and Gale would give depositions to Marlinga in exchange for immunity.

251

Marlinga reserved the right to take further action.

Marlinga said the deal was the same one he had offered Fieger weeks ago. Fieger said Marlinga had made concessions.

Marlinga said the ice was broken by chance two nights earlier. Marlinga was eating at the Gallery Restaurant, a half a block away from Fieger's office, when Fieger, Gale, Kevorkian and Janus entered. Marlinga said he apologized to Gale and, he thought, thereby broke the image that he was "a monster."

Fieger told the press that he had filed a $10-million lawsuit alleging that Richard Thompson, Lynn Mills, Patrick Mahoney, Andrew Burnett, Operation Rescue and various other groups had conspired to defame, humiliate and inflict emotional distress on Cheryl Gale.

The complaint alleged that the defendants implied "that Plaintiff either assisted, consented and/or acquiesced in the murder of her husband." It charged that Thompson "made mindless and gratuitous public statements concerning the death of Hugh Gale, including claims that Mr. Gale had been murdered and that Jack Kevorkian, MD, was 'Jeffrey Dahmer in a lab coat.' " Fieger said Thompson "made false statements to a circuit judge in order to obtain a search warrant" and falsely told Marlinga "that the piece of garbage had been found by a 'neighbor' of Neal Nicol's."

Thompson discounted the lawsuit: "Mister Fieger has really confused the playhouse with the courthouse. It's based purely on theatrics and fiction."

Mills, saying Fieger was acting liked a spoiled child, called the lawsuit "more Geoffrey hysterics." She pointed out that she was an unemployed housewife and added: "I don't know what they could take. Can you get water out of a stone?"

To increase her liquidity, Mills sent a fundraising letter to about 2,600 Right to Life supporters describing her battle with Kevorkian as "spiritual warfare" and pitching for donations so she could get photocopy and fax machines for her home office and a video camera to help in her surveillance of Doctor Death.

Andrew Burnett soon was back in front of Kevorkian's apartment, along with others. Mills told me they were "praying for Jack. Jack hasn't killed in—gosh—quite a long time, so maybe they thought he was going to kill again."

Fieger wanted the activists charged under the state's new "stalker" law: "It's harassment, it's terrorism, how else can you describe it? Everywhere he looks, they're there."

Outlawed, stalked and muzzled, Jack Kevorkian began to seem both ephemeral and ubiquitous—like Elvis.

"Sightings" were big news. One day, longtime *Free Press* tidbits columnist Bob Talbert reported: "I almost killed Doctor Death Monday afternoon." Talbert said he was driving down Main Street in Royal Oak, listening to news about the Marlinga inquest on the radio, when "as if by magic, Doctor Jack comes bounding off the sidewalk, running across Main headed onto the left front of my car. We both stopped at the same time, inches apart. He was standing at my open driver's side window.

" 'Doctor Jack! It's Bob Talbert,' I yelled.

" 'Bob Talbert! Bob!' he replied.

"We shake hands. He grins and then bounds off across Main."

The grinning, bounding denizen of 223 Main had international notoriety—name recognition in the same doctoral class as Timothy Leary and Benjamin Spock, the *Detroit News* concluded.

There was even a rock and roll song about him, by a Monterey, California, band named Tragic Humor. Against a thick dirge of electric guitars, the chorus begged: "Doctor Kevorkian/ Please, doctor, do me in/ Doctor Kevorkian/ Put an end to my suffering." The composer, Gerald Swisher, wrote Fieger a letter seeking publicity for the song. Fieger didn't exactly twist and shout at the request, and the *Billboard* charts had to get along without "Doctor Kevorkian."

The subject of all this attention still lived in his sparse walkup. Aside from royalties for *Prescription: Medicide*, which sold only a few thousand copies, Kevorkian had not made any money from his tremendous fame. He didn't charge patients for his services—and had to pay several hundred dollars each time he purchased the carbon monoxide, gas mask, tubing and other devices which routinely were confiscated by police. Donations did come in the mail; he said he put them into a special fund for the eventual expansion of obiatry.

"I don't care for fancy stuff," Kevorkian told a reporter. "I don't like fancy food, fancy cars. They don't mean much to me."

Kevorkian was not interested in fortune, and even fame was becoming a burden. No longer could he walk to the local library without risking harassment. And Fieger kept him on a short leash. Fieger made him back out of plans to speak at the American College of Forensic Psychiatry national convention in New Mexico in April 1993, even though 200 delegates were expecting him. Fieger said with "all these people out stalking him . . . the security problems are just too great." And so the pathologist who had long sought and failed to get professional recognition for his ideas now had to refuse a chance for that recognition because he was too famous.

As for assisting in suicide, Fieger had promised that Kevorkian would hold off until a ruling on the ACLU suit. But the ACLU took its time in filing briefs, and a preliminary ruling was a long way off.

As March ended, Janet Good confirmed another of Kevorkian's problems. As my cousins had told me, his carbon monoxide suppliers had been scared away. Good described her friend as "frustrated."

"He's working on something," she said cryptically.

On April Fools Day, I called the familiar number in Royal Oak and was astonished to find that Jack Kevorkian had an answering machine. Finally, Kevorkian was screening calls. And he wouldn't return mine.

Even more mysterious were his two assistants. Margo Janus and Neal Nicol did not respond to my letters and phone calls requesting interviews. Each had always shunned publicity.

Kevorkian implicitly trusted his two assistants, Fieger told me. They served as sounding boards for his ideas.

Fieger described Nicol thus: "He's a great guy. He's disarming because he's real bright but he comes across as very down-home. He's a super bright guy. He sort of reminds me how Andy Griffith plays the *Matlock* character. He plays him almost like he's gullible but he's sharp as hell. Neal is very, very down to Earth but very, very bright."

More clues to Nicol's personality might be gained from his acerbic answering machine message:

"Hi. . . . You know who this is, because you called me, but I don't know who you are unless you leave a name and number. You know the drill. At the beep leave a message and number. You'll be graded on originality and delivery. If you do a good job, I'll call you back. If you don't, go to your room without dinner. Hope you pass."

I failed, many times.

Faced with stone walls, there was one choice:

Dig.

CHAPTER THIRTY–EIGHT
THE *!@%*! VIDEOS

"Penumbra: 3. a: a surrounding or adjoining region in which something exists in a lesser degree: a marginal area: fringe b: a surrounding atmosphere (as of obscurity, emotion, meaning); aura, nimbus. c: an area containing things of obscure classification: an uncertain middle ground between fields of thought or activity: borderland, no-man's-land."
—Webster's Third New International Dictionary ❏

Geoffrey Fieger had advised me: *"The fucking videos—go look at them!"*

So I did.

Margo Janus shot videotapes of at least one pre-suicide consultation for each of Kevorkian's patients. Fieger had released to the press the tapes for Janet Adkins, Sherry Miller, Marjorie Wantz, Sue Williams, and Hugh Gale. When I asked to view tapes, those were the only ones Fieger would let me see.

Over several Saturdays, I watched the tapes in a library at Fieger's office. I watched Kevorkian trying to get Adkins to say the word "death." I watched Wantz asking to be cut up 10 ways. I watched Sue Williams saying she would never see God.

And I was amazed at how very little of this material had found its way into the popular Jack Kevorkian saga—much of which consisted of sound bites and Fieger's second-hand accounts. But the tapes that really stunned me were the ones that recorded the two visits of the Kevorkian team to the Gale residence in Roseville. Surrounding those oft-aired sound bites were conversations remarkable for the way they foreshadowed events that followed and shed new light on the people involved.

Kevorkian's demeanor—noticeably nervous in the early tapes—had changed to a very cool confidence by the time he visited the

255

Gales. Kevorkian sat back in a chair, tapping a clipboard with a pencil as if taking an inventory. And Neal Nicol oozed a glib self-assurance. They were two old pros.

On the evening of January 26, 1993, the tape records Gale sitting in a big armchair, his back arched and his large belly slumped forward. He has long white hair, a thin white mustache, tattoos on each arm, and an oxygen tube in his nose. When he talks, it is labored and he often gasps for air. His wife Cheryl is a diminutive woman who sits on the edge of her chair.

"Now, Mr. Gale, what is it that you wish?" Kevorkian starts out in his usual fashion. "Put it in plain English."

"Relief."

"What do you mean by relief?"

"Well. I can't breathe, of course, and every day it gets worse now."

"How do you want it relieved?"

"I know I'm going to die, but what I'm hoping for is I'll take my own way of going, and the easiest way out, I guess."

"You want help in ending your life? Is that what you want?"

"Right. By all means."

Gale admits he might have beaten emphysema if he had quit smoking when his doctor first told him to 20 years earlier. Now he is so weak he hardly can make it to the bathroom.

"That's why I got a hold of you, because it's getting close," he says. "... This, most of all, is what I want: To die with dignity. I don't want anybody to clean up after me. ... This is the time to do it because there's no sense ... to wait and take a lot of pain with it if you don't have to."

Nicol asks how long Gale has been thinking about suicide.

"It's been in my mind a long time, I guess. ... When I realized that there's only one way I'm going, I can't stop it and then, God love ya, you came, you rised up, and I said then: My God, that's the man I want. I want to meet you."

"Is there anything you could enjoy more if you went on longer?" Nicol asks.

"No. I've lost all interest. I guess the reason I've lost all interest—I don't know how to explain it—it just isn't there any more."

Gesturing to a landscape hanging on the wall above Kevorkian's chair, Gale says he can't paint anymore, he can't get to the garage to tinker anymore, he can't even get to the doctor.

He says he has been in the same chair for years.

"This is where you see me," he says. "This is my life right here."

Cheryl Gale says her husband has gotten steadily worse.

"Sometimes when he wakes up, he has so much mucus and fluid that he gasps and can't breathe. It's like he's drowning. He turns purple and shakes. It's like a seizure. It's very scary to go through and scary to watch. Then he'll say he can't go through any more of these, but then he falls asleep from exhaustion, wakes up more refreshed and says 'Let's keep trying, let's keep fighting it.' But he's grown afraid to go to sleep because of the hard wake-ups. . . . He told me it's like you're drowning, but your body will not give up. You can't get any air in."

"You're two people," Hugh Gale says. "One wants to live and the other says 'Leave me go,' but your body won't let you go."

"He's been praying to go in his sleep," his wife says. "He spoke to his doctor about wanting to die about a year and a half ago. His doctor said he needed more in his life, he needed to get out, to get an interest, to do something fun."

Hugh Gale says he tried to do what the doctor suggested, but there just wasn't anything to do.

Kevorkian asks Cheryl Gale: "Do you have any reservations about it?"

"I'm terribly scared," she replies. "Of what I really don't know. I'm not afraid of being alone, because he's going to pass away naturally sooner or later, and I'm an independent person and I take care of most everything now. I really don't know, I'm just very nervous about it."

Hugh has a fit of coughing, wheezing and gasping. "Goddamn it," he says, over and over. He finally asks for water and his wife hands him a plastic jug with a straw.

Cheryl explains: "He's always said to me, 'I'll know when the time is here.' He doesn't want to end up in a nursing home. His life has become so small. We've talked about it many times. The decision is totally up to him. It's very personal."

Cheryl says Hugh "started getting nervous before you came. I told him you don't have to decide anything. If you do make a decision, you can change your mind."

At great length, Kevorkian and Nicol confirm that Hugh Gale has that option.

Kevorkian: "You can change your mind right at the last minute and it won't bother us at all. We'll be delighted because we're here to help you...."

Nicol: "We'll be happy with it."

Kevorkian: "You run the whole show. If you say 'wait a minute'... we'll come back another day when you say. And nobody's upset, understand that. Don't ever think you're hurting our feelings or anything..."

Kevorkian then turns to religion.

"Do you believe in God?" he asks Hugh Gale.

"By all means."

"Do you think suicide is a sin?"

"I don't think so. I talk a lot to God. He sits by me like we're sitting here. And I say 'Dear God, I don't know, please forgive me if I'm doing wrong.' ..."

"Are you afraid at all?" Kevorkian asks.

"No," Gale says, then pauses. "I maybe have a little..."

"That's only natural," Nicol interjects quickly.

Kevorkian observes: "Well, we're all going to go there, it's just a matter of when."

Gale responds: "I've been saying that for three years. I won't know until I get there, and I just let it go at that and hope for the best."

Kevorkian then explains the procedure, saying they will use odorless, tasteless gas: "It's like breathing air. ... You'll breathe normally like you do now. You'll go to sleep with this. It varies with individuals from 30 to 45 seconds to 1 1/2 to two minutes—even 2 1/2 ... and then you'll go to sleep."

Hugh Gale looks confused. "And then I get the gas?" he asks.

Cheryl Gale explains: "He told me this is what he was worried about. This afternoon he was asking me, he said, 'If it's gas or something that you breathe,' he said, 'I'll choke on it.' "

"Well, no, you won't really choke on it," Kevorkian says, full of reassurance. "It's like breathing air."

Nicol also is very reassuring: "Any more than you now have the feeling that you're not getting enough oxygen, that won't get any worse. You'll just go to sleep..."

"I won't go into one of these ... just like I showed here?" Gale says, referring to his seizure a few minutes earlier.

"That could happen," Nicol says, "but not because of the carbon monoxide. That could happen just simply because you have a normal one. That could happen at that time but it won't be aggravated by the carbon monoxide."

"Well, people react differently to this," Kevorkian explains. "Some have no reaction at all. Some jerk a little bit when they're unconscious." He makes a jerking motion with his arms. "These are unconscious movements. Some will even snore. They go into such a deep sleep they just start snoring."

"We haven't really seen any patterns yet, where everybody does the same thing," Nicol explains matter-of-factly. "Different people react differently to the gas, and sometimes the medication that you're on will affect it. The low oxygen uptake, that may affect it. So there isn't any standard where you can say at two minutes you're going to be asleep, at five minutes it's going to be all over. Different people react differently."

From behind the camera, Margo Janus assures Hugh Gale in her quiet, steady, soothing voice: "But you won't feel it."

"You won't feel it," her brother agrees.

"You'll be unconscious," Margo says, "so these will be involuntary movements, if there are any."

"So the jerking?" Hugh Gale asks.

"That's an involuntary muscle reaction," Nicol assures him.

Kevorkian says: ". . . You'll be asleep and unconscious. This time you will not come out of it."

"There's no taste, no smell, nothing," says Margo Janus. "Just like breathing air."

"No color," says Doctor Death. "Like breathing air."

"And you'll still be breathing oxygen at the same time," explains Nicol, the medical supplies salesman. "It's just that you'll get carbon monoxide at the same time. There isn't any adverse effects of it. You just go to sleep."

"You know when you're in a stuffy room sometimes and you can't stay awake in a stuffy room?" Kevorkian asks. "That's the same kind of feeling. The same effect. The brain just gets little oxygen, the brain gets low. So you just get sleepy and fall asleep."

"But there's no pain involved," Nicol reassures him. "You shouldn't be worried about it."

"The gas is not irritating," Kevorkian says.

"Do you have all the medical history you need, Jack?" his sister asks.

"I think so," says Kevorkian. "We have a note that indicates the seriousness of his condition. Exactly what we need. Ethically, I suppose I should call the doctor and let him know, but they react negatively to this, and I don't want to bring any hardship on you and Mrs. Gale by calling the doctor."

"I don't want a funeral or anything," Hugh Gale says. "I just want—cremation."

Nicol and Kevorkian explain that the police will come and investigate and call the medical examiner, who will take the body to the morgue, do an autopsy and contact the funeral home.

"How is it gonna go for her?" Hugh asks, nodding to Cheryl.

"What do you mean?"

"The people, the damn people," Hugh explains.

Kevorkian reassures him that "in the other ones the reaction hasn't been that bad." He says the authorities handle it better now, they don't make a big deal out of it anymore.

"Well, what about Macomb County?" Cheryl asks. "Will they arrest you?"

"No," Kevorkian says. ". . . There's no risk for Mrs. Gale. There's no legal risk."

Kevorkian and Nicol say neighbors are usually supportive, though there's usually one who voices an objection.

"Just to get on TV," Margo says.

"You can't say anything to the media and we won't either," Kevorkian advises. "The media will want a story, but just don't say anything. Don't answer the door, and they'll lose interest. They didn't make a big deal out of the last one."

"The attorney will speak for all of us," Margo says.

"I like your lawyer," Hugh Gale volunteers.

"He doesn't take much from anybody," Nicol attests.

"I'd like to have him on my side," Hugh Gale says.

Kevorkian then asks Hugh Gale to sign Document A. Kevorkian apologizes for using "too many big words" in it. Cheryl reads the consent form, stumbling over the words "extrinsic" and "interminable." Kevorkian explains what they mean. She reads:

> I, Hugh E. Gale, the undersigned, hereby request of my own free will and without any reservations or extrinsic persuasion or duress, that my life of intolerable and interminable pain and/or suffering be ended in the most humane, rapid and painless manner with the help of a

competent medical professional. It is my understanding that I will end my life by breathing through a routine facial mask or plastic tent a lethal mixture of carbon monoxide and nitrogen gas. All details of procedures have been explained to me by the undersigned medical professionals, and I am fully aware of the implications and consequences of my voluntarily carrying them out. . . .

Nicol then reiterates that Hugh Gale can change his mind: "You have the right at any time to stop the procedure and say no. You will make the determination as to time, when you want to do it. Take the time, all the time that you need. . . . It's not something that you can say 'Oops, I made a mistake.' So we want you to be very well sure of what you're doing. And up until the time that you release the gas and even if you have released the gas, if you decide to call a stop, just say 'I don't want to do this any more' or 'Stop' or something like that, and the procedure will stop at that time. And there's no repercussions . . . We'd prefer that you went on with your life rather than end it like this. . . ."

"No, there's no, there's no reason to live any longer," Hugh Gale insists.

"But if you do feel good for a couple of days, go on a couple more days until you feel bad," Kevorkian says.

"You don't have to face time in a nursing home or being disabled," Nicol says. "You have the option to end it when you want to. Enjoy the life that you have as long as you want and then just call us."

"I feel marvelously well right now, just meeting you fellas and you, my dear lady," Hugh Gale says.

"That's good," Kevorkian says.

"Well, you know you have the option," Nicol says. "That seems to bring a lot of people peace of mind. . . . We've had a lot of patients who just go on and die naturally, and we don't do them at all, but they know that if things get bad, they can."

Kevorkian adds: "We would prefer that you feel so good now that you go to sleep one day and just don't wake up. . . . You know we're here. So don't ever hurry. There's no deadline on this. . . . You set the date . . . and try to enjoy these last few days, weeks, whatever it is."

"I'll run around a lot," Hugh Gale jokes. Everyone laughs.

Call whenever you want, Kevorkian invites him: "Let's hope it's weeks, let's hope it's a couple months."

"I feel so wonderful now, I really do," the dying man says. "This is an awful heavy load off my shoulders."

"That's wonderful," Kevorkian says.

"And if you go on and never utilize the service, we're just as happy," Nicol says.

"That's right," Kevorkian says.

◻ ◻ ◻

On the evening of February 11, Kevorkian, Neal Nicol and Margo Janus returned to the home of Cheryl and Hugh Gale. From the tapes, it seems clear that the Gales were expecting this session to be the final one, with the procedure to follow the next day. Document H, with "Feb. 12" atop it, suggests the same. But Kevorkian's team brought some distressing news, recorded on video at the outset.

"Some unusual developments have cropped up," Kevorkian says. "The authorities have pressured the companies to cut off our supply of gas. And it's in very short supply now. . . . So we're going to have to experiment with a new method. . . . And because of that, I think it's best if we wait several days before we try it, because there are another two patients that are also scheduled . . . and we're going to try to ration it off so that there's enough for everybody, and we're not taking any more patients."

"Until we get some more gas," Nicol picks up.

"Damn," Hugh Gale says.

"That's the way they are, Mister Gale," Kevorkian says. "These authorities really don't care about people."

"You don't have any gas at all, huh?"

"We have some," Kevorkian says. " . . . Don't panic. Don't worry. We have enough. We've just gotta ration it. . . . We're not sure what we're going to do. Neal and I were discussing it—to create a little tent over you, with a frame . . . in which you just breathe comfortably instead of a mask on your face. You'll probably feel better anyway that way. And then we can fill the tent up with the gas as needed. And that way we can conserve the gas . . ."

Nicol explains: "We feel that if there's a tent to capture that gas and you continue to breathe it, we can keep that from being wasted, and that should extend our supply."

"You'll go to sleep at roughly the same time," Kevorkian says.

Janus asks Gale if he can recline in his chair and lie flat on his back.

"Yeah," he says. They recline his chair some.

"Are you comfortable with that?" Kevorkian asks.

"Yeah," Gale says.

But his wife says: "He's telling you this because he wants to please you. If he stays like that for long, he starts coughing and choking."

Kevorkian says: "Oh, he'll be asleep within two minutes."

Margo asks Cheryl if her husband could lie like that for 10 or 15 minutes. She says he could.

"All we need is three or four, really," Kevorkian says. "You'll go to sleep and that's it. After that, it doesn't matter what happens. You won't know what happens after that. You won't wake up."

The tent will be made of clear material, Nicol says: "You won't feel trapped or anything."

"You'll breathe normally in the tent," Kevorkian says.

"We have been going out of our minds trying to figure out a way to serve everybody we promised and yet conserve the gas," Margo explains.

Cheryl Gale mentions that the *Final Exit* death prescription included taking barbiturates and putting a plastic bag on your head—the same method employed by Bertram and Virginia Harper.

"That's brutal," Kevorkian says. All agree it would be horrible to suffocate to death.

"Derek Humphry really had no business writing that book," says Margo Janus. "He's not a medical doctor."

"See, the tent is not like a plastic bag," Kevorkian says. ". . . with this you breathe in normally, so it's much more comfortable."

"Plus it's a more economical use of the gas," Nicol adds.

Hugh Gale says: "You don't want that person that's going out going out hard."

Kevorkian tells him: "We'll let you know. We'll work on it in the next couple days and devise this tent. We'll call you and we'll get together and do a final session then."

"Can't we make this the final session?" Hugh Gale says, "because I want to take my life, you know that."

"I know that," Kevorkian says.

"And you were kind of geared up tonight," Nicol says. "We really feel bad about that, because you were already geared up for it. And ordinarily there wouldn't have been a problem."

"They threw this curve at us today," Kevorkian says.

The discussion shifts to the Stanley Ball and Mary Biernat double suicide. Kevorkian and his sister say the two families really "hit it off" and had a party the night before the deaths.

"You meet the best people that way," Kevorkian says.

"Well, you have a common bond," Nicol says. "They're about to lose a loved one, you're about to lose a loved one. Yeah, they sent out for dinner and had a party the night before, stayed up late and talked about their lives and their attitudes about death and everything. When I got there the next morning, you wouldn't have known that they all didn't live in the same house. They were just great friends." The Balls even invited the Biernats to come back for boating and fishing.

Kevorkian concludes: "I'll let you know when we got it worked out, and we'll have a final session where Mister Gale can sign the final consent."

"Please make it as soon as possible," Hugh Gale says.

Nicol says to the man who had been planning to die the next day: "Well, we realize the mental and emotional hardship that this puts you under, but there's not an awful lot we can do."

"Yeah, you couldn't," Gale says. "I told my grandmother I was coming, see."

"She'll be mad at us if you don't show up, won't she?" Nicol remarks.

"Well, no, they got time to wait up there," Kevorkian jokes. "But keep your spirits up, because we're not abandoning you."

Kevorkian says the tent might be ready to try Monday on "a patient who needs help, it's a cancer patient and in really, really bad shape"—referring to Martie Ruwart. "So if you hear about it, don't worry. That way, we'll know the tent works anyway, and we'll contact you as soon after that as we can."

Nicol, Kevorkian and Janus say they're going to try to publicize the company's refusal to sell them the gas.

"In the long run, they're going to end up losing, because when this is accepted, they're going to look like wimps, they're going to look like weaklings who caved in," Kevorkian says.

Nicol adds: "I told Jack on the way over here: Really, I just feel like I'm challenged now, to see how resourceful I can be. And if I'm not smarter than the police departments, then I don't deserve to be in this anyway."

"What irritates me too is . . . the media, the way they portray you," Cheryl Gale says. "They make you sound so hard, Doctor Death and that."

"There have been no complaints. But then they ignore that," Janus says, "because it isn't to their financial benefit."

"Well, see, they're on the side of the authorities, all the press is," Kevorkian says.

Kevorkian concludes by telling the Gales: "We'll let you know as soon as it's available. It'll be several days, and then we'll contact you right away."

They leave Hugh Gale to wonder when his appointment with death might be. As it turns out, he would be the patient to die on Monday—because my uncle Bill Ruwart changed his mind about letting Martie use his house, and my cousin lost that slot in Doctor Death's schedule.

Later, I asked Fieger about the gas problem. He said it wasn't the first time companies had buckled to pressure and cut off the supply. But he pointed out that Roseville police confiscated the canister of carbon monoxide used in Gale's death. Kevorkian had enough gas to help Martie Ruwart and Jonathan Grenz, and in neither of those deaths was a tent used.

"They found gas, so they didn't have the problem subsequently" to Gale's death, Fieger explained. "They thought they were going to have a hard time getting gas but they didn't."

CHAPTER THIRTY–NINE
WHOSE BUSINESS IS IT ANYWAY?

"Penumbra: 4: a part of a picture where shade
gradually blends with light."
—Webster's Third New International
Dictionary ❏

On April 20, 1993, nearly 100 people came to the Community House in the well-heeled Detroit suburb of Birmingham to hear a debate on assisted suicide. Three years earlier, Janet Adkins was still alive, Jack Kevorkian was still a little-known eccentric, and it would have been hard to imagine 10 people coming to such a debate.

The doctor who couldn't even get a paramedic's job five years earlier had transformed the discussion over choice in dying from an academic parlor game to the number one topic of barber shop and coffee break bull sessions in Michigan and much of the nation. This night, Jack Kevorkian was presumably sitting in his apartment a few miles away, leaving half his dinner uneaten and enjoying the pleasures of J.S. Bach.

Local radio personality Warren Pierce moderated the panel: Hemlock's Janet Good, anti-euthanasia activist Rita Marker, legal scholar Yale Kamisar of the University of Michigan and ethicist Tom Tomlinson from Michigan State University.

Kamisar was an old hand at this. In 1958, he had written a land-mark law review article, "Some Non-Religious Views Against Proposed 'Mercy-Killing' Legislation." And 35 years later, he was still arguing many of the same points.

As director of the International Anti-Euthanasia Task Force, Rita Marker often had pitched me nasty comments about Kevorkian. Her organization's name made it sound massive and far-flung. In fact, I learned that the IAETF was one of the many tentacles of a little-known Ohio college, the University of Steubenville, that was something of a headquarters for right-wing Catholic extremists.

Marker had written a new book, *Deadly Compassion: The Death of Ann Humphry and the Truth about Euthanasia*, which had gar-nered her much more publicity and legitimacy. The book ostensibly

266

centered on Marker's friendship with the second wife of Derek Humphry, but served mainly as a vehicle for Marker's well-honed diatribes against assisted suicide. *Free Press* reviewer Susan Hall-Balduf noted: "Marker suggests that Janet Adkins may actually have died of her family's failure to protest when she suggested they'd be better off without her. 'Knowing someone wants you dead . . . is more lethal than cancer,' she writes."

Marker led off the night's debate by saying "all social engineering is preceded by verbal engineering." It is double-speak, she said, to call poisoning by carbon monoxide "aid in dying" or, as Judge Breck did, "medical treatment." It obscures the central issue, she said, which is whether doctors should have the power to kill their patients.

"I know that people like to steer clear of certain words, but what we're talking about is making people die, and the word for that is *killing*," Marker said.

Janet Good, seated next to Marker, was offended. Good said the subject of Marker's book never let herself be called anything other than Ann Wickett, her maiden name. If Marker hadn't known that, she could hardly have been her close friend, Good said.

Good said the Michigan ban was a creature of the "religious right," which she said was misnamed: "These people are not religious and they certainly are not right. They are radical fundamentalists who are slowly but surely taking over our places of worship, our schools, our governments and our rights to privacy."

Kamisar said the issue was not about refusing treatment. That battle was long over (he had been on the losing side of it). Americans now clearly had the right to order plugs pulled and even food and water withheld, on their own or through designated representatives. But assisted suicide was another matter.

"There is no right to commit suicide," Kamisar said. "One has the power, the capacity, to commit suicide. That does not mean one has the right." Granted, he said, suicide no longer was a crime. But that was only because government had realized it was senseless to punish the family if a suicide succeeded, and better to treat than punish the perpetrator if an attempt failed.

Tomlinson said attitudes toward assisted suicide stem from views on the morality of killing. Those who believe only God can give and take life would condemn all suicide, assisted or not, as a form of murder. Those who believe murder is wrong because it deprives another of autonomy could support assisted suicide if it were a freely chosen last-ditch alternative to awful suffering.

Tomlinson said it would be possible to have a workable policy that ensured people retained their autonomy in choosing death. But he admitted, echoing presidential gadfly Ross Perot, that "the devil's in the details."

Kamisar invoked his side's two main arguments: Pain Control and the Slippery Slope. Good pain management could alleviate most any suffering, he said, and thwart any need for suicide. As for the Slippery Slope, if assisted suicide were legalized, then the old, the infirm and the vulnerable would be next in line, he said.

"It becomes not only thinkable, but speakable," Kamisar said. "And as an old man, I have to wonder whether I am doing the cowardly thing by choosing not to cash it in."

Marker greased the slope further:

"Jack Kevorkian has rather an elitist view of who should live and who should die," she said, citing words she attributed to him from 1990: "The voluntarily self-elimination of individual and mortally diseased or crippled lives taken collectively can only enhance public health and welfare."

Marker translated: "In other words, get rid of the disabled and we'll all be better off.

"Jack Kevorkian appears to have this absolute certainty that he is the one that can be judge, jury and executioner. And I think Jack Kevorkian, while not getting money, does get a tremendous amount of power and jollies out of making other people dead."

Moderator Pierce interjected that many doctors quietly help patients die.

"There are many physicians every day who do a poor job," Marker rejoined, "many physicians who care more about managing their money market accounts than their patients' pain. There are physicians who do illegal acts. ... I don't think most physicians want to turn their medical licenses into licenses to kill, but you don't need a lot of doctors to kill a lot of people."

Tomlinson said Marker was getting the debate off track.

"We can spend all night, if we want to waste our time, talking about Doctor Kevorkian's character defects and his wacky statements, but that's a diversion," he said.

Kamisar said it was a diversion to talk about the terminally ill: Only two to three percent of all suicides are attempted by terminally ill people, he said, and 90 percent of those who try to kill themselves have diagnosable psychiatric illnesses.

Kamisar then invoked the Netherlands. (People on both sides of the debate often cited statistical evidence from Holland, where physician-aided death had been tolerated for more than 20 years.) Kamisar said 90 percent of the death certificates in the Netherlands were false, so it was not clear how many people there were being euthanized involuntarily.

Marker held up what she said was a card from a Dutch patients advocacy group. "Don't euthanize me," it read. People in Holland, she said, carried those papers like Americans carried organ donation cards.

When Pierce turned to the audience for questions, Don McNeil of Warren, a Hemlock stalwart, posed a stumper:

"If I'm terminally ill, incurable, in pain, and I ask my doctor to help me, and if my doctor is willing to do it, what business is it of yours? What business is it of the government's?"

Marker answered: "If it is a matter of autonomy that a person should be able to request that a doctor kill him . . . then any person for any reason should have a right to request it . . . we must allow it for anyone, anywhere.

"This is going to be offered as an option at first probably to those who want to die, killing the dying and then killing the costly. Then we will very quickly get to the point we are in Holland."

McNeil persisted: "But if I'm terminal, in pain, it's at my request and the doctor agrees, what business is it of the government?"

Marker conceded: "You can do whatever you wish, but you are asking that doctors have the right to do it for other people."

Tomlinson objected: "It's not sheer autonomy, it's a judgment about when your death would be the best outcome for you."

Kamisar rejoined: "The trouble is, if we pass a law, it covers thousands of cases and there'll be cases where the doctor or spouse or children suggested that assisted suicide is the best thing to do . . . Once we establish the principle that it's your business, then we have to extend it to everyone."

McNeil persisted: "That person in America makes his own decision. I have no right to tell him what to do, and you have no right to tell me what to do. That's freedom of choice, that's part of America."

"It's not part of America to kill people," Kamisar responded, "or to practice euthanasia."

A young man from the audience had the last word: "Ask what type of society we'll have in the future. If you allow assisted suicide, the future is open for question. Who will decide who will be allowed to have assisted suicide? Please remember what power the medical profession had in pre-war Germany."

Afterward, another reporter and I agreed that the debate, while provocative, was missing the sound and fury that could only be provided by Jack Kevorkian, the man whose words and deeds had gotten all these people fired up about this topic.

Chapter Forty
Brave New World

"Isn't it about time you took an honest look at
your stinking, miserable life?"
—David Letterman's "Top Ten Promotional
Slogans for the Suicide Machine" (#8) ❐

Being prosecutor of a rich, sprawling county with a million-plus population is a high-profile job. Richard Thompson's tough stance on crime had made him popular. His pursuit of Jack Kevorkian had increased his name recognition; it seemed, however, to be at odds with the wishes of a large percentage of the public. The man seemed to have little personality, apart from his job. Seated behind his huge desk for an interview, he began to slide down into his chair and became visible only from the neck up.

"What do you feel is at stake in this Kevorkian case?" I asked him.

"Brave New World is at stake here," he replied without hesitation. "I think it would be a disastrous mistake for our society to accept the premise that there are lives not worthy to be lived. And once we accept that, we are going down that Slippery Slope to an abyss of horrors where more and more groups of people will be placed in that category."

Thompson agreed that most people would support the right of terminally ill people to have help in dying, but pointed out that Kevorkian didn't limit his practice to the terminally ill.

"If everyone should decide when they want to die, why should we or why can we logically limit that right only when the patient is about to die? . . . Can't do it. It's illogical. So therefore anyone who wants to die ultimately will be allowed the assistance of a physician. . . .

"How do you define suffering? Is psychological suffering going to be acceptable as being as painful in certain respects as physical suffering?

"Once you make it a law . . . you're going to have a lot of abuses occurring, because there's no way to control the abuses.

"History repeats itself because we don't learn the first time. . . . All you have to do is look at what happened in Nazi Germany. When

271

they started out with physician-assisted suicide, it was the people that wanted it. . . . this whole genocide started with the small concept that there is such a thing as a life not worthy to be lived.

"Once you start that wedge, you can go right down the Slippery Slope, because there's no way to control it. And especially in our society where we're not a homogenous society, we don't have universal health care. Every day old people are being dropped off at emergency rooms at hospitals and people leave.

"It would be very easy for medicine, not this year but maybe 10 or 15 years down the road, to say: Their quality of life is no good, why waste the money? Why waste our scarce resources on this? Let's give them a lethal injection.

"Old people from the Netherlands are saying sometimes we know that we're being talked into wishing death, that we can't trust our own nursing homes, our own family physicians, that the yellow stuff in this needle, we don't know whether it's to help us out or it's to kill us.

"The idea that the state, or even the medical profession are going to make rules to ration health care, are going to determine who's going to live and who's going to die . . . there's that silent message that is being sent to ill people and to old people: Do us a favor. Don't hang around. We don't want to pay for you."

I asked Don McNeil's question: What business is it of the government if I make a decision to die with my doctor's help?

"If you ask a second party to help you out, then the state has an interest. . . . If a person wants to kill themselves, they can go into their garage and turn on their car, and they'll get the same kind of carbon monoxide poisoning that Doctor Kevorkian gives you out of a tank, but the state is not sanctioning it. I think the state still should have the policy that we hold life very sacred. . . .

"Many doctors say that if you allow physician-assisted suicide to be legalized, the entire dynamics of family care will change. Every time a patient is diagnosed as having terminal cancer, one of the considerations will be: Well, Mom or Dad or Grandpa or Grandma, should we spend the money on taking care of you, or should we save that money and have Doctor Kevorkian or someone else just zap you? . . . Aren't we going to be sweeping people under, under this guise of free choice, who really don't want to die but think others want them to die?"

Opposing assisted suicide is not an attempt to impose religious tenets on reluctant citizens, Thompson said: "In our society most laws are enacted on some fundamental moral principle. . . . That's a part of being in society, that we give up certain prerogatives that we might like to have.

"It's been traditional that doctors don't get involved in assisted suicide. I think they should have the burden of proving why we should now allow that to be a totally private affair.

"People support assisted suicide because they conjure up in their minds being terminally ill, suffering excruciating pain and having these doctors attach them to all the machinery. That doesn't have to happen. . . .

"There is a solution that is not as controversial, not as sexy, and that is hospice. Hospice assists thousands of people in dying with dignity, without a lot of tubes being attached to them, without all of the attendant publicity that Kevorkian has gotten in 15 deaths. I think that is the solution."

A real debate would get away from name-calling, Thompson said. In Fieger's attacks, he charged: "There has been a lot of anti-Christian bigotry. We would not tolerate one bit if those comments were made against some other religion."

The media, Thompson said, played into Fieger's hands.

"He has gotten away with making those outlandish attacks on every public official, and sadly the media has printed all these, very faithfully, and I think that has prompted him to do more. I think the television media is really to blame for a lot of the controversy because they love it, because he can give them a 10-second sound bite that we can't refute in 10 seconds."

Thompson said Fieger's charges of a conspiracy with Lynn Mills were outrageous. Thompson admitted he went to Right to Life meetings but said "I'm not involved" and had "never taken a position on the abortion issue." He said he did not know Mills before she called him.

Thompson said Macomb County officials delayed the search warrant on the Gale papers, and it was signed after the court closed because Judge Kuhn was in the middle of a trial.

Thompson predicted that public opinion in Michigan would change once a serious debate started. And he said the time and resources his office had spent battling Kevorkian were worth it.

"The issue is so important. We're on the cutting edge. The nation and the world is looking at Oakland County, at the state of Michigan, to see what we're going to do. ..."

If history could judge him, Thompson said he would like to be seen "as a prosecutor who is enforcing the law, doing his job, and happened to be in a county where Doctor Kevorkian decided he wanted to make the issue into a public debate.

"But I also believe, after I made my decisions and studied the issue, that it would be a disastrous mistake for our society to hold as a public policy that there is such a thing as a life not worthy to be lived."

CHAPTER FORTY-ONE
TAKING CHARGE

*"I will argue with them if they will allow them-
selves to be strapped to a wheelchair for 72 hours
so they can't move, and they are catheterized and
they are placed on the toilet and fed and bathed.
Then they can sit in a chair and debate with me."
—Jack Kevorkian, outlining his terms for a
debate with critics who charge he is too hasty in
helping people die (1993)* ❐

For four years, Janet Good would bring a bottle of pills to her mother's
nursing home bedside. Good wanted to give her dying mother a way
out of her agony. But her mother's voice inside her head—telling her
that only God gave and took life—drowned out her heart. She never
gave her mother the pills.

"I asked the doctors to put her out of her misery and they laughed
at me," Good said. "I'll never forgive those doctors."

Her mother's death was one thing that drove Janet Good to join
the Hemlock Society—and eventually to start a Michigan chapter.

In a small, neat office in her ranch home in Farmington Hills,
Good told me she could still recall how Tish Sommers, one of the
early leaders of the right-to-die movement, characterized the struggle.

"She called it 'taking charge of the end of your life.' "

For Good, a lifelong civil rights and feminist activist, being able
to choose the circumstances of one's own death was "the ultimate
civil right."

In the early days, her friends thought she was crazy to talk about a
right to die. The first time she showed her doctor a Living Will, in
1972, he told her to see a psychiatrist.

To Good, legalizing the right to assisted suicide was a matter of
justice. She said many doctors and other health professionals and
their families—and other people with connections or friends—had
drugs hoarded away as a suicide option.

"There is a select population who don't have to worry. That's not
fair. It should be available to everybody."

In fact, most people can't get the drugs prescribed in *Final Exit*, Good said. She said many desperate people contacted her asking her to send them hemlock. Though she had a hemlock tree in her back yard, she did not dispense its poisonous leaves, she said. Taking hemlock to die, like Socrates did, was a horrible way to go, she said.

Hemlock members, Good said, don't fear death, they fear losing control of the dying process. The Hemlock motto is "a good life, a good death."

The Slippery Slope was no danger, Good contended:

"We would not let older people be destroyed just because they are in the way."

In her living will, Good, 69, specified she wanted to die by lethal injection "when life is no longer meaningful for me."

One of her biggest fears was that her friend Jack Kevorkian would go to jail and starve himself to death, as he had threatened to do. Then he might not be there for her, she said.

"I hope both of us survive long enough in case I need him," said Good.

◻ ◻ ◻

At a Hemlock Society gathering in Southfield, I found several people younger than 60. I also found lunch, literature, speakers and a national Hemlock Society video.

On the video, a narrator begins talking over shots of rippling brooks and pine trees:

> We were born. We lived out our lives. And then when our work was done, it was time to simply die, usually after a short illness, usually at home. Death was a natural part of life.
>
> But it's not so simple now. In the span of a single lifetime, we've seen an explosion in science and medical technology. Wonder drugs, transplants, machines now make it possible to prolong the life of a dying person long past the point when any recovery is possible.
>
> Some say this is wrong. They say that when we prolong life this way, we really only prolong suffering and inevitable death, and to do so violates common decency and common sense. They believe that a dying person suffering terrible

pain, a person for whom life has lost all dignity and meaning, should have the right to say: "This is enough. It's time to die. Please help me." But we can't help them, not under the current laws . . .

The tape depicts several stories. A man speaks about how his wife, suffering from heart disease, took sleeping pills and placed a plastic bag over her head. A Hemlock volunteer talks about how her father, who had cancer, told his doctor not to prolong his death, but died "diapered, moaning in pain, moaning constantly, begging to die" because the doctor would not give him morphine. A man's daughter and granddaughter recount how he blew his brains out in the basement to end his battle with cancer.

"I wonder what he thought as he was facing that gun and pulling the trigger," the granddaughter says. "And I wonder how long he sat there before he pulled that trigger. And what his last thoughts were. And I'm angry he had to die such a lonely, violent death."

A physician, Warren Sparks, notes on the tape that many doctors routinely help people die: "It goes on all the time. It's being done without proper safeguards, because it's being done surreptitiously." Sparks predicts a future of "Baby Boomers getting older and technology getting better and better and better" and says the problem "is only going to be magnified greatly."

Ralph Mero, a Hemlock leader who subsequently left to start his own right-to-die group, is shown visiting and counseling a man on the eve of major surgery. The man says he has a drug stockpile and whiskey ready in case he needs it to end his life.

Mero comments: "People who are terminally ill often have no one who will be honest with them about what they're facing. . . . It's very common that if a person says, 'I can't take it anymore, I can't go on,' the physician says, 'Oh, but you'll feel better tomorrow.' If someone says, 'You know, I'm really thinking about bringing life to an end,' someone says, 'Oh, don't talk that way. That's not healthy.'

"But we're talking about people who are already dying. And people who every day experience continued degradation and loss of their body capacities. They know about the nausea. They know about the night sweats. They know about the continued diarrhea. They know about the ceaseless vomiting. . . . And when they say, 'I can't go on with this anymore,' I think someone should listen and say, 'You do have the right to make a decision for yourself which will enable you to die with dignity and self-respect.' "

The narrator concludes: "If you want to die with dignity, then you have to do something about it in advance. You have to accept that death is a part of life, and it will come to you later, later rather than sooner. We're talking about a concept that is the ultimate civil liberty: death with dignity."

Not once in the video did I hear the word "suicide" uttered.

After the tape was shown, Daniel Devine, a young attorney representing Hemlock, told the group about Hemlock's legal briefs supporting Kevorkian in his appeal of Judge Gilbert's injunction and opposing Thompson's appeal of Judge Breck's dismissal of murder charges in the deaths of Marjorie Wantz and Sherry Miller.

Breck, Devine said, "hit it on the head" in saying there was no difference between a doctor withdrawing life support and assisting in a suicide.

"It's really a distinction without merit," Devine told the group. "It's pure semantics, it's nonsense, because the effect is death, that's what the person wants and that's in fact what's occurring."

Devine said the high costs of caring for the terminally ill must be figured into the equation. "What could we do with that money if it was freed up by allowing competent individuals who choose to do so to leave on their own accord at a designated time? That would free those funds up for pre-natal care, for cancer research, for AIDS research, for breast cancer research. Wouldn't the quality of life be enhanced? Wouldn't the deficit be reduced?"

Devine said the penalties under the state's ban on assisted suicide didn't make sense. If it was really murder, why make it a four-year felony? Devine said the lack of a stricter penalty could tempt disgruntled spouses to risk four years in jail by killing their partner: "They're going to set up a bogus assisted suicide, go away for four years, and get 100 percent of the marital estate."

In debating the issue, Devine said it was time to separate the "nonsense and circus atmosphere from the reality of death and dying. The terminally ill person at the end of their rope doesn't give a hoot about Doctor Kevorkian or Geoff Fieger or Dick Thompson or Lynn Mills. All they know and have strength enough to know is that they're suffering.

"We're saying give them the right to be able to choose what they want for themselves and themselves only, and let's leave the personality conflicts for the soap operas."

CHAPTER FORTY–TWO
THE SLIPPERY SLOPE FLOW CHART

*A woman on a couch is talking on a phone. Jack
Kevorkian is sitting beside her, leering, with a
medicine bag nearby.
"Can't talk now, Mom," the woman says. "I'm
being treated for acute depression."*
—*Cartoonist Draper Hill of the* Detroit News ❐

Ed Rivet was so familiar with the terrain of the Slippery Slope that he had a computer-drawn flow chart depicting its various channels: the Kevorkian route, the Quill route, the Howard Brody route. He proudly showed me this nerdish philosophical map when I visited him in his cramped suite in a musty Lansing office building. Rivet, Right to Life of Michigan's legislative point man, knew the territory. And he never budged.

Rivet denied that Right to Life's interest in assisted suicide was a new cause to reinvigorate troops disheartened by the abortion battle. "We've tracked the euthanasia movement" since the early 1960s, he assured me.

At the suggestion of national Right to Life, Rivet said, he had prepared a draft bill against assisted suicide in December 1988, before Kevorkian even invented his suicide device.

"Our goal is to see that the law in our society protects innocent human life," Rivet said. "And that for us is the unborn, infants, handicapped, elderly, incompetent patients, those people who are most vulnerable to someone else's decision that they be dead. And that's why we focus specifically and always have on abortion, infanticide and euthanasia."

The euthanasia movement started by seeking the right of patients to have treatment withdrawn. Right to Life had no problem with that, Rivet said. But next on the agenda was the Living Will, which extended that right to a patient advocate. Rivet said a Living Will is "sort of an oxymoron, to talk about controlling your medical care after you're out of control." Largely because of Right to Life's opposition, Michigan remained in 1993 one of a few states that had not codified Living Wills. The next step on the Slippery Slope, Rivet said, was "the substituted judgment"—a ruling that even in the absence of a Living Will, an interested party could request the withdrawal of treatment if it could be demonstrated that the patient would have agreed.

If assisted suicide were legalized, Rivet said, the same steps would occur. The right to die would be extended first through a Living Will, then via substituted judgment, and then, "we're right to the involuntary euthanasia that we've got going on in the Netherlands now."

I asked Rivet the Don McNeil question. He answered with his own question.

"How are we going to know when the next person dies that they're not incompetent or they're not vulnerable or they're not coerced? . . . I mean, we can start killing people left and right and saying it was an assisted suicide. . . .

"One of the terrific distortions we have in our 1980s and '90s culture is that everything has become a right. And it's not. . . .

"If we allow legalized assisted suicide, there's virtually no way we're going to stop involuntary active euthanasia, the killing of incompetents, mentally ill people, mentally retarded people, severely handicapped people that are incompetent, handicapped newborn babies: They will be euthanized."

Why wouldn't society be smart enough to prevent the slide down the Slippery Slope? I asked.

"Because we have to lie to ourselves in order to justify legalizing assisted suicide," Rivet said. "The criteria don't really exist in a practical fashion that are going to prevent healthy people from killing themselves."

Wherever you drew the line, Rivet said, someone on the other side would argue he had the same constitutional right. Rivet said no one had ever answered his questions: Where do you draw the line? And who draws it?

For Rivet, the devil in the details was an omnipotent demon.

"I have yet to see any advocate of assisted suicide put forth a plan that doesn't get chopped to ribbons by somebody or by everybody else," Rivet said " . . . If it's a privacy right, then it's going to extend a lot further than I think the average citizen wants it to go. And that's exactly what we saw with the abortion debate, too."

When people examine specific guidelines for assisted suicide, their support for the concept erodes, Rivet said. The vote in Washington, "the most unchurched population of any state," showed that opposition was not fueled by religious fundamentalism, Rivet argued.

Rivet said people want the right to determine for themselves when they should be allowed to have a doctor help them die, "but they can't look at a system that's going to work where they feel it's going to be good for the society overall."

Rivet said the slide down the slope already had begun.

"When we debated the durable power of attorney, one of our arguments was if you start taking away basic levels of care, like food and water, and starve a person to death, then you can euthanize them, because it makes more sense to let them die in 12 seconds rather than 12 days. . . . Oh, don't be ridiculous, they told us, that's just your fanatical paranoia. We're not going ever to be having a discussion about legalizing euthanasia or suicide. The medical profession would never accept that as part of their ethical standard. . . . We had a bill introduced less than three years later to legalize assisted suicide and euthanasia."

Rivet said Right to Life was defending "a legal, moral, ethical and medical standard that's been in existence for this nation's entire history. Assisting in a suicide has always been deemed to be an inappropriate, illegal, immoral, unethical action. And yet we're the ones who are said to be pushing the wrong agenda or trying to change the status quo or do something contrary to the American way."

It was Jack Kevorkian who was acting "contrary to the American way," Rivet said, by "writing the laws for himself." Kevorkian was the best thing that had happened to the anti-euthanasia movement in a long time, he said. Were it not for Doctor Death, Rivet said, "that draft of a bill would have still been sitting in my file."

CHAPTER FORTY–THREE
JIM JONES ON MAIN STREET

Superman lies on the ground. A woman tells a
man: "I just sent him to Doctor Kevorkian
for a physical."
—*Editorial cartoonist Chip Bok in the* Akron
Beacon-Journal ❐

Geoffrey Fieger's favorite TV dance partner, State Senator John Kelly, said he had no problems with assisted suicide under proper guidelines. He had a problem with Jack Kevorkian.

"Most of the people in this state, including myself, support euthanasia under some conditions. In fact, it has always taken place. The question remains: Who do we want to draw the line for the various circumstances under which it can be done?

"There's no social consensus on when someone should be euthanized. There is no majoritarian point of view. So we must have a greater debate on this whole issue.

"In the interim, Kevorkian doesn't respect the process. He doesn't lobby his representatives. He just says: The hell with everybody.

"He just goes out and recruits people in pain, either psychological or real, induces them to come to him—an untrained, unprofessional non-clinician, with no background in psychology or psychiatry or oncology or anesthesiology, who has a mind-set about what he's going to do before he's objectively analyzed the condition—and he takes the law into his own hands.

"I just find that outrageous."

So when push came to shove, John Kelly voted with Right to Life—the group he had fought tooth and nail for 15 years.

"Occasionally even monkeys on typewriters can write something legible," he told me. "In this case they're right."

Kevorkian's patients, Kelly said, "lack the capacity to arrive at a judgment about the termination of their life, and he is not trained to see that. . . . We have no way of knowing what their state of mind was. The videotapes don't prove anything.

"The situation itself is coercive. He uses his doctor degree the same way Jim Jones in Guyana used his reverend title: to induce these people into a position of confidence and trust.

"In Kevorkian's world, he's the sole arbiter. He makes all the decisions. If you say it's terminal, that's good enough for him.

"Who in the hell put him in charge?

"And then the horror of it all is he gives these people a reason for dying. You're now a martyr in the greater cause, your pain means something for other people. What lies, what hypocrisy!

"Here's a guy who's been preoccupied with this issue his whole life. He goes through all these permutations. First he was an inventor and then an angel of mercy. Next he becomes this kind of willy-nilly unguided executioner. He constantly redefines his purposes.

"He's a rogue. You take the profiles of these women to a psychiatrist who specializes in serial killing and ask him what kind of person is doing this. I bet it comes out as a sociopath.

"My problem is what happens if you have a 20-year-old high school dropout with a low IQ and bad complexion, he's lost his job, his girlfriend walks out on him, he's in extreme depression and he walks into the Kevorkian suicide parlor and says 'I know what I'm doing. I just want to end it'?

"I don't want to see that kind of a world. It bothers me. It just offends every part of me.

"There's a value to existence. People shouldn't have their lives extinguished without some thought. Depression is not a basis for euthanasia."

Kelly said it was not a matter of privacy.

"Nothing is to prevent people from taking their own lives. A handful of over-the-counter sleeping pills with a couple of glasses of whiskey will do it. A .38 slug in the mouth will do it. But to give another person legal permission to kill a person in no way can be equated with privacy. It's about when do you surrender your autonomy to another person. When do you allow that person to make decisions that are irreversible?"

Kelly said: "There are good, quiet, ethical doctors who are out there every day doing this with clean consciences. With medical technology, people can be kept alive longer. There are more treatable diseases, more people in long-term care facilities. We're going to have to come to terms with it. . . . We have to have a social debate on these questions.

"But Kevorkian is the worst-case example of who you would want to see implementing this.

"You add Fieger to it, and it's even worse. He intimidates everyone. His whole purpose is to bully and humiliate the other parties. He's not addressing any of the germane issues."

What if Jack Kevorkian were Marcus Welby and his lawyer were Robert Redford?

"It would be a totally different debate. The Legislature is just like everybody else; they deal with what they're given.

"I doubt you would have the same law on the books."

Chapter Forty-Four
The Right Credentials

"People say, 'Well, you're just a pathologist.' My specialty is death. And if not a pathologist, who? Would you have a pediatrician do it? Or let's get more absurd. What if I was a urologist? Could I help only men end their lives?"
—Jack Kevorkian (1993) ❏

"Doctors do this all the time," Jack Kevorkian told Ron Rosenbaum. "It's just done in the shadows."

Respectable doctors did it all the time, John Kelly said.

Dr. Murray Levin confirmed that. Levin, Kevorkian's old colleague at Pontiac General, was a respectable doctor. He was an official with the Oakland County Medical Society, which in 1989 rejected Kevorkian's initial advertisement for obiatric services. When Janet Adkins died, Levin told the press that Kevorkian had crossed the line.

When I interviewed Levin in his cluttered office at the end of his busy day of seeing patients, Levin told me that Kevorkian's very public crusade was making things difficult for respectable doctors. Some of those doctors, Levin volunteered, occasionally hastened the demise of patients in hopeless straits by giving them lethal doses of pain medication.

"This is done," Levin said. "I don't know how much it's done. These deaths are not advertised, they're not talked about, they're not emphasized. You can understand the uproar, you know, just from the pro-lifers. It's something that's got to be handled between the doctor and the family—and the patient if they're competent."

I asked Levin if Kevorkian was just being more honest by assisting openly in suicides.

"He probably is, in a sense, but it's something that has caused so much publicity. The publicity itself interferes with the process. It's something that's so personal, and it should be handled very quietly."

When Kevorkian assists in a suicide, Levin said, "it's done outside of the mainstream. Of course, he can't do it in any other way. Doctors are doing it in a hospital setting, under people who have the right credentials and the right circumstances."

Doctor-assisted death was nothing new, Levin said. In the 1960s, when Levin had just started his practice, a doctor he knew helped a terminally ill neighbor die. The stricken woman could hardly breathe because disease had so weakened her respiratory system.

The family begged the doctor to end the suffering of the woman, who was unconscious and on a respirator. The doctor gave her a shot of morphine and she died, Levin said.

"I think others do it," he told me. "The intent is to relieve anxiety or pain or suffering. As a by-product, the patients happen to get respiratory depression and die. Somewhat different from Jack's, but it's a direct effect.

"It's done, and that's why he's caused doctors a lot of trouble, a great deal of apprehension. This atmosphere is now charged. It's brought in all this assisted suicide business, and made doctors very frightened of legal consequences that shouldn't be there."

Levin spoke of another case: A close friend of a doctor was in a car accident, suffered severe head injuries and became a vegetable. The victim's wife and two children got together with the victim's doctor, and they all agreed to accelerate the death by giving extra morphine.

"It was the right thing," Levin said. "That's what I would want to have done to me under those circumstances. There was no hope for any recovery, he had irreversible brain damage. Yet he could, with tube feedings, have gone on for a very long time."

In another case he knew personally, the wife of an acquaintance of Levin entered the hospital.

"She came in with a severe stroke, irreversible. She was through. She could breathe and her blood pressure was maintained, but nothing above that level, no mental activity. Totally stroked out, no hope for recovery. The kids lived out of town. They had families, they had activities. There was no point in waiting around God knows how long for the inevitable to occur. So they did this—the family and her doctor. They gave a morphine drip to allay anxiety, and of course she was in a coma, there was no anxiety. It was death by appointment, so the families could go back to their lives."

I asked Levin about the ethical distinction between the acts of respectable doctors he described and what Kevorkian had done.

"The ethical part blurs. Our position years ago was much clearer: We don't go out killing people. But it's done in the circumstances I have talked about. It's just accelerating the inevitable. And that's probably unethical from our point of view, but doctors do it. Our Hippocratic Oath says you don't do this. But some doctors come to the belief that just to let people suffer till the normal inevitable circumstance is a disservice. But doctors don't say that publicly, they say it privately within the confines of the family, because people misinterpret this. When it gets out into the public, we get people who believe in life at all costs. But they haven't seen the suffering that can go with a tragedy, with terribly ill people."

The backlash Kevorkian created—and the new Michigan law passed to stop him—had made doctors afraid, Levin said.

"If I were to give someone 30 sleeping pills, if they took all 30 they wouldn't die from it, they'd get a good sleep. But if they took them with alcohol, they could kill themselves. I could be accused of assisted suicide because I gave them the pills. . . . So now I'm a little more reluctant to do these things."

Requests for aid in dying were rare, Levin said. Much more common were demands by family members for costly treatments to prolong the lives of brain-dead relatives.

"Jack's problems are minuscule compared to the problems that I face every day. . . . Usually what happens is there's three out of the four children who say 'Look, it's time nature took its course, you know, let's withhold treatment,' and the fourth one, who usually lives in California and who probably had some estrangement with the family, says 'I want everything done.' So we do everything. That is a huge problem. It's an economic problem. Here I'm saving hopelessly ill patients."

He told of one case where two sons said goodbye and left their brain-dead mother but her daughter refused to give up.

"I'd talk to her every Sunday when I made rounds. I'd say, 'Would you like to live like this?' She said, 'No, I wouldn't like to live like this.' 'Then why are you letting your mother live like this?' 'I just have to do this for her.' She had some psychological need. So she's in our intensive care costing about a quarter of a million bucks for six or eight weeks.

"That occurs every day probably in every hospital 10 times a day. And that's a huge problem."

CHAPTER FORTY–FIVE
THE HANDLER

"I could put him on a book tour tomorrow and he could make a million dollars in less than six months! And he won't do it!"
—*Geoffrey Fieger* ❏

Geoffrey Fieger was reckless, but he always seemed to land on his feet. Always ready for a fight, never worried about choosing words judiciously, Fieger sprinted confidently across mine fields in his personal and professional life.

On April 22, 1993, we talked for nearly three hours in his office. For the first two hours, he spoke mostly about himself—his youthful love of rock and roll, his mature love of the law, his legal record of Ty Cobb proportions, even what kind of governor he'd make. Running for office had crossed his mind, he said. Name recognition would be a plus. Of course, "They would say, look at this guy, equanimity isn't his strong point, which is true. They would say he's not well-suited for politics, because he tends to be explosive, which is also true." But, he said, "I would bring intelligence and creativity" and "I would get things done. And I wouldn't sell out to anybody."

With few exceptions, Fieger said, current officeholders, including Michigan Governor John Engler, were "wormy, undistinguished people."

"I'm not saying I'm a great man or anything, but the best and the brightest are not going into politics. . . . There's an overwhelming abundance of really just stupid people who are clearly unqualified to do anything and who are making their living either getting their palms greased or feeding off the public trough or both, like Engler, who I find to be not only undistinguished but unqualified to do anything."

I asked Fieger if he might run as a Libertarian.

"*No!*" He laughed. "I'm not a Libertarian! I think those guys are nuts, too. They go off the deep end. They say we can't have income taxes and stuff like that, too."

I asked him if he was a liberal.

"Labels are for stupid people," he said. "Frankly, on this issue, on the Kevorkian issue, I'm a conservative. If a true conservative means the pre-eminence of the individual over government intrusion, if it means less government, not more, if it means that, then this is truly a conservative issue. . . .

"I've got no bones to pick with anyone. I don't care if you're a religious fanatic as long as you don't try to impose your religious views on everybody else."

But the religious fanatics, Fieger warned, were trying to do just that on assisted suicide.

"What the Kevorkian issue is about is an ongoing development in this country of an attempt to impose a theocracy on the United States. . . . When you got Jerry Falwell, when you got these guys trying to take over the Republican Party, when you got the Lynn Millses, and you got what happened here in Lansing making assisted suicide a crime for no reason other than these religious fanatics who want it to be a crime, because nobody got murdered, everybody did exactly what they wanted to do and it was totally justified in every one of the cases. . . ."

If Right to Life were concerned about suicide, Fieger had a suggestion: "Tomorrow ban handguns. You would find a significant decrease in suicides. One hundred to 200 Americans a week blow their brains out. If you really wanted to stop suicide."

I asked Fieger if he believed there was any rational non-religious opposition. He guffawed, and called Yale Kamisar a "shaman."

Kamisar, Fieger said, reasons "that because historically there's always been a prohibition against suicide and that society has the right to . . . make you suffer, society therefore has the right to enforce a ban against assisted suicide, and therefore a ban against assisting a suicide passes constitutional muster for those reasons.

"Maybe. But it's not acceptable." Fieger laughed. "Maybe. *So what*?" he screamed.

"Obviously there's nothing in the Constitution that says anything about abortion. We protected it under the catch-all of the First Amendment. . . . Roe versus Wade made a clearly unprotected right protected . . . by creating the legal fiction of the penumbra of the right to privacy. That is the way you protect this right also.

"I agree with Kamisar that there's nothing constitutionally defective about a law outlawing assisted suicide or abortion for that matter. . . . But certain things must be protected against lunatics. And these lunatics will inveigle themselves into our lives and deaths and they'll make us suffer. We are less than animals. I mean, no logical person can possibly say that a mentally competent dying adult is entitled to less beneficence than an animal!"

Who should qualify for this service? I asked.

"Kevorkian has set forth the most assiduous criteria that anyone could suggest. It's obviously a medical decision. . . .

"This society celebrates your right to say I'm having a bad day, go down to the gun store, blow my brains out. We don't raise an eyebrow about that, and we won't do anything to stop you. But if you say I'm dying from a disease, I want to go to the end, get everything out of life and then when life has lost its meaning—and I can't pick up the gun—I would like some assistance to end my suffering, society says 'Well, no, we can't do that because, you know, we'll be killing children and then, you know'. . ."

The Slippery Slope.

"That's a lie. That's a bullshit lie. Hey. Do doctors have the right to prescribe medication? Absolutely. Are drugs a bane on society? Are they fucking ruining this society? Absolutely. Do doctors abuse the right to prescribe drugs? Absolutely. *Does that mean we take it away from them? No!!!*

"Do doctors make decisions regarding life and death every day that we never blink at? Kidney dialysis. Not nearly enough kidney dialysis machines to go around. Every hospital has its own criteria for who gets 'em and who doesn't. You get 'em you live, you don't get 'em you don't. OK? Anybody say anything about that? *No!*

"Heart transplants, kidney transplants, lung transplants—It's a gift of life or death. Who decides?" Doctors are bribed for organs, Fieger said. "That happens all the time. And the criteria are all different in every hospital. OK? Do we change that? *No! So what's the problem with this?* . . .

"I mean, Martha Ruwart, she was going to die. Do you need to be a brain scientist to know that she had a right to decide? No!"

Fieger said that, except for Marjorie Wantz, every patient Kevorkian treated was terminally ill, including Janet Adkins. Though Adkins's death wasn't imminent, "she had the worst fatal disease I can imagine, losing your mind, and then losing every bodily system you have."

Eventually, our conversation turned to Jack Kevorkian himself.

I asked Fieger how he thought Kevorkian had managed to become famous.

"Because he's a great man. . . . That doesn't mean he's not a son of a bitch, that doesn't mean he doesn't have major character flaws. But . . . this guy is one of the real bright guys I've ever met in my entire life. . . . There is a certain quality in great people that Kevorkian has. Maybe it's that son-of-a-bitch quality, maybe it's those weird quirky things that allow him to take the stances that he takes, because I would be much more self-protective. Would I be prepared to die in jail the way he is prepared? *No!* No, definitely not. It takes somebody like him to do this.

"Do you understand that if Derek Humphry or the Hemlock Society was still the only one proselytizing this issue, we wouldn't be here talking about it, you wouldn't be writing a book, and nothing would have been done?

"Would we be better off not having a law against assisted suicide and having it still done in the shadows and have Kevorkian never having existed? Clearly not. He's done nothing to hurt the issue. If anybody says that, they're crazy. . . ."

Fieger said Kevorkian's qualities were "probably not the best qualities to have in interpersonal relationships, but they are qualities that allow people to rise above the rest of us.

"He's a zealot in his own way. . . . He's uncompromising in his position, he does not give. He's got a great deal of courage. Could some of that courage be foolishness? Yes. He's got a childlike innocence about him . . .

"He's a very good person. He's the most honest person I've ever met. I mean, I'm talking honest, I mean, brutally honest. And he's right. *That's like the bottom line, he's just right.* . . . There isn't any debate, and everybody knows it. . . .

"He's a *real good guy.* I mean, he's a wonderful friend. . . . He's challenging intellectually. I love talking to him. His knowledge far exceeds this issue. If anybody thinks he's some kind of morose guy who is consumed by death, they're just crazy. He's not at all. He's fun to be with. I mean, he likes women. I mean, he likes girls; we like looking at girls. . . .

"I don't know where they get these caricatures of Jack as somebody strange. They must be watching a couple of news snippets, because he's not at all like that, really. . . . He makes me laugh, and I find him very easy to be with. Except when he is going off and he's got to do what he's got to do—then he's an immovable force. And at that point I want to strangle his turkey neck. At that point I never want to see him again. I want to take a baseball bat and thump his head in. Not that he's saying something wrong, but he's just refusing to look at another side of it that would make him more palatable.

"The reason I've become his spokesman is because he's become the issue himself, and therefore it's unseemly for him to have to defend not only the issue but himself. Also, when pushed, he becomes very, very rigid, strident. And in the technology of today they use the sound bites that make him appear to be other than he is and make him appear unflattering. . . .

"I know more about communicating what he's really saying than he does because he's involved too much in it. . . . That happens to be one of my talents. So like it or not, for better or worse, I have gotten him kicking and screaming to the point he's at. He's not in jail. I think if any other lawyer'd ever handled him he'd be in jail right now, and this thing would not have gotten as far as it did. We were lucky to find each other in that respect. We're a very, very good match. We're much more alike than we are different. . . ."

I observed that some people would find it funny to imagine Geoffrey Fieger as the voice of restraint.

"Even when I'm strident, I'm in total control of what I'm doing. He's not. . . . The hardest thing I've ever had to do is to convince Jack that he is not a public relations genius. . . .

"At first it was extremely hard. He wouldn't accept anything. And it's come to the point almost that I said, 'Jack, I don't care what you think, we're not going to do this.' Because he understands that I've put myself on the line for him, too. And I have as much to lose in terms of the issue as him."

So that's the true test for him? I asked Fieger. He's got to know that you're going to be there for him, because a lot of people haven't been?

"Oh, yeah. I don't talk to him a lot, but I would guess that just from my experience with him, because somebody must have hurt this guy bad at some point."

Why do you say that? I asked Fieger.

"Because it's not natural to be as untrusting and as suspicious as he is. . . . I can't explain it myself, because he's literally adored by his two sisters, who are like mother hens around him. And he absolutely trusts them. And from as much as I can tell, he was his parents' favorite, too. So maybe his attitude is that of a spoiled child. I don't know. ..."

Fieger said Kevorkian was "very, very creative."

"We're sitting in court once. He takes two pens, and he can write a sentence the correct way, and then write its mirror image backwards with his left hand. ...I said, 'Man, Jack, that's scary.'"

Painting, movie-making, sports cap inventing, limerick-writing—these were all testaments to Kevorkian's creativity. And he was a heck of an engineer, too: "You should see the updated real versions of the Mercy Machine. ...Those are technological marvels."

Noting Kevorkian's many failed projects, Fieger said:

"One of his worst qualities is he's a quitter. .... This issue is very unusual for him in terms of his life. In fact, it's unique, because up to this time Jack, whenever he met resistance, quit. Now that's a common trait for most people, frankly. Maybe it's his old age that he just said, 'I'm gonna finally do something in life.'"

Fieger said Kevorkian's personality also figured into the famous Hugh Gale "typo."

"Normally people would just throw the goddamned piece of paper away and start again. But not Jack. He's too cheap. And this was like an intellectual game for him. .... He figured out exact words to put in there that fit it, just as a mental challenge to him."

Kevorkian changed the document "solely for himself. I mean, who's gonna know? I mean, if Hugh Gale really did say that, I mean, who's gonna know?"

Also, Fieger said, Kevorkian's attention sometimes wandered.

"He can absent-mindedly put things down that aren't exactly right. That happens regularly with Jack." In fact, Fieger told me, *Free Press* columnist Bob Talbert recently had warned him that Jack regularly had been leaving important documents in copiers at a Royal Oak copy center.

I recalled that a few weeks earlier Kevorkian couldn't answer a question I posed him over the phone about the Janet Adkins case.

"I think I'm getting Alzheimer's," he joked.

At least, I thought it was a joke.

❏ ❏ ❏

Fieger told me Neal Nicol and Margo Janus would not be present at Kevorkian's next assisted suicide, since it was now clearly illegal.

And Fieger told me the promise to hold off until after the ACLU suit was settled was Fieger's idea.

"It was a promise I made without consulting him, and I convinced him that was the best way to go. . . . I said 'Jack, you're gonna do that, you're not gonna betray me, 'cause how long do you have to wait, I mean, not very long.' . . ."

In fact, it had been nearly seven weeks since Fieger made that vow—and it would be another four weeks before Kevorkian broke it. Many of Kevorkian's cases had not lasted that long from initial contact through death—Martie Ruwart's, for one. What was happening to people who were seeking Doctor Death's help now? Kevorkian had always said the suffering patient came first. What was he telling people who contacted him? That he couldn't help them with their agony because his lawyer had made a promise to hold off?

Fieger commented that the ACLU had better hurry up its case.

"I will be eating a lot of crow if they make it too much longer because I promise you: He ain't gonna wait forever."

CHAPTER FORTY–SIX
THE CHRISTMAS PRESENT

*"The Legislature and some of these groups that
are fostering this law banning assisted suicide,
they're ignoring the ultimate reality, that death
occurs to everyone here. Death is really the only
reality, because everything else is just perception
and discussion."*
—*Hemlock attorney Daniel Devine* ❒

The Hugh Gale case, a matter of screaming headlines in late February, almost had vanished from the news by the time I visited Carl Marlinga on April 26.

In his airy office in Mount Clemens, the soft-spoken Marlinga told me he was not going to press charges against Jack Kevorkian. Cheryl Gale's testimony had exonerated Doctor Death.

"She's got the least to gain or lose from a false version of events," Marlinga told me, "and she's very persuasive in her testimony. My own subjective view of things is that she accurately remembers the way that things happened, and Doctor Kevorkian just had a terrible glitch in remembrance to write down things the way he wrote them down the first time."

Marlinga said Cheryl Gale told him under oath that her husband's discomfort after getting the carbon monoxide was just like his usual emphysema attacks.

"Maybe it was the fear, maybe it was something else," Marlinga said. "But there wasn't enough time for the carbon monoxide to be the explanation."

Marlinga said he would have brought manslaughter charges if there were any testimony that Hugh Gale said "Take it off" a second time. But failing that, he had no evidence of a crime.

"I have one document that was changed. In one sense the alteration is evidence that somebody is trying to hide what went on. On the other hand there is the innocent explanation that a mistake was made in the writing of the document."

Marlinga admitted:

"I don't have a good explanation for that document. Doctor Kevorkian wrote what he wrote. It was his first impression of the events and therefore probably more believable than the later advice that he got from Neal Nicol and Margo Janus that what he wrote was wrong.

"Those are very tough words to find an explanation for, other than that it happened that way. But you can't build a prosecution on simply one document."

Marlinga said the investigation could always be reopened.

"If Doctor Kevorkian said to somebody else, 'I changed the document only because Neal Nicol insisted I do it, but what I wrote was the accurate way,' then I probably would bring charges," Marlinga said.

At first, Marlinga said, he had trouble believing Document H was for real. He told an assistant: "This document is simply too good. It's too cute. They're something odd about this. Doctor Kevorkian would not write such a damning document about himself."

Marlinga scoffed at Fieger's characterization that Thompson had manipulated him:

"This is part of Fieger's routine, where he just makes things up to suit his own purposes. Geoff Fieger is given to so much exaggeration and hyperbole that I believe he loses credibility because of his antics. I really stopped worrying about Geoff Fieger ever since the time that he put the clown nose on Dick Thompson's picture."

But Marlinga said that he found the man who screamed at him on radio and TV "affable and charming on a personal basis."

Marlinga said he was dismayed that Fieger and Schwartz went to the media right after Gale's death "criticizing me that this was some sort of politically motivated witch hunt, when they knew that . . . my charging Doctor Kevorkian for assisted suicide was not likely. As a lawyer it would be my instinct to try to keep my client out of trouble no matter what, not try to goad the prosecutor into bringing charges."

❏ ❏ ❏

Marlinga had taken depositions from Cheryl Gale and Neal Nicol on March 28 at Geoffrey Fieger's office.

Neal Nicol's deposition confirmed that he was the person who got the gas for Kevorkian's assisted suicides. Marlinga said Right to Life activists had harassed Matheson Gas of Indiana into not selling any more carbon monoxide to Nicol.

Nicol also revealed that it was a half-hour after Gale's death before police were called. When police arrived, no tent was found. It was later determined that a pressure regulator on the valve of the gas tank had been removed. Nicol explained he and Kevorkian didn't want the $200 item to be confiscated.

"The physical evidence at the scene was disturbed," Marlinga noted. "It certainly did raise our level of suspicion."

Nicol's deposition also provided a rare glimpse of Kevorkian's mystery right-hand man—and shed new light on some of the mysteries surrounding Hugh Gale's death.

Marlinga asked Nicol if he and Kevorkian had any contingency plan if a patient requested a halt in a suicide.

"Just common sense," Nicol replied.

"What do you mean by that?"

"That the effects of carbon monoxide toxicity can be reversed if you stop the flow and it just—you know, you allow the oxygen to flow again, and those steps were taken."

"What's your educational background that allows you to know about carbon monoxide effects?"

"I'm an ex-med tech from the service who worked in hospitals for seven years or so after starting in medical technology." Nicol said he had a high school education and "some college."

"You never became precise as to who would do what if he wanted to stop?" Marlinga asked.

"No, no, we didn't become very precise, although he had the option, he had the use of his facilities . . . he certainly had sufficient strength to take off a mask."

Nicol testified that he turned the gas on when Gale was ready and said Gale's request to "Take it off!" referred to the tent, not the mask. "It was hot in there," Nicol reported Gale saying.

Lynn Mills had claimed the signatures of Nicol, Janus and Cheryl Gale verified Kevorkian's account of the death. At Fieger's urging, Nicol confirmed under oath that those at Gale's death all signed only the top part of Document H, indicating their presence, and that Kevorkian wrote and signed the "Procedure" section later.

"Contrary to the lunatic's statement that you are verifying the middle part," Fieger said. "Make it very clear, when a lunatic gets that statement and the lying sacks of shit that they are, they are lying about it."

Marlinga sounded offended: "Anything can be said in the course of a deposition and I'm not here to—"

"I am," Fieger persisted. "If you are going to get this public, I want it to read, 'these lying sacks of shit.' "

"I again will simply ask that we use appropriate language."

"That is appropriate to describe these people."

Marlinga asked why Kevorkian would write "Take it off!" twice. Nicol replied:

"If you want me to tell you what Doctor Kevorkian was thinking, I can't do that." Kevorkian offered no explanation, Nicol said. "I didn't think an explanation was needed. He made a typographical error and he corrected it."

"Except that we are talking about a typographical error four lines long, of course," Marlinga observed.

Fieger responded: "No, we are not. We are talking about a typographical error of one thing. You see, it's the perception, not the reality. If he writes something down, if he stands in front of the world and says assisted suicide is OK, nobody wants to listen to him. But if he writes the words 'Take it off' in error, everybody says that's an exact truth. It's not everybody who says it, only religious lunatics."

Was it Kevorkian who whited out the words? Marlinga asked.

"As far as I know," Nicol answered. "I don't think it was Margo Janus. I believe it was Doctor Kevorkian."

Marlinga asked why Kevorkian didn't rip up the document and start over with a new one.

"Because he is cheap," Fieger replied, "because he is real cheap."

Nicol said that if Kevorkian started fresh, he would have to get the signatures all over again, and "knowing Doctor Kevorkian, I would have to agree with Geoff that it was cheap, it was easy and it was quick."

Fieger asked what Nicol would say to people who say he helped murder Hugh Gale. His answer was cool and understated:

"Well, my reaction is that not having been there, they wouldn't know whether we murdered him or not. Everyone is entitled to their own opinion."

In her deposition, Cheryl Gale told Carl Marlinga that the last six months of her husband's life were terrible.

"It got to the point where he had faced death so many times from these seizures that he wasn't afraid anymore. He would pray not to wake up. He would pray that his body would not bring him back again to go through it over again."

They had talked about suicide often, she said.

"He was very concerned that what he did did not affect me. He talked about a gun, but he didn't know where to get a gun and he said that was too messy and that would be too hard on me."

Cheryl Gale said her husband first brought up Kevorkian in December.

"It was just before Christmas and I said: 'I don't know what to get you . . . what would you like for Christmas?' And he said 'I would like an appointment with Doctor Kevorkian.' "

She testified that her husband told her "God was not keeping him alive, that if God had taken him in his own time, it would have been a long time ago. He said what was keeping him alive was pulmonary machines and the oxygen concentrator and that he couldn't go on with that anymore, that he wanted to go."

Gale said Hugh was so calm the night before his death that he slept the whole night for the first time in years.

"Once he found out that Doctor Kevorkian would help him, a tremendous peace came over him and he was a different person."

She said that when Kevorkian arrived on the morning of February 15, he said to her husband: "You seem to be feeling better today. You are not wheezing. . . . Why don't you wait and give me a call when you are feeling really bad?" But Hugh Gale said: "No. . . . I want to do it today."

Gale said she sat on a chair beside her husband. Hugh took his oxygen canula out of his nose and put the gas mask on. Kevorkian helped him put the elastic behind his head.

"After he pulled the clip, it was a very few seconds that he became very red in the face. . . . He grabbed the arms of his chair and he kind of pushed himself back and he became very red and his face looked sort of puffy. . . . Then he said: 'Take it off, take it off.' I don't know if he had started to go into a seizure or if the gas was causing the lungs to lock, but he acted like he did when he would have these seizures and he had the fear of suffocating. And that is why he said 'Take it off, take it off,' meaning the tent.

"Doctor Kevorkian jumped up immediately and took the tent off of him." With his nasal oxygen back in, her husband slowly came back to normal.

"Doctor Kevorkian said, 'Mister Gale, I know that was very uncomfortable for you. Let's just stop this right now. If you want to I can come back another day.' And I remember his words very clearly in my mind, that Mister Gale said to Doctor Kevorkian: 'Please don't go. Just let me sit for a minute. I don't want you to come back another day. I want to do this. I want to do this today.' "

Cheryl Gale said they sat for 15 to 20 minutes relaxing and talking about other things, and then her husband said to Kevorkian, "OK, let's get on with it," and then Hugh put the mask on again. This time the nasal oxygen stayed: "Doctor Kevorkian said he would have to leave the oxygen on because his lungs were bad.

"It seemed like a very few seconds that he . . . again flushed and turned reddish-blue in the face and he became very rigid and pushed himself back into the chair. And then it was just a few seconds after that his breathing was very short breaths and not rhythmic and then he relaxed. His body relaxed and I knew he was unconscious.

"I waited a few seconds after that and then I had to leave the room because his eyes were still open and I couldn't stay any longer. . . . I went into the kitchen and Margo followed me . . . to see if I was OK and then . . . Margo went back into the living room and I went to the living room doorway and I stood there for a few minutes. And then somebody had closed my husband's eyes . . . Then I went back into the kitchen. I was not there when he took his last breath."

Marlinga noted that Cheryl Gale had told a Roseville police officer who arrived at the scene: "This wasn't supposed to happen like this." Gale replied: "I don't recall saying that, but if I made that statement I was probably referring to what happened after the death and also the way that the police and detectives invaded my home and I felt like I was a hostage in my own home."

Fieger asked her how Lynn Mills's accusations made her feel.

"It made me feel like they believed that I watched my husband being murdered, being murdered. I can't really tell you in words how it made me feel."

CHAPTER FORTY–SEVEN
LOST TREASURES AND ABIDING MYSTERIES

"9. The Mesh Parachute.
8. Clorox Coladas.
7. The Rickety Ladder.
5. The Steel-Bristle Retina Brush.
3. The Tub Toaster.
1. The Popeil Pocket Suicide Machine."
—From David Letterman's "Top Ten Other
Inventions by the Suicide Machine Doctor" ❒

The morning after I saw Marlinga, I was in Geoffrey Fieger's library searching a court file for the lost treasures of Jack Kevorkian's life. When I told Fieger that Marlinga had issued his statement on the Hugh Gale case, Fieger scolded me for not bringing him a copy. Ten minutes later, he came storming in, waving a sheaf of paper, and yelled:

"You're not paying attention!"

He pointed to Marlinga's statement, just received via fax. In it, Marlinga had written that Richard Thompson originally had told Marlinga's chief assistant Joseph Cozzolino that the Hugh Gale document "was found by a neighbor who had rummaged through Nicol's trash."

"A neighbor!" Fieger yelped. "I told you! Thompson just got his fucking ass fucked!" Fieger stomped from room to room, bouncing off secretaries. His arch-enemy had been caught in a lie and Fieger was giddy. "Finally I got somebody with the balls to do something!" he said, referring to Marlinga.

He yelled at the receptionist: "Marlinga just exonerated Kevorkian. I'm going to get a lot of calls from the media today!"

He handed me a copy of his lawsuit against Thompson and Mills and bellowed: "See? Everybody said I was making this all up! See?"

As it turned out, the newspapers and TV noted Marlinga's exoneration of Kevorkian, but did little with the "neighbor" statement. Fieger wasn't swamped by media calls. Later, Richard Thompson gave me his version of his conversation with Cozzolino:

"My statement to him was that this person had been at a neighbor's house and had seen the trash go out. Either I misspoke myself or he misunderstood. I think he misunderstood."

◻ ◻ ◻

In the mini-morality play that centered around the death of Hugh Gale, many questions remained unanswered. So did other mysteries about the life of Jack Kevorkian.

When I first heard about Kevorkian's lost paintings, I didn't realize the magnitude of the loss. But as I learned more about the life of Doctor Death, I came to realize how much was missing from that Royal Oak apartment—and why Kevorkian himself had characterized his life as a failure.

In 1985, Kevorkian put his most valuable possessions into storage at the California Freight Company in Long Beach. They included all 18 of his oil paintings, his electronic organ and harpsichord, a video camera, VCR, stereo, 50 copies each of his diet book and his two books published by Philosophical Library, plus reference books and business correspondence—and two prints and two videotapes of his full-length movie about Handel's *Messiah*.

On September 14, 1990—three months after the death of Janet Adkins had propelled him onto the world stage—Kevorkian requested delivery of the goods. On October 4, representatives of California Freight told him there had been a mixup and the shipment had been sent to Australia. Later, they said his possessions had been lost.

Fieger sued California Freight, but two years were wasted because Fieger filed in Michigan and Michigan courts eventually ruled he should file in California. Fieger did so early in 1993. Officials at California Freight refused to talk about the lost shipment, and the case remained pending.

The movie was about the only topic in his open-book life that Jack Kevorkian steadfastly refused to discuss with anyone. Fieger said Kevorkian had invested his life savings in making it. Why then did he lock it away in a storage facility? Was it another dismal failure? Was it ever shown? Kevorkian refused to say. Cursory checks in Hollywood failed to unearth anyone who knew anything about the project.

Why had Kevorkian turned his back on the movie and his fantastic paintings for five years before trying to retrieve them? Was the explanation as simple as a lack of funds? Or had Jack Kevorkian, upon leaving California, committed a form of demi-suicide, cutting off a large part of himself?

Penumbra Inc.—the corporation Kevorkian had set up in 1976 to produce the movie—continued to file annual reports with the State of Michigan. The latest, filed March 3, 1993, listed among the corporation's assets a motion picture valued at $99,941 and Kevorkian's famous rusty van, valued at $1,689. The van remained parked behind 223 Main Street in Royal Oak. Fieger told me Kevorkian did not want to sell it for fear it would turn into some macabre collector's item, and that Kevorkian would junk it if it finally died.

At the end of our three-hour interview on April 22, Fieger showed me color photographs of Kevorkian's paintings. I was not prepared for their impact. I returned a few days later to rummage through the California Freight files and to get a closer look at the photos of the paintings. The 18 canvases are as bold and strident, as critical and unforgiving, as pointed and dramatic as Kevorkian's own fighting words. They are strikingly well-executed, stark and surreal— and frightening, demented and/or hilarious, depending on one's point of view.

The paintings are full of disembodied organs and limbs, skulls, skeletons, ghostly faces, blood and guts. Many of the faces and figures are "Everyman" representations, resembling the kind of theater poster art that was popular circa 1960. Several works feature duality: split figures, divided faces. Cannibalism is a theme in several works, and snakes appear in a few.

Art critics and psychologists might say much more, if they could see the works. Given Kevorkian's notoriety—and the morbid nature of the paintings—their release would cause a sensation.

Fieger knew full well their value, at least monetarily.

"I told Jack if he made reproductions of these, I could sell them at an art auction for $100,000 apiece!" he told me. "But he won't do it. He doesn't care about money."

Fieger believed he had the only illustrations of the lost paintings. But in the California Freight case file I discovered a flyer announcing a 1980 exhibition of the paintings sponsored by the Midland Arts Council in Midland, Michigan.

When my colleague Tom Ferguson inquired at the arts council, the staff was surprised and intrigued. Once slides of the paintings were found in the council's files—apparently along with Kevorkian's own written commentaries on his works—the council director started to sound as if she possessed a ticking H-bomb.

After a month of repeated inquiries, director Maria Ciski finally told Ferguson: "I don't think it would be appropriate to open the files at this point." She refused to share Kevorkian's commentaries or even send copies of press releases announcing the exhibit.

"I'm going to leave this file closed, and that is it," she said.

CHAPTER FORTY–EIGHT
ALL POWER TO THE DOCTORS

*"Ethicists don't belong in this decision. The doc-
tor can philosophize as well as any theologian
can, but a theologian can't know medicine like a
doctor. It takes training and experience."*
—Jack Kevorkian (1990) ❏

Howard Brody, MD, longtime chair of the Michigan State Medical
Society bioethics committee, sat in a very cluttered office at Michigan
State University. A huge string of books on medical ethics lined a
shelf behind him.

Since June 4, 1990, Brody told me, his ethics committee had
talked about little but assisted suicide. Kevorkian's crusade, he said,
had been a profound revelation to doctors.

"The public doesn't have much confidence in us. There's a feeling
that if I put my death in the hands of doctors in the hospitals, I'll
lose control, and anything I want will be trampled on."

Patients' rights to choose treatment had been accepted in medical
ethics for 20 years, Brody said. The problem remained in getting
doctors' practice to conform with the ethical standard.

George Annas of Boston University's School of Medicine told
Time magazine that Kevorkian "is a total indictment of the way we
treat dying patients in hospitals and at home. We don't treat them
well, and they know it."

But Brody said Kevorkian's alternative to standard medical treatment of death did not necessarily heighten patient autonomy.

"One of the most fascinating and distressing things about the
approval rating that Doctor Kevorkian gets is the lack of recognition
of the underlying theme running through everything he does: That
this is all power to the doctors.

"If Doctor Kevorkian went on TV and said: My mission, my crusade, is 'All power to the doctors,' I don't think he'd get the time of
day from anybody. And yet when he says 'I'm Doctor Death,' everybody says: Great, this guy's a savior. I don't think people are looking
under the surface to see how incredibly medicocentric is everything

that Kevorkian has always proposed throughout his whole career, and what he's now proposing."

Brody said decisions on tough questions of medical ethics were best made by involving many disciplines, but Kevorkian adamantly opposed any involvement by non-physicians.

"As far as he's concerned, anybody else doing medical ethics, well, it's some kind of religion or mumbo-jumbo, it's not rational or logical—only doctors are real scientists.

"When I see that side of Kevorkian so prominent in everything he writes and I see the public opinion polls, I just can't rationalize those two things."

But, I pointed out, Kevorkian always said he was only doing what the patient wanted.

"That's what he says, and in that regard he's bringing a value of patients' rights front and center. But when you look at how he proposes to implement that, what structure he wants to create, it's necessary to get one step below the rhetoric.

"He's basically saying that doctors should decide what they're going to do. He would say the law has absolutely nothing to say about medical practice. In his framework, doctors are really not accountable to anybody outside of medicine for what they do. One on one, we're accountable to our patients, but in terms of societal accountability, it's zero.

"The other thing I think is really rather strange is how he described in detail his plan for obitiatry. He has these forms, and it supposedly is this foolproof system; there's going to be no abuses if you fill out these forms. Well, the forms are essentially blank spaces. There's no indication of a protocol for how you are going to evaluate patients or accept them. The only thing going on is that people who have certain kinds of degrees after their name are going to determine this based on their expert wisdom. So if a psychiatrist looks at you and says you're sane, the fact that he had psychiatrist, MD, after his name is what makes that OK. Whether he figured that out by tea leaves or whether he figured that out by doing a three-hour interview or whether he figured it out by doing a brain scan is irrelevant.

"There's almost no appreciation for the actual technique of finding out something and almost naive faith that, if you've got the right letters after your name, whatever you say will be true."

But, I pointed out, Kevorkian constantly called doctors hypocrites.

"That fits, too. He's saying to doctors the reason you're a bunch of hypocrites is because you have let other people in society tell you what to do. Now if you were all my kind of doctors you would be making these decisions on your own ... The real bone he has to pick with the doctors is they are turning over the control of medicine to people outside medicine."

To get away from being under the control of bad doctors, Brody maintained, Kevorkian asked patients to put their trust in true doctors like him.

CHAPTER FORTY-NINE
THE COURT OF TRUE JUSTICE

Ron Rosenbaum: "I think you have a self-defeating harshness toward the rest of the world."
Jack Kevorkian: "Absolutely. You're right. My dad used to say that." ❏

Judge Alice Gilbert wouldn't allow Jack Kevorkian to invoke his intellectual superstars in her courtroom. Perhaps no judge ever would. But Kevorkian submitted his defense anyway—to *Health Care Weekly Review*.

The small Detroit area weekly published an "Exclusive: A final statement from Jack Kevorkian, MD" on April 27, 1992. An editor's note explained Kevorkian delivered the statement to the paper on April 22. At the time he was awaiting trial for the deaths of Sherry Miller and Marjorie Wantz, and he figured on being in jail soon, said George Adams, the paper's publisher.

Kevorkian told Adams that his pledge of non-cooperation with the authorities would be total: He would take no food and no water.

"I've always wondered what it would be like to starve to death," Kevorkian told Adams.

An editor's note accompanying the "final statement" explained: "The opinions expressed are those of the author, and do not necessarily reflect the views of this newspaper."

But Adams had never concealed his support for Kevorkian, and the accompanying headline was something less than objective:

"Great Minds Rule from the Grave:

"Dr. Kevorkian Is Right"

The jeremiad began: "The following testimony in the Court of Reason and True Justice is in response to authorities who oppose medically-assisted suicide for agonized and incapacitated human beings."

There followed a series of quotations from Albert Einstein, each targeted specifically to Kevorkian's enemies. Kevorkian fantasized Einstein lecturing to Governor Engler and Senator Dillingham about tyrannical government. Einstein scolded "those who control the communications media" on how control by "private capitalists" brainwashed citizens. Einstein lectured Archbishop Maida on the superiority of scientific to religious morality. Einstein berated the medical profession.

Kevorkian invoked other great Western minds—Abraham Lincoln, Montesquieu, Voltaire, Samuel Johnson, Edmund Burke, Tacitus, Alexis De Tocqueville, Justice Felix Frankfurter, Mark Twain and Thomas Jefferson, and of course St. Thomas More.

For "the poltroons of the Michigan State Medical Board, of the Michigan State and county medical societies, of the editorial boards of 'prestigious' medical journals, and all the craven sophists called 'ethicists,' " Kevorkian cited the doctor-assisted suicides of Sigmund Freud, King George V, and Dr. William Harvey, the physician who discovered blood circulation, and quoted Dr. Walter Alvarez, a leading physician of the early 20th Century, who favored euthanasia.

This all served as a preface to "Dr. Jack Kevorkian's final statement and unalterable position."

That also began with a quote from Einstein on how scientists should refuse to cooperate with reactionary politicians. Finally, the writer himself spoke his mind:

> Now, I, Dr. Jack Kevorkian, am being repeatedly called before one of those evil committees facetiously dubbed "courts of justice." I have infringed neither a duly enacted statute nor a *secular* moral tenet. I am a blameless citizen steadfastly committed to the re-implementation and unconditional preservation of the basic human right of any mentally competent adult to avoid and curtail intolerable and irremediable pain and incapacitation—reimplementation, because such a right was available and guaranteed in the more genuine democracy of ancient Hippocratic Greece.
>
> Because I know that Einstein was much wiser than are any of the critics who ruthlessly operate those evil committees, I will heed his counsel. His warning, together with the illustrious examples of Thoreau, Gandhi, Martin Luther King Jr., Nelson Mandela, Susan B. Anthony and Margaret Sanger, reinforces the wisdom of my own conscience in unflinching determination to refuse to cooperate in any way in socially criminal behavior mandated by

our cryptic totalitarian state.

Therefore, I will obey no injunction with regard to my humanitarian intent and actions, especially one that was maliciously inflicted by means of character-assassinating vituperation spewed by a morally outraged Alice Gilbert. Such conduct in a so-called judge is unseemly at best.

Furthermore, I will not cooperate in any trial, be it before a legitimate petit jury or a sham monstrously orchestrated by a no less morally outraged prosecutor who calls it a grand jury.

Finally, in accord with the intent of the Nuremberg Tribunal cited by Einstein, I now invoke the superior authority of my own affronted conscience and its dictated sense of justice. I repeat: I will not obey or respect any statute, injunction, or arbitrary regulation which interdicts my obligation as a physician and as a rational and compassionate human being. My contempt for the farcical "justice" ineptly mimicked by Gilbert, Kuhn, Sheehy, and O'Brien will sooner or later—and most likely sooner—be vindicated by history as the verdict of *true* justice. If the travesty concocted by Dillingham, Ciaramitaro, and all their socially immoral co-conspirators in the Michigan Senate passes through an intimidated House and is signed into law by an equally immoral governor, I will never obey it, no matter what the consequences.

My position and attitude are not the results of naive egoism or self-righteous megalomania. It is only by default that I am in the vanguard of unarguable right, that I alone represent the feckless intellectuals whom Einstein addressed. By default, because even though many of them know and only privately (and timidly) admit that I'm right, not one authoritative so-called intellectual in the country dares speak out forcefully enough to matter.

Yet, I am not really alone; for I have the rare honor of representing a host of truly intellectual giants—indeed, geniuses—now dead, who did speak out courageously. I am honored that from their graves they once again speak and act through me in a way that surely does matter and will make a difference. Heretofore, brute coercive power made it easy for despotic authorities to toy with Dr. Jack Kevorkian and amuse themselves by vilifying and slandering him. But things have changed. From here on you benighted inquisitors will have to contend with the invincible mentality and superior moral character of the illustrious personages quoted above who are testifying posthumously in my behalf.

Go ahead, all you "judges": try to argue with Thomas Jefferson, Justice Frankfurter, and with King George V and the Royal family. See if you can do it without looking as ridiculous as you really are. Go ahead, governor, and all you prosecutors, senators, and newspaper editors: you, too, try to convince the Royal family, and then argue with Mark Twain (what a mismatch!). And all you "benevolent" doctors controlling the AMA, the AOA, the medical societies, and the journals, go ahead: argue with Doctors Harvey, Freud and Alvarez (if you dare). And I dare Archbishop Maida to try arguing with Saint Thomas More. If it's merely a matter of opinion, whose would be the most authoritative? Would the Archbishop dare to answer?

From here on, any spiteful attack or purposeful injustice and calumny inflicted on me is inflicted on the esteemed memory and legacy of these intellectual giants. But then, that would be of concern and shameful only to an honorable individual.

Einstein ended his short letter of 1953 with this terse warning: "If enough people are ready to take this grave step (of non-cooperation with obvious injustice) they will be successful. If not, then the intellectuals of this country deserve nothing better than the slavery which is intended for them."

The slavery intended for me is here. I will not submit to it. As a freedom-loving physician, scientist and ordinary man, I will take the recommended grave step and break it—or die trying!

V

ACCEPTANCE

"I wake to sleep, and take my waking slow.
"I feel my fate in what I cannot fear.
"I learn by going where I have to go."

—Theodore Roethke, "The Waking"

CHAPTER FIFTY
THE UNDERTAKER

"For some, Doctor Kevorkian seems quite magical, a true angel of death. . . . By going to this man, they may be saying, 'I've put myself in this wonderful person's hands and now I don't have to go through any more of this pain of deciding whether to live or die."
—*Psychologist Dr. Joseph Richman* ❐

To my great surprise, State Senator Fred Dillingham looked like a grown-up Beaver Cleaver.

Geoffrey Fieger's number one religious fanatic didn't have the slicked-back hair of a fundamentalist preacher nor the smooth-talking jive of a glib politician. He had a soft voice, an easy manner, and a firm handshake. And he had a large corner office across from the Capitol full of sunlight and photographs of children.

When I asked Dillingham why the public supported Kevorkian's position, he rejected my premise.

"The media seems to perceive that there's strong-based public support," he said. "What they don't take into account is there's an awful lot of people who don't write letters to the editor, who don't participate in talk shows but are quietly very conservative on this issue—and they show up at the polls."

But what about the scientific surveys?

"You can find a scientific poll to show anything," Dillingham scoffed. "Liars participate in polls and polls lie."

If there were so much public support, he wondered, why hadn't the other side mounted a campaign for a ballot proposal?

"Very frankly, if the public is so supportive, that's what they ought to do," he challenged.

I asked the man who had wanted Kevorkian's lights punched out why he felt so strongly about the issue.

"I have a very strong conviction that the role of government is to preserve, protect and enhance the quality of life. I took an oath to follow that conviction, and not create public policy that would sanction the taking of human life."

Dillingham said he was consistently pro-life, opposing abortion and the death penalty. As a Republican, he stuck out like a sore thumb, he said, in voting for pre-natal programs, health care, funding for hospices and other "liberal" causes.

"I happen to feel that pro-life is a liberal position," he explained.

"People who disagree with me call me names, attack me as being a religious zealot—I don't know what that is—identify me as part of the religious right—I don't know what that is—and apparently attack me for having some belief in a Creator. I am not about to tell them whether I am a person who is active in any particular church. And I've never had them check. They have made that assumption and created the perception, which tells me that they're all smoke. And unfortunately that's what has characterized an awful lot of this debate, because the facts don't support what they're doing."

Dillingham said he was raised Catholic, but was no longer active in the church.

"I laugh when they accuse me of being part of the religious Right or of being a pawn of the pope or the bishop, because frankly I told all the bishops and also told [former Detroit Archbishop Edmund] Szoka on the front page of the *Detroit News* that he was a horse's rear because they weren't active enough in helping me fight abortion in the Legislature."

So what business was it of the government, I asked, repeating Don McNeil's question. To my surprise, Dillingham didn't take me down the Slippery Slope.

"Suicide I think is the ultimate act of depression," he said. "If we are aware that someone is about to take their own life, I think government has the responsibility to do what they can to save the life. I've talked to many people who've attempted suicide and they're darn happy that someone stepped in and prevented them from doing away with themselves. ...

"If you told me that the pain had reached a point where your life was worthless, I would say: No, I think that there is some value to your life. I feel I have some responsibility to add something to your life, not to agree with you that your life is worthless and should come to an end.

"Government has to have a constructive role, not a destructive role, in working with its citizens. And if we start sanctioning in public law suicide and assisted suicide, then what we're doing is we're saying that government has taken on a destructive role."

Besides his Catholic upbringing, there were some personal experiences that Dillingham said contributed to his views.

On several occasions, Fieger and Kevorkian both had confided to me, cackling about the irony of it all, that Dillingham was an undertaker.

Dillingham told me his father was the funeral director for the small town of Fowlerville, near Lansing, so Dillingham grew up in the business. In high school, he ran an ambulance service. He said he dropped his mortician's license in 1989.

"Being brought up in close personal touch with death is probably giving me a greater respect for life," he said, explaining that he'd seen most of his friends go through the suffering and grief that are part of dying and death. "Being exposed to that part of life always reminded me of the importance of living out each day, and being thankful for that.

"And there's another personal thing too. When I was getting involved in public office I had a special daughter born to me. And that has given me an even greater appreciation for life, because she is severely physically and mentally impaired. For the last several years I've raised her basically as a single parent. That has enhanced my feeling for appreciating life. . . . It makes me an advocate."

Dillingham concluded: "This is a very, very important debate. . . . I think we need to talk about this. And I think in talking about it we may reach social understandings, social growth that doesn't really need government's intervention."

CHAPTER FIFTY-ONE
BACK IN BUSINESS

*"It's unstoppable. It may not happen in my
lifetime, but my opponents are going to lose."*
—*Jack Kevorkian (1993)* ❐

Eighty-seven days after Martha Ruwart died, Detroit police went to a
real estate office on the east side of the city and found Jack Kevorkian,
Geoffrey Fieger and a corpse.

The dead man was wearing a mask with a tube attached to two
tanks of carbon monoxide.

Police arrested Kevorkian and took him to 1300 Beaubien, the
cavernous, musty police headquarters. They fingerprinted him and
held him for two hours. He and Fieger passed the time watching a
basketball game on TV. Then police let them go.

So much for the confrontation of liberty versus tyranny that
Fieger long had predicted. For months, Fieger had conjured up the
image of Richard Thompson putting Dr. Kevorkian in chains and
throwing him into a prison cell, where Doctor Death would starve
himself to death.

The death of Ronald Mansur was more like an elaborate game of
hide-and-seek. Mansur, the cancer-stricken man who became
Kevorkian's 16th suicide patient, lived in Southfield, in the heart of
Thompson's turf, Oakland County. But Mansur died in his dingy real
estate office in Detroit, in Wayne County, the territory of Prosecutor
John O'Hair, who had looked the other way after Jack Miller's death.
Mansur's death, on a Sunday morning, was the first Kevorkian-aided
suicide in Detroit—a city in which juries are notoriously sympathetic to criminal defendants.

Kevorkian had vowed he would openly defy the assisted suicide
ban. But Fieger made it sound as if Kevorkian had been an innocent
bystander at Mansur's death. Fieger created an air of mystery about
who supplied the gas, who turned it on and even whether Kevorkian
had been counseling Mansur. There were no videotapes, no letters
from the deceased.

"Mister Mansur, as I understand it, turned on the carbon monoxide canisters, put on the mask, unclipped the mask, and died," Fieger told reporters. "As simple as that."

Fieger said Mansur, 54, was so crippled by lung cancer that bones in his arms were breaking apart. To dull the pain, Mansur carried a morphine pump with him wherever he went.

"He was in hell," said Donna Cady, a longtime friend. Cady told *Time* magazine: "I know that when he put that mask on his face he had his finger sticking up in the air to say: Screw you all for the laws that made me suffer like this."

But how could Mansur possibly have died unaided? He was too weak to carry the heavy tanks of gas. And how did Mansur and Kevorkian get to the real estate office? Mansur could not drive, and no vehicle—other than Fieger's—was at the scene.

"I really don't know where he got the canisters, and I think it's fairly insignificant," Fieger said.

And how did Fieger, who adamantly insisted he did not know about Kevorkian's assisted suicides in advance, get to Mansur's office before police arrived? Fieger's home and office were at least 30 minutes away from the death scene.

A few days before Mansur's death, Margo Janus, Neal Nicol and Kevorkian came to Fieger's office and met behind closed doors with Fieger and Schwartz.

A month earlier, Fieger had told me Janus and Nicol would not be present at the next suicide. They certainly weren't there when police arrived.

Mansur's death set in motion a familiar train of events.

There was Jack Kevorkian, in a powder blue sweater, blue tie and striped shirt, walking head down from police headquarters as cameras clicked. There was Fieger beside him, one hand on his shoulder, wearing blue jeans, a plain white polo shirt, no tie, and a sports coat, looking like he'd been roused from a quiet Sunday brunch.

And there was a picture of the two on the front page of the next day's papers.

Hours after Mansur died, there was Fieger in the parking lot outside his office, taunting the authorities in front of the TV cameras.

"If the Wayne County prosecutors want to get in a fight with me and have a three-ring circus in the Recorder's Court while I kick their butt around the block and no jury in the world will do anything but acquit Doctor Kevorkian and laugh at the prosecutors, go right ahead. I'm ready . . . Anybody who thinks they want to charge

Doctor Kevorkian is going to come to me and fight with me, and they are going to get their butt kicked."

There was the usual reaction from Richard Thompson: "We are a government of laws, and everyone should obey the law, regardless of whether they think it's a good law or not. At this point, it is no longer a public debate on the issue of assisted suicide. I think the question is rather whether we're going to keep letting Jack Kevorkian take the law into his own hands."

And Archbishop Adam Maida: "We can only hope and pray that the fact that, at this time, such actions are also illegal will help bring a permanent ban and end to this . . . deadly behavior."

And an outraged state senator, this time Republican Jack Horton: "The man has proven he has no regard for the law. He is a criminal with a mission, and I think he intends to test the limits of humanity. What will we tolerate?"

And there was Fieger on the six o'clock news, parrying questions with his own punches.

TV moderator: "No paperwork, no picture, no witnesses—Is this the new premeditated strategy to bypass the law?"

Fieger: "I don't know about that, but it sure focuses your viewers' attention on the fact that this law, if it was enforced the way these sadists want it to, would have made Ron Mansur be screaming in agony right now. . . . These people like Engler would have him suffering even tonight. What kind of people are these? . . .

"I'm certainly ready to get it on with guys like Engler and this Wayne County prosecutor . . . I can't believe this is the United States 1993 and we've got guys out there threatening people with jail if they even think about ending the suffering of dying people. That's nutty! . . .

"Let's take away the focus from Kevorkian and indeed myself. Let's put the focus on these sadists who really want to enforce their own morality on the rest of us. Let's get these people out of our sick beds."

And the next day, there was the *Free Press*, still castigating Lansing in an editorial:

"Had lawmakers resolved to do the job they were elected to do after Dr. Kevorkian took part in his first assisted suicide, nearly three years ago, Michigan might have a workable, humane system in effect today that could serve as a national model.

"Instead, we have the suicide doctor, still a law unto himself."

And, the next day, there was the ass-kicking Fieger again—on the

Channel 7 noon news, shocking staid anchor Erik Smith.

"Did Doctor Kevorkian violate the new law, Geoffrey?"

"No way. And anybody who tries to charge him has got another think coming, plus a boot up their rear end."

"Well, alright, uh—that's graphic." Smith was flustered.

"It is, it is. Figuratively, you'd think after 16 cases there's been enough boots up the rear end of some other prosecutors that Mister O'Hair does not want to get involved in a fight with me."

And there was *Free Press* columnist Hugh McDiarmid, referring to Geoffrey Fieger in passing as a "lawyer-clown." And the Barracuda, Michael Schwartz, snapping back in a letter to the editor: "There are many sobriquets that may apply to Geoffrey Fieger, but 'clown' is not one of them. A clown does not emerge victorious in virtually every attack waged by an entrenched establishment. . . . A clown does not win millions of dollars in verdicts and settlements for his clients."

On Thursday, May 20, eight days before Kevorkian's 65th birthday, there was another familiar scene. While Fieger's staff and his famous client were on a dinner train excursion, Detroit police raided Kevorkian's apartment, looking for evidence to link him to Mansur.

That raid—and the Detroit police investigation—became moot a few hours later, when Wayne County Circuit Court Judge Cynthia Stephens granted the ACLU's request for an injunction against the state's assisted suicide ban. After months of procedural delays, Stephens swiftly batted down the law. Her ruling rested heavily on technical grounds. Lawmakers, she said, had violated the state Constitution by passing the two-headed monster that made assisted suicide a crime while creating a panel to study if it should be a crime.

According to Michigan law, bills were supposed to have a single purpose, and Stephens ruled that the hybrid law did not. Stephens also reserved the right to challenge the bill on broader grounds, writing: "This court finds that the right of self-determination . . . includes the right to choose to cease living."

Fieger lauded Stephens, calling her "one of the most intelligent judges in Wayne County."

The previous fall, Fieger and his wife had donated $3,000 to Stephens's unsuccessful campaign for the state court of appeals—making them among the biggest donors to her $100,000 campaign.

Detroit police dropped their investigation.

Opponents vowed to pass a new law.

And there was Fieger again on the six o'clock news, saying the ruling wouldn't make any difference to Kevorkian.

"The law didn't affect him one way or the other," Fieger told Channel 7. "There's an opportunity now for physicians to come forward. And if they don't, there's no excuse."

And there was John Kelly on TV, citing Kevorkian's writings:

"Here's an individual who envisions a society where those with arthritis, those with bronchitis, those with neurological disease, those who are crippled, those who have minor problems, can actually be put to death. ... I can't go along with that. He also envisions a society where he can then auction off and then sell those body parts for commercial profit. Is that the world you want to have? Not me."

And there was Lynn Mills back on Main Street in Royal Oak, praying for another interview.

"He belongs in jail and I live for that day," she told a TV reporter.

Mills predicted that, like abortion, the fight over Jack Kevorkian and assisted suicide would take many more years.

And there, on the 11 o'clock news, was Fieger again—and Bill Bonds. Fieger was in a jocular mood.

"If Lynn Mills ever had an idea in her head, it would be in solitary confinement," he quipped.

Bonds asked if Fieger thought the Legislature would try again.

"Oh, of course. Listen, they're on a moral crusade, Bill. They're doing God's work. And when you're doing God's work, you can do some unholy terror upon us all."

"Where does that leave Doctor Kevorkian?"

"They're going to go after him still. Of course he'll continue because he's right. But what it really should do is open a window of opportunity now for the medical profession to step in and say: Wait a minute. We're not having the Legislature legislate morality. We're not having the governor tell us how much we have to suffer..."

"Geoffrey, you know and I know as we sit here tonight that the medical profession is not going to take a stand on this. They've never done it and they're not going to do it."

"You're right. You're right. Then we're going to have to have Kevorkian be the scapegoat for these moral crusaders and we're going to have a Scopes trial, because they're going to get him and we're going to have a trial..."

Fieger was still hoping to be the Clarence Darrow of the 1990s.

In closing, Bonds observed:

"I suspect that Doctor Kevorkian is going to resume his work. Is that right?"

"Well, do you think he's gonna stop?"

"No, I don't."

And there, on Jack Kevorkian's 65th birthday—the day people with regular jobs retire—was his smiling face on the cover of *Time*.

The unemployed pathologist was back in business.

A month later, a three-judge panel of the state Court of Appeals stayed Judge Stephens's injunction and reinstated the assisted suicide ban pending a full hearing. Kevorkian had not assisted in any suicides in the interim, even though it would have been legal to do so.

Driving past Kevorkian's apartment in Royal Oak, I noticed that the 1968 Volkswagen van—in which Janet Adkins had died three years earlier to start a new epoch in human history—was gone.

I called Geoffrey Fieger, who informed me that Kevorkian was completely obsessed with something new. Every day now, Fieger said, Kevorkian drove his van to someplace green and beautiful and remote.

Doctor Death was playing golf.

On August 4, the *Detroit News* proclaimed across the top of its Metro section front: "Dr. Death Takes a Holiday." Reporter Robert Ourlian noted that Jack Kevorkian had never assisted a suicide in the summer.

Indeed, it had been a quiet June and July. Geoffrey Fieger was busy with other high-profile cases, including a lawsuit on behalf of a former Mrs. Michigan beauty queen who had been stripped of her title after stripping for *Playboy*. Noir Leather, the kinky sex paraphernalia emporium down the street from Kevorkian's apartment, was selling "Doctor Death" T-shirts. The shirts had a ghoulish rendering of Kevorkian holding a needle and the inscription: "He has the solution."

Kevorkian was busy chasing little white balls down fairways, and had been playing table tennis at attorney Michael Schwartz's house, the *News* reported.

"You have to remember that Jack's like other people," Schwartz told Ourlian. "He's not always all the way out there."

Police officers on Belle Isle, Detroit's mid-river park, could have been reading the *News* story at 8 a.m. when Geoffrey Fieger burst into the station. Fieger said he needed directions to a place where he had arranged to meet Jack Kevorkian.

Most Detroiters knew the layout of the huge park. On summer days, cars cruised the island blaring rap music at picnickers, bicyclists, swimmers and fishers.

Following Fieger's directions, police pulled over a beige 1968 Volkswagen van near the giant slide in the children's play area. Jack Kevorkian was at the wheel. His only passenger was a dead man.

So much for taking the summer off.

To avoid TV cameras, Kevorkian lay down in the back of an unmarked car as cops drove him down to headquarters. Other authorities drove away the van bearing the body of 30-year-old Thomas Hyde. As the *News* was hitting doorsteps with the story of Kevorkian's hiatus, Doctor Death was questioned for hours and then released.

Detroit Police Inspector Gerald Stewart said the case differed from the death of Ron Mansur and other Kevorkian assisted suicides because "he was at the scene in other cases. He was *with* the scene this time. He was taking the scene with him."

Hyde, Kevorkian's 17th and youngest suicide patient, had been diagnosed only a year earlier with Lou Gehrig's disease. His doctor said Hyde had great trouble breathing, swallowing and speaking, and had only very limited use of his left hand.

Hyde was a former construction worker and landscaper who had served a few years in prison for armed robbery. He lived in an apartment in suburban Novi with common-law wife Heidi Fernandez and their 18-month-old daughter.

One week before Hyde's death, Bob Pavkovich had come from Florida to visit his friend in Novi. He found Hyde outside, struggling to turn on a garden hose to clean dried feces from his legs.

"I would like to thank you for helping Tom die with some of his dignity left," Pavkovich later wrote Kevorkian.

Not only was Doctor Death back in business, for the first time in three years he had used his much-maligned vehicle as a suicide parlor. At an afternoon press conference, Fieger defended the van: "I think it's apropos that Thomas Hyde died in a beautiful park setting in . . . what's been described as a rusty old white van, but actually is truly a really kind of nice van, and there's nothing ignominious about that."

Evoking memories of Michael Modelski's 1990 comparison of Kevorkian's suicide practice to a pizza delivery service, Doctor Death had picked up Hyde and driven him to Belle Isle. Why there?

"Because it's a beautiful island," Fieger replied to a reporter. But it was an island most white suburbanites avoided. Hyde, like all of Kevorkian's suicide patients, was white. This time, it seemed, Kevorkian had his own reasons for picking such an unusual site. This time, Kevorkian and Fieger were daring Wayne County Prosecutor John O'Hair to respond.

To the surprise of reporters, Fieger's long-muzzled client gave a statement in Fieger's parking lot only hours after Hyde died.

"I assisted Thomas Hyde in a merciful suicide," Kevorkian declared. "I will always do so when a patient needs it because I'm a physician. I'm a pathologist but also a physician. . . .

"This is our business. It has nothing to do with religion, philosophy or ethics. . . . You have medicine and personal autonomy, and that's all that's needed. You don't need press releases, press conferences, you don't need laws, you don't need any kind of persecution or prosecution or arrests or fingerprinting. You don't need any of that."

Kevorkian challenged the medical profession "to stop talking, stop all this jostling, get down to business, declare that it's a medical service, then it's covered by law like all medical service, and then you sit down and lay down the guidelines and the rules how you'll operate, and you'll change them every week as you learn more and more."

Kevorkian clarified his definition of terminal illness:

"Any disease or affliction that limits life from its natural ending is terminal. Alzheimer's is terminal, ALS is terminal, multiple sclerosis is terminal, and even strokes are terminal."

Fernandez stood silently next to the man who had helped her husband die. She was dressed in shorts, a T-shirt and a baseball cap. Later, she told reporters that Hyde had wanted friends and relatives to have a good time at his memorial service:

"Tom told me, 'I want it to be outside. I want everybody to have a good time, drink beer and wear shorts.' "

In response to reporters' questions, Fieger said Kevorkian was no longer playing cat-and-mouse: "He is confronting this face-to-face, and if someone wishes to charge him, he stands ready."

Kevorkian recast his threat of a hunger strike if jailed, making it sound more like he was considering suicide:

"I don't want to be a martyr, that's silly. It's rather kind of childish. . . . But I do not choose to live in a society that's still in the Dark Ages. I put it on record that I, for one, am enlightened enough to say I am out of the Dark Ages. Now if the rest of this society upholds that silly thing called a law, which is really a despotic ukase, it's not a law at all . . . to continue the agony of people like Thomas Hyde, I don't want to live in that kind of society."

The next morning, Fieger told WJR's J.P. McCarthy, Detroit's morning radio king, that O'Hair was a "respected jurist" who "understands the inherent deficiencies of the law" against assisted suicide and how unpopular that law appeared to be in Michigan.

In the next hour, O'Hair told McCarthy that Kevorkian's admission wasn't specific enough.

"The magic words were not there. . . . If Dr. Kevorkian is genuinely interested in challenging this law, all he has to state is . . . that I, Jack Kevorkian, turned the gas on, knowing that Mr. Hyde wanted to cause his death, or I provided the means knowing that Mr. Hyde was going to use this equipment to cause his death. That's all he has to say."

Later that afternoon, the poker-playing pathologist called O'Hair's bluff. In front of TV cameras, Kevorkian said the magic words:

"I connected the tubing to the tank. I put the clip on the tubing. I put the mask over Mister Hyde's face because he could not move that much. . . . I turned on the gas by the main valve on the tank.

"I asked him one more time if he was sure what he was doing. I couldn't get an intelligible reply, but there was a small smile you could see crack his lips. And he looked up with a sort of pleasant face and pleasant eyes and a moan or two, and I thought I heard him say, 'I'm fine.'

"He then pulled the string and the clip came off the tubing. It was a slow flow of gas, very slow volume.

"He then went on and died."

Kevorkian told reporters he wanted to help O'Hair: "I want to do everything possible to make his job easier."

Fieger declared:

"Let a judge and a jury end this charade once and for all. Personally, I do not long for a showdown, but this has to be ended."

Lynn Mills told reporters:

"I look forward to Jack's permanent incarceration."

□ □ □

Kevorkian got his wish—and Mills came a step closer to having her dreams fulfilled—on August 17, 1993. That morning, O'Hair called an unusual press conference to announce he was prosecuting Kevorkian for violating a law that O'Hair personally opposed.

O'Hair said that if he were in Thomas Hyde's shoes, he would have done the same thing.

"If I was enslaved in the body, having led a full life, and I came down with Lou Gehrig's or something like that, where I reached the point where I had to lay in bed, have people feed me, whatever assets I had go out the window to medical providers rather than to my family ... I wouldn't have a moment's hesitation in making that decision. Not a moment."

O'Hair thanked Kevorkian for performing a public service by forcing the issue. The prosecutor, a member of the legislative commission created to recommend a permanent state law on assisted suicide, proposed legalizing the practice for terminally ill people. But he said it was his duty to prosecute Kevorkian so the current law could be tested in court.

"If it takes a criminal trial of Dr. Kevorkian to bring this issue to a resolution, so be it," O'Hair said.

That afternoon, three years to the day after Kevorkian had tried to get Aristotle, Einstein and other great dead men to speak in his behalf but was muzzled by Judge Alice Gilbert, history's most outspoken pathologist stood mute in Detroit's 36th District Court before Magistrate Robert Costello. Kevorkian smiled as Costello scheduled a preliminary hearing and then released the accused on $100,000 personal bond.

Kevorkian went straight to the parking lot behind Fieger's office, where he compared himself to Galileo, whose heretical discoveries about the solar system were repressed by religious authorities for 250 years.

"I can't wait two and a half centuries, and neither can patients like Thomas Hyde," Kevorkian declared before returning to Royal Oak for a poker game. "I will continue to help suffering patients no matter what, as long as I'm free to do so."

Fieger anticipated another Scopes trial.

Free Press columnist Hugh McDiarmid pointed out that neither Galileo nor John Scopes "gleefully employed gas masks, rusty Volkswagens and exhibitionist lawyers to promote themselves (although Geoffrey Fieger may think he sees Clarence Darrow from time to time when he peers into his curved, vainglorious private mirrors)."

But even Kevorkian's longtime enemies conceded the legal showdown could have enormous impact nationwide.

"I would predict the Kevorkian trial would be the start of a major debate that will take anywhere from five to 10 years to resolve and will push abortion aside as the major social issue facing Americans," said ethicist Arthur Caplan.

Alexander Capron of the University of Southern California's health ethics center said a trial would "make Doctor Jack Kevorkian into a hero, a martyr or both in certain circles and in other circles even more the devil than he's seen as being."

But Kevorkian said the trial wouldn't be about him at all.

"It isn't Kevorkian that's on trial," he told reporters. "It isn't assisted suicide or euthanasia that's on trial. You know what's on trial? It's your civilization and your society that's on trial."

On September 9, 36th District Court Judge Willie Lipscomb denied Fieger's motion for a dismissal and ordered Jack Kevorkian to stand trial for helping Thomas Hyde end his life.

Eight hours later, police in Redford Township, a Wayne County suburb, responded to a 911 call reporting a suicide at a residence. They found Kevorkian, a tank of carbon monoxide and the body of Donald O'Keefe. O'Keefe, 73, was a retired Ford Motor Co. worker suffering from bone cancer.

It seemed that nothing short of jail was going to stop Jack Kevorkian's Death Rounds.

CHAPTER FIFTY-TWO
BREAKING THE SILENCE

"We all want to go on. We want to
postpone death."
—Jack Kevorkian (1993)

"I'm as scared of dying as you are."
—Jack Kevorkian (1991) ❐

Jack Kevorkian has had a tremendous impact on the medical profession, Howard Brody told me.

"Before June 1990 there were doctors saying: We've got to make sure that patients understand they have rights. We've got to make sure that patients are encouraged to fill out Durable Power of Attorney. There were doctors saying pain control is a scandal, we've got these wonderful drugs and we don't use them to control pain. There were people out there pushing these agendas—I was one of them—before June 1990. But we couldn't get a microphone to tell the world about this like we can today, thanks to Kevorkian. Kevorkian gave us the soapbox.

"It's kind of amazing that a guy like him, this pathologist, this out-of-work fringe kind of character, has been able to accomplish this much."

❐ ❐ ❐

In the 1960s, Jack Kevorkian wrote this copy for the dust jacket of his book *Beyond Any Kind of God*:

"Who has not at least once in his lifetime asked himself: What is this thing called 'life'? What does it mean to 'be'? How and why do we 'live'? What is this great and sinister unknown 'death'? An instant of meditative stargazing may prompt any of these questions. ...

"As it ends thus for us on Earth so too will 'death' end this discourse. The knell will not be so much a dirge as it will be a harmonious synthesis of a grand unity—the undissectable fusion of death, life and existence into an inscrutable scheme that might be cogent and imposing enough to cause one to look beyond his idols and icons to the essence of his being and his non-being."

◻ ◻ ◻

I talked to my Aunt Grace on the phone about two months after my cousin Martie Ruwart's death. She said the last time she had talked to her niece was when Martie was recovering from her operation in the hospital in Grand Rapids. Martie had sounded real hopeful, Grace said.

"I feel Martha should have had the chance to do what she wanted to do," Grace said. But she said she keeps thinking about how sad it must have been for Martie to take that last car ride from Kalamazoo, to go all that way to die.

"I think about what she must have been thinking: I'll never see grass again or trees or the sky.

"To me it's like a public execution. I can't think of any other situation where you know the exact moment of your death in advance."

◻ ◻ ◻

Geoffrey Fieger told me a week after my cousin died:

"It was the first case that really got to me. I tell you what, I go in afterwards, I'm pretty stoic and I'm pretty steeled to the events now, so the bodies really don't bother me anymore. At first they did, but they really don't anymore.

"It's not a macabre scene, it's very pleasant actually. The family's all there. There's a sense of really strong relief. There's a real close bond and there's almost a sense of elation that they're out of their pain—I can't describe it to you, OK?—and there's an overwhelming sense of love, which is always interfered with by the police. The Ruwart family was particularly close. As I recall, there were three sisters there and the two friends. And she looked terribly sick."

Fieger's voice went very soft.

"I looked at her, you know, she was 41 years old, and I said, wow, I mean, because I'm 42. That bothered me a lot. And then they gave me her picture. I saw her picture, and that just tore me apart because she was a really beautiful girl. And she didn't look anything like that anymore. I mean, what that cancer had done to her! It was the first one that really got to me, not that she died from Jack, it's that she was 41 years old, and it could happen to any of us. This could be me."

❏ ❏ ❏

In a rare interview, Margo Janus told *Time* magazine:

"Our mother suffered from cancer. I saw the ravages right up to the end. Her mind was sound, but her body was gone. My brother's option would have been more moral than all the Demerol that they poured into her, to the point that her body was black and blue from the needle marks. She was in a coma, and she weighed only 70 pounds. Even then I said to the doctor, 'This isn't right, to keep her on IV,' but he shrugged his shoulder and said, 'I'm bound by my oath to do that.'"

❏ ❏ ❏

Jack Kevorkian once wrote:

"Most physicians would agree that birth and death are the two most important events in the existence of any human being. But in reality, their importance is not equal, simply because once having been unconsciously experienced, a person's birth is no longer part of his or her life. Therefore, death, which is not yet experienced, becomes paramount because everything in life is terminated by it. No other experience in life has such a devastating effect. . . .

"Not too long ago the important event of birth was not a part of honorable or acceptable medical practice. The 'demeaning' activity of obstetrics was left to abject midwives and was deemed far beneath the exalted status of noble physicians. . . .

"Currently, we blaspheme the process of exiting—the most important event—by not according it even the indignity of comparable 'midwifery.' Such brazen inconsistency is inexcusable. . . . The medical profession must take the lead immediately to shorten the deplorable evolution of this last unjustified taboo by elevating the most important life event called death to the place of honor in the hierarchy of ethics it has always deserved."

❏ ❏ ❏

Dr. Howard Brody made these observations to me:

"We live in a society that has an incredible death phobia. But if our whole society's afraid of death, then why is Doctor Kevorkian a hero? Why is Doctor Death a hero in a society that fears death?

"Well, it's complicated. We live in a society that has a profound unease and ambivalence about dying. It just has not assimilated the notion that dying is a part of life and dying is natural. When you get that, you get irrational behavior, since if everybody dies but our culture can't make sense of everybody dying, then you get a culture that acts in bizarre ways. And one bizarre way is to try to say: Well, if we just get all the machines hooked up to all the people all the time, nobody will die. And if you die, it must be because some doctor committed malpractice. It must be technological failure or bad faith. Something was evil. There's got to be a villain to blame out there if you die, you know, as opposed to: You die because that's what kind of beings we are.

"One kind of bizarre behavior is: A 94-year-old person in the last stages of a terminal illness, instead of dying at home surrounded by family, will die in an ICU hooked up to machines. And they drive up a tremendous bill and they suffer and the family ends up anguished . . . instead of the kind of death that we can all envision as a more normal, healthy, natural death.

"A lot of people today don't die the way they would have chosen had they really thought about it. So that's one bit of phobia.

"But the other bit of phobia or craziness is the American penchant that says: If there's a problem, if you just get the right machine it will solve the problem for us. We fear death, we fear the loss of control that comes with death, we fear death as an unknown, we fear death as something we can't handle, we can't control. And then along comes Doctor Kevorkian and he says: I've got this machine. And it's a lovely American solution to the problem. I'll just hook myself up to Doctor Kevorkian's machine, I'll be in charge, everything will be fine. And I don't have to struggle with any of the deep spiritual turmoil that I would feel if I actually thought about dying.

"If I really, really took seriously the kinds of choices I am making when I think about my death, and what effects this could have on my family, what does it mean in terms of what I've been able to do in my life, what does it mean in terms of what I have not yet done that I wish I had done, and all that stuff, and all that baggage—and instead of dealing with all that stuff and going through the spiritual turmoil and anguish it would take to work through it, I say: Ah. The machine. Hook me up, push the button and it's fine. Technology comes to my rescue."

◻ ◻ ◻

At the end of a day spent doing interviews for this book, I came home and found a message on my answering machine from an assistant at my doctor's office:

"The doctor wants you to call."

Too late. The office was closed and wouldn't reopen until noon the next day.

A week earlier, I had undergone the second part of a colon cancer screening test. Because colon cancer killed my father at age 58 and there's evidence of a hereditary link, I get tested regularly. Part one of this year's test was a sigmoidoscopy—a code word for having a doctor insert a long black tube with a camera on it up your rectum and halfway through your intestinal system. I got immediate results from that: My lower intestines looked great. Part two was an upper GI to examine the rest of the intestines. That consisted of a barium enema followed by an elaborate series of painful maneuvers on an X-ray table.

I figured the doctor's office was calling to tell me the results of part two. Chances were excellent the results were good. But, being fully enlisted in the American death phobia, I plunged into worry.

I was putting my seven-year-old son Patrick to bed when he suddenly started telling me the story of how he had chosen me to be his father: He was a star child and had come down from his star to check out adults on Earth. The way it's done is you turn into a mosquito and then you land on people's skin to see which one you like. Patrick said he chose me and his mother right away, on the first day.

I told him I was glad he had. He said he was glad, too. Then he said: "Dad, you know how you said some people believe we might come back as other animals, or other things, after we die? Well, no matter what, I'm going to choose you to be my dad—even if we come back as pencils."

I slept well.

And the next day when I called the doctor's office, I found out that my intestines were healthy.

◻ ◻ ◻

I once asked Geoffrey Fieger what he had learned from his two years with Jack Kevorkian.

"We're normally fearful of death. But there is a point when that fear utterly goes away. And death becomes a desirable portal from which to end your existence. That's what he says. There comes a point at which not just you accept it but you desire death. Every single patient has not had any second thoughts, but has said 'Let's go! Now! Let's do it.'

"I can't imagine it. We can't imagine it. And these people aren't crazy. They're saying: It's time. Let's go. None of them has ever expressed any second thoughts. None of them has ever expressed any fear."

❐ ❐ ❐

About her friend Sherry Miller, Sharon Welsh told me:
"She was not afraid to die. She was afraid to go on living."

❐ ❐ ❐

Fred Dillingham told me this about his special daughter:
"I live on a day-to-day basis with knowing that I could lose her. She's 19 years old and weighs 40 pounds. She has to be catheterized, her bowels have to be worked with, she has to be fed.

"If I wanted to describe all the negatives and not look for the positives of the way she affects my life and her life, I could subscribe to any of the arguments that have been made in terminating some 15 different lives with assisted suicide. I don't believe that. She has a quality life. She's happy. She provides me with a great deal of love and a great deal of work and a heck of a lot of responsibility. And my other four children have been touched by all the blessings that she has brought with her. And they all can care for her, and there isn't one of them—and I know without ever having asked—that would say that we as a family, they as an individual or she as a person would be better off if she were dead."

❐ ❐ ❐

Sharon Welsh also told me that Sherry Miller's death has changed her life.

"I have a different outlook on life. Sherry has taught me not to judge people. I used to see news stories on TV and say 'How could someone do that?' I don't do that now.

"Sherry's decision to end her life was her decision. It was the right thing for Sherry. For me, maybe not. I lost a friend. And I miss her a lot. It would be nice if she were still here—but at what cost?

"A lot of people have judged her decision. That makes me angry, and it hurts me. Because until you've lived in her shoes and had to experience a day in her life, how could you judge?

"I feel that she was a pioneer. I think she was brave. She made a decision and she went through a lot of obstacles. A lot of people tried to talk her out of it and change her mind and she continued to say: This is for me. This is what I want. I don't care what everybody else says."

When Sharon Welsh goes for long walks, "I do a lot of thinking about Sherry. What she did was right for Sherry. And I don't feel we have any right to say she can't do this."

❑ ❑ ❑

Mary Ruwart told me this about her sister and my cousin Martie:

"She had always said she wanted to make her death beautiful like Mom's. I think she succeeded."

❑ ❑ ❑

By age 50, Kenneth Shapiro of East Lansing, one of the plaintiffs in the ACLU's challenge to the assisted suicide law, had been through six major surgeries and countless "minor" operations. He had been told several times that his condition was hopeless.

But the most traumatic result of 15 years of cancer was that his employers told him he could no longer work.

"Not having a job, not being a contributing member of society, that's tough," Shapiro told me. "It's hard to keep going when you have no sense of productivity, no sense of usefulness.

"That's worse than fighting cancer."

❑ ❑ ❑

Howard Brody also told me:

"Kevorkian has played a positive role in raising the issue and making sure the issue is not going to go away. There's no way we can play hide-and-seek any more with physician-assisted suicide, thanks to Doctor Death.

"He's played a somewhat negative role in presenting himself as the knight on a white horse. If they don't like him, a lot of people will simply brush aside the whole topic area by saying, 'Well, that's Kevorkian, I don't like Kevorkian, so I don't want to think about that.' So to the extent that he's personalized the issue and to the extent that he has some non-endearing personal qualities or Fieger has some non-endearing personal qualities, that skews the debate over the personality and not over the issue."

Largely because of Kevorkian, Brody predicted, "within the next five years a state someplace will legalize something like this. That state will then have two or three or four years' worth of experience and a variety of stories will come out of that state. If the stories are generally reassuring stories, then I think a few more states will try it and more stories will come out of those states, and we'll sort of see which way the wind is blowing. If those stories are horror stories, then people will react very negatively, that state will repeal its law and laws like this will not be enacted in any other states."

◻ ◻ ◻

I knew hardly anything about my cousin Martie's adult life until her sisters sat down with me one afternoon and told me her story. After her death, I got to know her better than I ever had during her life.

The silence among my relatives following Martie's death was awkward. The lack of a service for Martie didn't seem right.

As I finished this book, I decided: I would take the lead and organize a service.

Not for Martie Ruwart's sake. But for mine.

So there wouldn't be such a silence anymore about death in my family.

We finally had the service six months after Martie's death. Some of my relatives gathered in a small room on a Saturday afternoon. My cousin Mary Ruwart showed a moving sequence of slides depicting Martie's life from infancy to the night before she died, when she looked emaciated but resolute and serene.

Then Mary showed the videotape taken the night before Martie's death.

When Kevorkian asked if she had any message for those who might later be watching the tape, Martie replied:

"I hope they understand that I love them and I'll miss them."

Then she turned in her bed, faced the camera, and said to us:

"I hope you'll understand why I'm doing this."

❏ ❏ ❏

Jack Kevorkian told Ron Rosenbaum:

"That's the biggest misunderstanding about me, that I'm obsessed with death. I'm really pro-life. My writings are all about trying to get medical benefits from death. Life back from death."

❏ ❏ ❏

Very Still Life is the painting Jack Kevorkian did at an art class in the early 1960s to shock and sicken his conventional classmates.

It is a painting of a large gray skull, its top leaning back a little, its jaw twisted. The skull is on a red velvet cloth. Around it and under it are bones and a broken femur. Tacked on the wall behind it is a piece of pasty yellow-green skin.

Out of the eye socket of the skull, a delicate, beautiful iris reaches toward the heavens.

Out of the skull, a flower.

NOTES ON EPIGRAPHS

Part I. From philosopher Ivan Illich's 1974 lecture at the University of Edinburgh, reproduced in *Toward A History of Needs* by Ivan Illich (Pantheon Books, 1977).

Chapters 4, 16, 40, and 47. *An Altogether New Book of Top Ten Lists*, by David Letterman, Pocket Books.

Chapter 5. San Diego psychologist and right-to-die advocate Faye Girsch is quoted in "Choosing Not to Die Alone," by Pamela Warrick, *Los Angeles Times*, March 30, 1993.

Chapters 6 and 49. "Angel of Death: The Trial of the Suicide Doctor," by Ron Rosenbaum, *Vanity Fair*, May 1991.

Chapters 7 and 48. From Kevorkian's testimony of June 8, 1990, before Judge Alice Gilbert in Oakland County Circuit Court.

Chapters 8, 10, 18, 22 and Part IV. From "The Odd Odyssey of 'Dr. Death,' " by Gloria Borger, *US News & World Report*, August 27, 1990.

Chapter 9. Ron Adkins, responding to Ron Rosenbaum's question about whether he'd tried to change his wife's mind about suicide, is quoted in Rosenbaum's *Vanity Fair* article, May 1991.

Chapter 11. From Timothy Quill, "A Case of Individualized Decision Making," *New England Journal of Medicine*, Vol. 324 No. 10 (March 7, 1991), p. 694.

Chapter 13. George Annas, "Killing Machines," *Current*, November 1991.

Chapters 14, 29, 41, 44 and 51. Quoted in "Rx for Death" by Nancy Gibbs, *Time*, May 31, 1993.

Chapter 15. From a personal interview, April 2, 1993.

Chapter 19. Ronald Maris is director of the Center for the Study of Suicide, University of South Carolina. The quote is from "Choosing Not to Die Alone," *Los Angeles Times*, March 30, 1993.

Part III. The folk wisdom is included in *Walking the Medicine Wheel Path in Daylight* by Donato Cianci "Pathmaker" and Suzanne Nadon "Sunshine" (Maplestone Press, Owen Sound, Ontario, 1986).

Chapter 24. Kubler-Ross is quoted in the *Detroit News*, Dec. 29, 1992.

Chapter 25. From a letter Collins wrote to Senator Fred Dillingham, December 2, 1992.

Chapter 27. Personal phone interview, January 1993.

Chapter 31. Quoted in April 1993 Associated Press profile of Fieger by Julia Prodis.

Chapter 33. Personal phone interview, February 1993.

Chapter 36. "Tale of the Terminator," *Chicago Tribune*, February 21, 1993.

Chapter 45. From a personal interview, April 22, 1993.

Chapter 46. From his talk at a Michigan Hemlock Society meeting, April 3, 1993.

Part V. Janet Adkins selected Roethke's poem to be read at her memorial service.

Chapter 50. Joseph Richman is a New York psychologist and author of several books on suicide. He is quoted in "Choosing Not to Die Alone," *Los Angeles Times*, March 30, 1993.

Chapter 52. The first quote is from *USA Today*, February 22, 1993; the second from Rosenbaum's *Vanity Fair* article.

SOURCES

<u>Books and Journal Articles</u>

Anonymous, "It's All Over, Debbie," *Journal of the American Medical Association* 259 (1988), p. 372.

Bender, Leslie, "A Feminist Analysis of Physician-Assisted Dying and Voluntary Active Euthanasia," *Tennessee Law Review*, Vol. 59 (1992).

Brody, Howard, "Assisted Death—A Compassionate Response to a Medical Failure," *The New England Journal of Medicine*, Vol. 327 No. 19 (Nov. 5, 1992), pp. 1384-88.

Kamisar, Yale, "Some Non-Religious Views Against Proposed 'Mercy-Killing' Legislation," *Minnesota Law Review*, Vol. 42 (1958).

Kamisar, Yale, "When Is There A Constitutional 'Right to Die'? When Is There No Constitutional 'Right to Live'?", *Georgia Law Review*, Vol. 25 (1991).

Kevorkian, Jack, "The Fundus Oculi and the Determination of Death," *American Journal of Pathology*, Vol. 32 (1956), pp. 1253-69.

Kevorkian, Jack, and Glenn Bylsma, "Transfusion of Postmortem Human Blood," *American Journal of Clinical Pathology*, Vol. 35 No. 5 (May 1961), pp. 413-19.

Kevorkian, Jack, Neal Nicol and E. Rea, "Direct Body-Body Human Cadaver Blood Transfusion," *Military Medicine*, Vol. 129 (January 1964), pp. 24-27.

Kevorkian, Jack, *Slimmeriks and the Demi-Diet*. Southfield, Mich.: Penumbra, Inc., 1978.

Kevorkian, Jack, "A Brief History of Experimentation on Condemned and Executed Humans," *Journal of the National Medical Association*, Vol. 77 No. 3 (1985), pp. 215-26.

Kevorkian, Jack, "Medicine, Ethics and Execution by Lethal Injection," *Medicine and Law*, Vol. 4 (1985), pp. 307-13.

Kevorkian, Jack, "Opinions on Capital Punishment, Executions and Medical Science," *Medicine and Law*, Vol. 4 (1985), pp. 515-33.

Kevorkian, Jack, "A Comprehensive Bioethical Code for Medical Exploitation of Humans Facing Imminent and Unavoidable Death," *Medicine and Law*, Vol. 5 (1986), pp. 181-97.

Kevorkian, Jack, "The Long Overdue Medical Specialty: Bioethiatrics," *Journal of the National Medical Association*, Vol. 78 No. 11 (1986), pp. 1057-60.

Kevorkian, Jack, "The Last Fearsome Taboo: Medical Aspects of Planned Death," *Medicine and Law*, Vol. 7 (1988), pp. 1-14.

Kevorkian, Jack, "Marketing of Human Organs and Tissues Is Justified and Necessary," *Medicine and Law*, Vol. 8 (1989), pp. 557-565.

Kevorkian, Jack, "A Controlled Auction Market is a Practical Solution to the Shortage of Transplantable Organs," *Medicine and Law*, Vol. 11 (1992), pp. 47-55.

Kevorkian, Jack, "A Fail-Safe Model for Justifiable Medically-Assisted Suicide ('Medicide')," *American Journal of Forensic Psychiatry*, Vol. 13 No. 1 (1992) pp. 7-42.

Newman, Stephen A., "Euthanasia: Orchestrating 'The Last Syllable of . . . Time,'" *University of Pittsburgh Law Review,* Vol. 53 (1991), pp. 153-91.

Quill, Timothy, "A Case of Individualized Decision Making," *New England Journal of Medicine,* Vol. 324 No. 10 (March 7, 1991), pp. 691-94.

Quill, Timothy, Christine Cassel and Diane E. Meier, "Proposed Clinical Criteria for Physician-Assisted Suicide," *The New England Journal of Medicine,* Vol. 327 No. 19 (Nov. 5, 1992), pp. 1380-84.

Ruwart, Mary J., *Healing Our World: The Other Piece of the Puzzle.* Kalamazoo, Mich.: Sun Star Press, 1992.

Wanzer, S.H., et. al. "The Physician's Responsibility Toward Hopelessly Ill Patients," *New England Journal of Medicine,* Vol. 320, No. 13 (1989), pp. 844-49.

Watts, David T., and Timothy Howell, "Assisted Suicide Is Not Voluntary Active Euthanasia," *Journal of the American Geriatrics Society,* Vol. 40 No. 10 (October 1992), pp. 1043-46.

Most Important Newspaper and Popular Magazine Articles *(in chronological order)*

"A Vital Woman Chooses Death," *People,* June 25, 1990.

"The Odd Odyssey of 'Dr. Death,'" *US News & World Report,* August 27, 1990.

"Mercy or Murder?" *Michigan Law,* February 1991.

"I Am Not Afraid," *Detroit Free Press Magazine,* Feb. 3, 1991.

"Angel of Death: The Trial of the Suicide Doctor," *Vanity Fair,* May 1991.

"In Matters of Life and Death, The Dying Take Control," *New York Times*, August 18, 1991.

"Killing Machines: Doctors and suicide," *Current*, November 1991.

"Would it have made a difference if they were MEN?" *Detroit Free Press*, Nov. 4, 1991.

"Why help? 'You've got to do something with your life,'" *Detroit News and Free Press*, Feb. 9, 1992.

"Great Minds Rule from the Grave: Dr. Kevorkian Is Right," *Health Care Weekly Review*, April 27, 1992.

"Come and Watch, Kevorkian Offers," *Detroit Free Press*, July 24, 1992.

"Living in the State of Death," *Detroit Free Press*, July 25, 1992.

"Kevorkian has danced to his own tune since childhood," *Detroit News*, Dec. 28, 1992.

"Mercy's Friend or Foe?" *Time*, Dec. 28, 1992.

"Doctor Who Assists Suicides Makes the Macabre Mundane," *New York Times*, Feb. 22, 1993.

"House at the End of Life's Road," *USA Today*, Feb. 22, 1993.

"Dr. Kevorkian's Death Wish," *Newsweek*, March 8, 1993.

"Choosing Not to Die Alone," *Los Angeles Times*, March 30, 1993.

"Rx for Death," *Time*, May 31, 1993.

"Sisters of Mercy," *Time*, May 31, 1993.